Statistical Reasoning in Medicine
The Intuitive *P*-Value Primer

Second Edition

Lemuel A. Moyé

Statistical Reasoning in Medicine
The Intuitive *P*-Value Primer

Second Edition

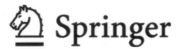 Springer

Lemuel A. Moyé
University of Texas
Health Science Center at Houston
School of Public Health
Houston, TX 77030
USA
moyelaptop@msn.com

Library of Congress Control Number: 2006930252

ISBN-10: 0-387-32913-7
ISBN-13: 978-0387-32913-0

Printed on acid-free paper.

© 2006 Springer Science+Business Media, LLC
All rights reserved. This work may not be translated or copied in whole or in part without the written permission of the publisher (Springer Science+Business Media, LLC, 233 Spring Street, New York, NY 10013, USA), except for brief excerpts in connection with reviews or scholarly analysis. Use in connection with any form of information storage and retrieval, electronic adaptation, computer software, or by similar or dissimilar methodology now known or hereafter developed is forbidden.
The use in this publication of trade names, trademarks, service marks and similar terms, even if they are not identified as such, is not to be taken as an expression of opinion as to whether or not they are subject to proprietary rights.

Printed in the United States of America.   (EB)

9 8 7 6 5 4 3 2 1

springer.com

To Dixie and the DELTs

Preface

You and I have some important and interesting conversations coming up shortly. However, I propose that we postpone those for a moment while I share with you my motivations for writing this book.

The frustrations of doctors, nurses, judges, legislators, and administrators that arise as they interpret healthcare research efforts are the unfortunate and predictable products of their meager research backgrounds. It is only human for them to grab for whatever supporting grips are available; one such handhold is the ubiquitous p-value.

This reduction of a research effort to a single number is regrettable, but quite understandable. The complexity of a modern healthcare research endeavor requires a clear understanding of the circumstances in which one can generalize results from relatively small samples to large populations. Even though the concept of generalization is nonmathematical, many researchers are not its master. Recognizing their disadvantage, they latch onto the p-value, believing that it neatly binds these complicated features into one tidy package.

However, like continually substituting desserts for nutritious meals, the habitual replacement of p-values for clarity of vision is unfulfilling and dangerous. This book reaches out to these principle-starved people. Specifically I want to use the ubiquity of the p-value as an overture to the discussion of statistical reasoning in medicine.

Statistical reasoning in medicine is the process by which one determines whether sample-based results can be extended or generalized to the population at large. The concepts are straightforward, intuitive, and quite precise. However, their application requires thoughtful consideration.

For many years the tendency in the research community has been to replace this deliberation with a quick and simple assessment of the p-value's magnitude. The research community, in its quest for significant results, has created a polluted sea of p-values in which we all restlessly swim. Although p-values were designed to make a simple statement about sampling error, for many they have become the final arbiter of research efforts.

Investigators often gnash their teeth over this entity's value at their study's conclusion: is it less than 0.05 or ≥ 0.05? To these workers, p-values are the switching signal for the research train. If the p-value is less than 0.05, the research-train moves down the main track of manuscript publication, grant awards, regulatory approval, and academic promotion. However, if the p-value is greater than 0.05, the switch moves the other way, directing the research train off to the elephant's graveyard of discarded and useless studies. Replacing the careful consideration of a research effort's (1) methodology, (2) sample size, (3) magnitude of the effect of interest, and (4) variability of that effect size with a simple, hasty look at the p-value is a scientific thought-crime.

P-values continue to be the focus of research discussions in academic centers, remaining a staple of the medical community's research effort. The approval of a new medical intervention commonly includes consideration of the *p*-value, and arguments in courts of law for the scientific basis of an assertion frequently concentrate on the size of the *p*-value. Clearly, many researchers, journal editors, regulators, and judges cling doggedly to its use. It is therefore all the more curious that so few of these specialists understand either what the *p*-value is or precisely what information it is designed to convey. Although they understand the message that the *p*-value "had better be less than oh five," there is little understanding of either the source or justification of this ubiquitous mantra.

I don't think we statisticians have been as helpful as possible. A biostatistics professor at a school of public health once asked a statistics student sitting for his qualifying exam (that must be passed to enter the Ph.D. candidacy phase), "Explain what a *p*-value means." The professor never received a satisfactory response.[*] When biostatisticians do respond to this question, we often give the following response, "the *p*-value is the conditional probability of rejecting the null hypothesis in favor of the alternative hypothesis when the null hypothesis is true." I fear that to the non-statistical world, this answer smacks of Orwellian double-speak.

This text emphasizes an intuitive understanding of the role of the *p*-value in sample-based research, deemphasizing the underlying mathematics. This nonmathematical approach is available when the foundation principles of statistical reasoning in medicine are clearly articulated. Our purpose here is to clearly state and develop the principles that govern when and how one takes results from a small sample and applies them to a larger population in healthcare research. The enunciation of these principles brings the roles and limitations of *p*-values into sharp focus.

Lemuel A. Moyé
University of Texas
School of Public Health
April, 2006

---

[*] Related by Dr. Sharon Cooper, Chair of Epidemiology and Biostatistics, Texas A&M Rural School of Public Health.

Acknowledgments

Approximately 8,000 North Carolina Cherokee are descended from those who did not take the *Nunadautsun't* to the Oklahoma reservations; one who remained was my grandmother. An important lesson she taught her grandchildren was never to begin the day until you have given thanks to God for the people He has placed in your life to guide you.

I owe a special debt of thanks to the leaders and members of the Cardio-Renal Advisory Committee of the Food and Drug Administration, with whom I served as a statistician from 1995 to 1999. They are Ray Lipicki, JoAnn Lindenfeld, Alastair Wood, Alexander Shepherd, Barry Massie, Cynthia L. Raehl, Michael Weber, Cindy Grimes, Udho Thadani, Robert Califf, John DiMarco, Marvin Konstam, Milton Packer, and Dan Roden. The public sessions held three times a year are among the best training grounds for cardiovascular research epidemiology and biostatistics. I am also indebted to Lloyd Fisher, with whom I have often disagreed and from whom I have always learned

I am indebted to my alma mater, The University of Texas School of Public Health, and to public school education in general, which has provided much of my education. To all of you, and especially Asha Kapadia, Palmer Beasley, Robert Hardy, Charles Ford, Barry Davis, Darwin Labarthe, Richard Shekelle, Fred Annegers, and C. Morton Hawkins, consider this book an early payment on a debt too large to ever repay. I would also like to thank Craig Pratt and John Mahmarian, who have been patiently supportive in the development of my ideas. Furthermore, I would like to express my gratitude to Marc Pfeffer, Frank Sacks, Eugene Braunwald – you have been more influential than you know.

To the fellow classmates and friends known as the "DELTS"— Derrick Taylor, MD, Ernest Vanterpool, and Tyrone Perkins. Ever since high school in Queens, New York, we have pushed and prodded each other to excellence. You are a part of all my worthwhile endeavors.

Additionally, I have been blessed with friends and colleagues who were always willing to share from their wellspring of good sense with me. Four of them are James Powell of Cincinnati, Ohio, John McKnight of Washington D.C., Joseph Mayfield of New York City; and Gilbert Ramirez, now in Iowa.

John Kimmel, the reviewing editor, and many chapter reviewers have provided good questions and additional references, improving the book's structure. In addition, Dr. Sarah Baraniuk, Dr. Yolanda Muñoz, and Dr. Claudia Pedroza each suggested important improvements in the last chapters of this book. Dr. Steve Kelder provided some especially helpful insights for the chapter on epidemiology.Lisa Inchani, a graduate student of mine, selflessly volunteered her time to patiently review and copyedit this text. Its readability is largely due to her steadfast efforts.

Finally, my dearest thanks go to Dixie, my wife, on whose personality, character, love, and common sense I have come to rely, and to my daughters Flora and Bella, whose continued emotional and spiritual growth reveals anew to me each day that, through God, all things are possible.

Lemuel A. Moyé
University of Texas
School of Public Health
April, 2006

Contents

Introduction

I sat quietly, awaiting the one question that would utterly destroy my career. It exploded in a gasp of exasperation from the great man...

Like every new fourth-year medical student at Indiana University School of Medicine in 1977, I thought hard and carefully about life as an M.D. With an undergraduate degree in applied mathematics, I had decided to begin graduate studies in statistics after I graduated from medical school. However, several practicing doctors convinced me to postpone my formal education in statistics for a year to first complete a one year medical internship upon graduation from medical school.

My personal life required that I stay in Indianapolis for any post-medical school work. Thus, while my classmates applied to many hospitals across the country and around the world, I applied to only two, and was interested in only one of those — Methodist Hospital Graduate Medical Center. Studying their response, I was stunned to learn that one of my questioners would be Dr. William Kassell, Chairman of Obstetrics and Gynecology.

This was terrible news! My performance in obstetrics and gynecology as a third year medical student the year before was not auspicious. As my first clinical rotation after psychiatry, Ob-Gyn was a rude awakening to the ceaseless and pressing responsibilities of surgeons. I awkwardly tried to juggle 6:30 AM rounds, patient responsibilities, demanding surgeons, steep learning curves, and long overnight hospital hours. Now, I would have to meet with the tough-minded chairman of that department, a man known for his quick appraisals and blunt critiques.

Self-inflicted brutality characterized the night before my interview with Dr. Kassell. Reluctantly pulling out my old Ob-Gyn notes, I again reviewed colposcopy findings and cervical cancer treatment procedures. Re-memorizing the workup of pre-eclampsia, I rubbed my brain raw with the sequence of gynecologic examination procedures.

By the next morning, I was jammed full of gynecologic and obstetrics information. However, while I bullied myself into believing that my head was ready, my heart dreaded the coming confrontation scheduled to begin shortly. Driving to the hospital, I paid no attention to the fall foliage, distracted by a new, persistent smell of defeat that now spoiled the crisp, clean air.

Arriving five minutes early, I stood alone in his huge office, the bright light from the open curtains illuminating my anxiety. Heart racing, shirt sticky with nervous perspirations, I waited his arrival with growing dread.

Suddenly, Dr. Kassell burst into the room, gruffly throwing a greeting in my general direction and waving me to a seat facing him. He was tall and clean-shaven, with large expressive eyes and a thick mane of silver hair. He carefully scrutinized me over his expansive desk, heaped high with textbooks, papers, and hospital charts. I sat, quietly awaiting the one question for which I had not prepared the night before — the one question that would send my career plans crashing into ruin. It exploded in a gasp of exasperation from the great man:

"Dr. Moyé, will you please tell me where a *p*-value comes from?"

"What!" Well,…It….I mean…." I stammered, trying to catch my intellectual breath.

"I asked you," he repeated impatiently, raising his voice for emphasis, "to tell me what a *p*-value is. Can't you do that? What's all of this 0.05 business about? What's so special about that number?" the doctor continued, his frustration conveyed by the boom in his voice.

Just prior to my interview, the chairman had reviewed a manuscript for his journal club (the author and topic I have long since forgotten) in which *p*-values served as the yardstick against which the results were measured. It seemed to Dr. Kassell that these *p*-values were like some unfeeling arbiter, dispassionately determining if study results were positive or negative. Having reviewed my record with its annotation of my undergraduate statistics background, he had decided to spend our interview time discussing this research issue, and not the details of Ob-Gyn.

This book is for everyone in healthcare who requires a nonmathematical answer to Dr. Kassell's question. *Statistical Reasoning in Medicine: The Intuitive P-value Primer* focuses on both the underlying principles of statistical thought in medicine and the ethical interpretation of *p*-values in healthcare research.

A physician confronted with a new finding in her field, a director of a pharmaceutical company analyzing a series of experiments, an expert sitting on an advisory panel for the government, or a judge assessing the scientific aspect of a lawsuit must have an understanding of *p*-values and the underlying statistical thinking that guides their interpretation. If you are a decision maker without in-depth training in statistics, but now find that you must grapple with the thorny theory of statistical reasoning and the nettlesome issues of *p*-values, then this book is for you.

With an emphasis on patient and community protection, *The P-value Primer* develops and emphasizes the *p*-value concept while deemphasizing the mathematics. It also provides examples of the *p*-value's correct implementation and interpretation in a manner consistent with the preeminent principle of clinical research programs: "First, do no harm".

The *P-value Primer's* prologue, describes the controversies that have engulfed statistical reasoning for 400 years, providing a brief history of the development of the concept of data analysis. In Chapter One, the concept of sampling error, and the reasons that physicians have such difficulty understanding the population perspective that is so prevalent in research is discussed. The requirement of sample-based research is developed from basic principles, building up the reader's nonmathematical intuition of the notion of sampling error. The natural, intuitive, and nonmathematical notion of study concordance (in which an experiment analysis plan is immune to incoming data) versus study discordance (in which an analysis plan itself is severely perturbed by its own data) is introduced in Chapter Two.

Chapter Three reviews the statistical hypothesis-testing paradigm and introduces the concept of p-values and power from the sampling error perspective. Stressing the concept rather than the mathematics permits the development of a useful definition for the p-values in laymen's terms. Chapter Four discusses the principles of epidemiologic research and the role of p-values. Progressing from there, the longstanding debate over the propriety of p-values is discussed in Chapter Five. This chapter reveals that the concern about p-value use is not simply whether they are interpreted correctly, but about the proper role of mathematics in healthcare research.

The *P-value Primer* moves from there to discuss relevant issues in the applications of hypothesis testing for the investigator. Chapter Six provides a modern discussion of the issues of power and sample size. Discussions of how the courts view scientific evidence in general and statistical inference in particular is offered in Chapter Seven. Chapter Eight focuses on one-tailed versus two-tailed hypothesis testing. I then describe the basics of alpha allocation in the research effort that has multiple clinical measures of interest and combined endpoints (Chapter Nine). Subgroup analyses are data dredging are developed from first principles in Chapter Ten. Chapter Eleven discusses the interpretation and utility of regression analysis. Finally, an introduction to Bayes analyses is presented (Chapter Twelve). The book's conclusion provides concrete advice to the reader for experimental design and p-value construction, while offering specifics on when the p-values of others should be ignored.

The unique feature of *The P-value Primer* is its nonmathematical concentration on the underlying statistical reasoning process in clinical research. I have come to believe that this focus is sorely lacking yet critically needed in standard statistical textbooks that emphasize the details of test statistic construction and computational tools. I quite consciously deemphasize computational devices (e.g., paired t-testing, the analysis of variance, and Cox regression analysis), focusing instead on the nonmathematical features of experimental design that either clarify or blur p-value interpretation.

There is inevitable tension between the mathematics of significance testing and the ethical requirements in medical research; this text concentrates on the resolution of these issues in p-value interpretation. Furthermore, the omnipresent concern for ethics is a consistent tone of this book. In this age of complicated clinical experiments, in which new medications can inflict debilitating side effects on patients and their families, and where experiments have multiple clinical measures of success, this text provides concrete, clear advice for assembling a useful type I error structure, using easily understood computations, e.g., the asymmetric apportionment of alpha and the intelligent allocation of alpha among a number of primary and secondary endpoints in clinical experiments.

The *P-value Primer* is written at a level requiring only one introductory course in applied statistics as a prerequisite; the level of discussion is well within reach of any healthcare worker who has had only a brief, introductory statistics background. It will be valuable to physicians, research nurses, health-care researchers, program directors in the pharmaceutical industry, and government workers in a regulatory environment who must critique research results. It is also useful as an additional text for graduate students in public health programs, medical and dental students, and students in the biological sciences.

So, how did I answer Dr. Kassell back in 1977? Fortunately, I answered him accurately, but unfortunately, I gave the knee-jerk response many statisticians give, "A p-value is the conditional probability of rejecting the null hypothesis when the null hypothesis is true," I most certainly confused him. Even though my response hit the technical nail on the head, I failed in providing the clear, direct answer that would have more usefully answered his query. Over the years, I could never shake the feeling that, after listening to this terse, reflexive reply, a nonstatistical listener remains befuddled about what these p-values really are. Like the newcomer to a foreign language who gets a verbose reply to his short and hesitant question, the inquisitor is frustrated and overwhelmed. This book's goal is to dispel much of that confusion.

Prologue
Aliis exterendum

It is difficult to appreciate the bitter contentions probability and statistics engendered when introduced to Western society. Considered unnecessary in a world where all events were predetermined by higher powers, the study of the relative frequency of events was discouraged for centuries. The nascent field of statistics (not known by that name when first introduced) was all but torn apart by the political and religious controversies its initial use sparked. While some resistance to these areas can be found in jealousies that plague the human heart, an important source of this active resistance was the inability of an unprepared society to first grasp, and then be transformed by the illumination these fields provided.

Thus, an understanding and appreciation of the role of statistics—past, present, or future—can be found in an examination of the culture in which it operates. The Persian practitioner Avicenna in the eleventh century provided seven rules for medical experimentation involving human subjects [1]. Among these precepts was a recommendation for the use of control groups, advice on replication of results, and a monitory against the effects of confounding.* These observations represented a great intellectual step forward; however, this step was taken in relative isolation. While probability, statistics, and the principles of reasoning from data first require a set of data to evaluate, data was available for centuries before these fields developed. An additional 500 years passed before the line of reasoning that led to the concepts of modern probability in applied healthcare emerged; and it was another 300 years before statistical hypothesis testing and p-values were produced. In order to understand the initial twists and turns of the development of this curious discipline, we need to take a quick diversion to life in Europe 500 years ago.

Europe's Emergence from the Middle Ages
Ensuring society's survival before developing society's statistics was the necessary order of progress. The continent struggled, unevenly emerging from the provincialism and ignorance of the Middle Ages in the sisteenth century. Although the majority of Europeans subsisted in the abject rural poverty, groups of Europeans were coming together in numbers. Naples, Lisbon, Moscow, St. Petersburg, Vienna, Amsterdam, Berlin, Rome, and Madrid each contained more than 100,000 people in the

---

* Confounding is the observation that the effect of one variable may confuse the effect of a second variable. For example if only women are exposed to an active therapy, and only men are exposed to the control therapy, then the effect of the therapy is confounded, or bound up, with the effect of gender.

1

1500s, with London and Paris being the largest of these new urban centers [2]. This movement to urbanization accelerated, albeit slowly, creating new links of interdependence among the new city-dwellers. However, with little knowledge about themselves, the residents of these new cities remained blind to their own corporate needs, and could therefore not direct their social progress.

Although rural inhabitants vastly outnumbered urban-dwellers, the contrasts between the large city with its incipient education system and exciting culture on the one hand, and the surrounding, poverty-stricken countryside, on the other, were striking. The one-sided economic relationships between the two environments reflected the undesirability of rural life. Although towns required the resources of the countryside, these agrarian products were not purchased, but instead, were extracted through tithes, rents, and dues. For example, the residents of Palermo, Sicily, consumed 33% of the island's food production while paying only one-tenth of the taxes [2]. While peasants often resented the prosperity of towns and the ensuing exploitation, the absence of rural political power blocked attempts to narrow the widening disparity of wealth.

However, the attraction of cities was only relative; they had their own share of maladies. The unstoppable influx of unemployed rural immigrants looking for work generated a great job demand. Since cities proved no professional paradise for these unskilled workers, poverty emerged as a serious problem in the eighteenth century [2]. Additionally, this rapid arrival of destitute immigrants produced overcrowding that sparked a new round of disease. Despite an end to the most devastating ravages of plague, cities continued to experience high death rates (especially among children) because of unsanitary living conditions, polluted water, and a lack of sewage facilities. One observer compared the stench of Hamburg (which could be smelled from miles away) to an open sewer.

Why was this intolerable situation tolerated? One explanation was the lack of opportunity for most people to reflect on the quality of urban life. Consumed with work, sleep, church, or illness, citizens had little time for considered thought on how life could be improved. Additionally, there was no quantitative measurement of the problems of poverty and illness on a societal level. While each citizen had his or her own poignant anecdotal experience, these personal stories and examples provided conflicting views of the state of urban affairs. No group or person was able to assemble a corporate sense of the quality of life. Thus, there was no way to determine exactly how much poverty existed in a city, and therefore no procedure to track its level over time. The only widely accepted standard for urban life was rural life, and this, everyone agreed was worse than the current city conditions. Finally, the prevailing view was that living conditions improved exceedingly slowly, with progress measured over centuries rather than within a lifetime. This progress rate was far too slow to either track or influence.

Poverty was ubiquitous in the new urban centers, with as much as 10% of the population dependent on charity or begging for food in England and France. Earlier in Europe the poor had been viewed as blessed children of God, and the duty of Christians was to assist them. However, this point of view was replaced with a newer, darker suggestion that the poor were slovenly and unwilling to work themselves out of their lot in life. These opposing points of view produced a contentious search for the cure to poverty. From this emerging cauldron of social conflict came a fervor for change and the need to understand environmental and social influences on human culture. Since the cities were made up of individuals, were there not some features of the whole urban unit that could be influenced?

The first, natural place for people to turn for answers was not data, but the ruling class, seated at the pinnacle of European power.

Absolutism

The religious and social tragedies of the sixteenth and seventeenth centuries sparked the rise of the absolute king. The reformation in the early sixteenth century had been relatively and remarkably free of bloodshed. However, the growing division between the Christian churches in Europe, driven primarily by Protestant dissatisfaction with Catholic kings, unleashed a series of armed conflicts that would rage across Europe for more than 100 years. These vicious international and civil wars produced the deaths of tens of thousands of civilians in the name of religion. The institution of absolute monarchies was originally proposed as a solution to these violent religious disorders, and many in Europe were pleased to exchange local autonomy for peace and safety [3].[*]

With the exception of England, which experienced the replacement of its omnipotent monarchy by first a republic and then a weakened king, the rest of Europe supported the institution of supreme monarch. The icon of these monarchs was the "Sun King", Louis XIV of France, who under the claim of Divine Right, centralized the government, the civil bureaucracy, the legislation, and the judiciary [3].

Following his example, continental Europe moved in mass to the concept of an absolute monarch. Brandenburg, Prussia[†] would become one of the most powerfully centralized states in Europe under Frederick the Great. The Hapsburg emperors worked (ultimately, in vain) to consolidate the Czech-speaking territories into what would become the Austrian–Hungary empire. Tsar[‡] Peter the Great of ruled Russia until 1725, brutally centralizing and westernizing its unique culture. Each of these empires converted from loosely governed autonomies to centralized states.[§]

---

[*] Europe with its history and memory of Roman rule intact, understood the problems that came with acquiescing to the power of an absolute monarchs. However, people were desperate for respite from the current civil slaughter underway. In March, 1562, an army led by the Duke of Guise attacked a Vassy Protestant church service Champagne province of France, slaughtering men women and children—all of whom were unarmed. Thus began the French Wars of Religion which were to last for almost 40 years and destroy thousands of noncombatants [3]. Ten years later, on August 24, 1572, the day before St. Bartholomew's Day, royal forces hunted down and executed over 3,000 Huguenots, in Paris itself. Within three days, soldiers under the direct command of disciplined officers systematically executed over 20,000 Huguenots in the single most bloody and systematic extermination of European civilians until World War II [3]. The war would last another 20 years.

[†] This would become modern-day Germany.

[‡] The words "Tsar" or "Czar" are taken from the Latin "Caesar" [3].

[§] An interesting historical irony is that the most absolutist states in history (Third Reich, Soviet Union) would not be created until the twentieth-century.

The monarchs of these new kingdoms wielded absolute authority in their nation-states, diminishing local rule of law. It was only natural that the people would turn to these super-rulers for wisdom on how to improve their lot. However, by and large the response was subjugation to the will of the king, and the requirement to pay national taxes to support new standing state armies.

A natural tax system was required to support the growing centralized superstructure. However, since a tax system would be unenforceable without at least the façade of equity, a census was required to raise revenue to support the new large standing armies. Thus, the first modern issues in statistics were issues not of statistical hypothesis testing, but of simple counting – the basis of demography.

Refusing to be Counted

The idea of counting individuals had its roots in antiquity and was described in the New Testament [4]. However, the notion of counting citizens fell into disfavor during the Dark Ages. The earliest modern attempt has been traced to a fourteenth century parish in Florence, Italy where births and deaths were recorded by beans (black for boys and white for girls) to determine the sex ratio [5].*

Early demographers in seventeenth-century England faced a daunting challenge, since anything approximating modern census machinery was nonexistent. Fearing that their involvement would lead directly or indirectly to higher taxes, many in the population actively refused to be counted. Additionally, the national government, recognizing the potential military value of a count of men available for service in the new national army, labored to keep whatever demographic data it had a secret. Thus, the first demographers lacked both a counting methodology and reliable data on which to base previous population size claims. Facing an unwilling population that actively resisted enumeration, the demographers' ingenuity was tested as they labored to create indirect estimates of the population's size, age and sex distribution. Multiplying the number of chimneys by an assumed average family size, or inferring age distribution from registered information concerning time of death were typical enumeration procedures [6].

On these basic estimates, taxes were collected, guaranteeing the existence of armies. These, in turn, guaranteed wars, as another lethal era of armed conflict began in the eighteenth century [2]. The Seven Year's War, involving the five great European powers, which spread from the Far East, across Europe and into the New World can legitimately be viewed as the first world war. As the new scale of conflict and terror rapidly drained resources, the demand for new taxes increased. These strident calls for new levies in the absence of the monarchs' interest in learning of the needs of its citizens, fueled cries for change. New, virulent diatribes against the privileged orders caught these ruling monarchs unprepared. This social ferment, created by sustained population growth, abject poverty, and more rapid communication through trade, created disruptive tensions that undermined the foundations of the old order [2].

---

* No one knows the name of the priest who attempted to use church records for counting.

Thus, the restricted use of early data tabulations indirectly added to the burdens of the increasingly impoverished and desperate populations. New calls for tax relief generated more extreme cries for restructured social order. The monarchs' inability to deal meaningfully with these stipulations led to a revolutionary outburst at the end of the eighteenth century, heralding the beginning of the end of absolute royal law. Attention to technology and profit replaced fealty to kings. And with the appearance of leisure time, people began to play games of chance.

No Need for Probability

Games of chance have been recorded throughout history. They had a prominent place in ancient Greek literature and society [7].*The idea of casting lots is mentioned in the Old Testament of the Bible. This concept spread across the Western world, and was converted into games that were played throughout the Middle Ages. The ubiquity and popularity of these diversions would have been a natural proving ground for the laws of probability. However, despite the long-standing existence of these games, people dismissed the idea of developing rules to govern their outcomes. There was a manifest absence of concerted effort to use mathematics to predict the results of games of chance for hundreds of years.

The explanation lies not only in the immaturity of mathematics, but also in the culture in which the mathematics would be viewed. For thousands of years, up through the fourteenth-century, not only was there no clear idea of a random event, but the need for such a concept did not exist. The prevailing perspective viewed all outcomes as determined by either man or deities (benevolent or malevolent). Thus, for many, a "game of chance" was played not to watch random events, but to observe supernatural forces at work. When biblical characters cast lots, they commonly did so not to gamble, but to engage in a process that removed man from the outcome, directly invoking the action of the supernatural. Many thought-leaders of the time believed that all events were pre-determined, further banishing the idea of random events.

Thus, for many, winning a game of chance in an otherwise brutal and unforgiving world equated with receiving, if only for a moment, the undeserved favor of God. The idea of predicting the outcome of the game, thereby diminishing the perceived role of the supernatural, was both anathema and anti-cultural. Such prediction activities flirted with lewd conduct at best† and witchcraft at worst.

---

* Aristotle said, in a justification of gambling, "Amusement is for the sake of relaxation and relaxation, must necessarily be pleasant, since it is a kind of cure for the ills that we suffer in working hard." Aristole. *Politics* VIII5, 1339b;15–17, trans. T.A. Sinclair.

†The conversion of harmless games of chance to gambling by the injection of money tarnished the spirituality of the pasttime, and the practice was seen as less benign. As the recognition grew that gambling attracted the seamier side of cultural elements, attempts were finally made to limit its practice. For example, nobles who chose to fight in the Crusades were permitted to gamble, but the games they could play and the number of attempts they could make were strictly regulated.

Such prevailing opinions pushed the idea of the random events and their predictions beyond the reach of mathematics.[*] Many generations would pass before culture could openly embrace the reasoning of workers who argued that some results appeared to be governed by chance. This acceptance, which first appeared in the 17th century, permitted society to be illuminated by the development of new natural laws.[†]

Intellectual Triumph: The Industrial Revolution

The instigating activity of the industrial revolution substituted inanimate energy forms for organic (human and animal muscle) ones. This replacement transformed society as never before. Unlike the prevalent ethereal forces directing peoples' loyalties to the old order of monarchies, this energy conversion required direct, information-based, cerebral activity. The Industrial Revolution's knowledge-based approach to productivity required quantitative data in ever-increasing amounts. A triumph of the intellect, the Industrial Revolution represented not just a one-time jump in productivity and wealth but a process of ever-accelerating change.

England of all European countries was the best poised for this thrust forward. Its low interest rates, stable government, available lending sources, (relatively) low taxes and the a weakened guild structure sparked enterprise. Once created, this environment catalyzed a cascade of innovation as one invention sparked another.

The development of the flying shuttle, the spinning jenny, the water frame, the power loom, and the spinning mule in the eighteenth century were just a few of the technical innovations that increased productivity. As iron and steel production became a reality, large-scale mechanization was possible for the first time.

The product of this innovation was either sold at home or easily shipped abroad. Demand from larger markets led to improved transportation systems. New agricultural techniques decreased the vulnerability of food crops to bad weather. There were improvements in fodder crops, with a subsequent rise in meat production. Coal was used as fuel, and the implementation of fire-resistant materials (brick and tile) produced by coal heat led to a drop in the frequency of disastrous city-based fires. Consequently, resources needed for rebuilding were conserved. A new belief in the principle of resource conservation paralleled the development of both insurance and government-sponsored food surplus stockpiles.

Quarantine measures helped to eliminate the plague after 1720. The population of London increased from 20,000 in the year 1500 to 500,000 by 1700. A relatively wellfed workforce, now using these technologies for achieving unanticipated new levels of productivity, began to alter its perspective. People became healthier, stronger, better-rested, and more comfortable. Looking anew at their surroundings, the citizenry wondered about the true limits to growth. Although meas-

---

[*] During the Middle Ages, trying to use mathematics to predict an outcome made as much sense as it would now to use modern probability to predict the winner of an election 100 years from now.
[†] Even Albert Einstein, criticizing the statistical approach to particle physics, said, "God does not play dice with the universe."

uring quality of life was generations away, a collective sense suggested that it could and must be evaluated.

The productive climate and the improved standard of living excited intellectual initiative. No longer seen as heretical, the enterprising spirit was now respected and encouraged. As opposed to the closely guarded estimates of population size, technical know-how in the marketplace and the incipient halls of science were not restricted to a few geniuses, but shared by many. These new industries excited artists e.g., Turner and the Impressionists. This was a time when old facts long accepted without proof were unceremoniously discarded. Now, new thinkers would endeavor to answer questions by querying nature directly, bypassing the traditional appeals to monarchs. However, even the most basic information on the citizenry of England itself was absent.

Reasoning from a Sample

The rise of capitalism with its need for market-size estimates required new knowledge of the population's demography. However, in the mid-seventeenth century, even the most basic of facts remained out of reach For example, no one knew the size of London's population; some believed that the city had over two million residents (an exorbitant estimate). The monarchy had a particular interest in this question because of their need to tax the citizenry at a rate the public could bear.

John Graunt's (1620-1674), *Natural History and Political Observations on the London Bills of Mortality* in 1662 was the first modern work in demography. Prior to its appearance, data on the number of deaths in London had been available in the *London Bills of Mortality* [8]. However, no one had actually undertaken a study of this data. Graunt's reviews of these records, and his subsequent careful deductions based on his analyses, revealed new observations and generated novel hypotheses about London death rates. Graunt's singular contribution was to establish the value of careful observation of imperfectly collected human data.[*]

He produced several unique computations, e.g., the process of counting burials to estimate the proportion of deaths. From this preliminary work, Graunt showed that the widely circulated but unsubstantiated speculation that millions of people lived in London was a profound overestimate. His effort established a universal registration of births and marriages, not for religious purposes, but for the purposes of accurate reports on population size to the government and citizenry. Graunt initiated work on the first lifetable, and was honored by nomination to the Royal Society [9].[†]

William Petty received impetus from Graunt's early tabulations, and together they labored to develop lifetable methodology, a procedure that permitted a crude estimate of death rates in London. Under their auspices, information was collected on both the number and causes of deaths, producing the first scientifically

---

[*] The data for the bills was collected by women who were commonly elderly, inebriated, open to bribes, and ignorant of medicine. See Sutherland, referenced at this prologue's end.
[†] It is alleged that King Charles II himself nominated Graunt for fellowship in this august group. See Sprat T. (1722) *History of the Royal Society*, London, p 67, or, more recently, Kargon, R. (1963) *John Graunt, Francis Bacon, and the Royal Society: The Reception of Statistics. Journal of the History of Medical Allied Sciences.* **18**: 337–348.

based cause-specific death rate estimates. Finally, the number of deaths from bubonic plague, consumption and "phthisis" (tuberculosis) could be quantified and followed over time [5].

This was a seminal time in statistics. Prior to the determinations of Graunt, the purpose of counting was simply to take an inventory, with no interest in, nor methodology for, inference. The work of Graunt and Perry held out the idea that there were circumstances in which one could extend results from samples to populations. This notion, so critical to the application of statistics to medicine generated rapid development in the new field. Huddes book *Annuitties* appeared in 1671. Petty's *Political Arithmetic* appeared in 1699, and Greogeory King's *Nature and Political Observations* in 1696. Charles Davenaut's *Discourses on the Public Revenues* (1698) [*] was followed by the first census in modern times, which took place in Ireland in 1703 [10]. Thus a period of slow development produced a critical mass of new thought, producing an eruption of new concepts and products. This cycle of slow development followed by rapid, indeed, sometimes chaotic and unchecked growth can be seen most recently in the development of air travel and the evolution of the modern computer.

Political Arithmetic

However illuminating these first demographic investigations were, the innovative workers behind them were not known in their contemporary world as statisticians. That term, derived from the Italian *statistica* for "statesman" was reserved for constitutional history and political science [5]. The contemporary term for the incipient demographic work of Graunt and Perry in the early 1700s was *political arithmetic* [5], defined as "the art of reasoning by figures, upon things related to government.[†]

It was John Sinclair who argued that the term *statistics* should be usurped to describe the process by which one inferred new meaning about the state of human affairs and interrelationships:.

> the idea I annex to the term is an inquiry into the state of a country, for the purpose of ascertaining the quantum of happiness enjoyed by its inhabitants, by the means of its future improvement...

However, the political arithmeticians at the time soon found themselves embroiled in an intellectual controversy that endures to the present.

The Role of Religion in Political Arithmetic

The collection of this first vital statistics data by Graunt and Perry instigated not merely a new collection of queries but controversy as well. The very nature of their work shattered the old order of looking to the monarchy or diviners for insight into the social order of culture. However the inquiries of these "political arithmeticians"

---

[*] It remains a point of contention as to whether this political arithmetician was a grandson of William Shakespeare.

[†] From Charles D'Avenant, taken from Karl Peasons *The History of Statistics in the 17th and 18th Century*. See references.

declared that social issues could be addressed through the examination of data. This new approach was fraught with major political consequences that became clear when some suggested that a new list of questions could be addressed by the demographers.

Although the initial sampling work started as simple tabulations of the total number of people in London by gender, other more interesting questions rapidly followed: "Why are there more burials than christenings? How many men are married? How many are fighting men? How long does it take to replenish housing after a wave of the plague? How many men ignore their civic duties? In what proportion do men neglect the orders of the church?" The techniques used by the demographers went through a series of refinements in attempts to answer these questions. However, the consequences of sample-based answers to these politically volatile questions produced a series of hotly debated answers. These debates generated the question of who was best able to provide the interpretation of this controversial data, the political arithmeticians, or the cultural thought leaders who had vested interests in the answers.

It is impossible to understand the world of seventeenth to eighteenth century England without paying explicit attention to the overwhelming issue of religion [6]. Religion was not seen as a private matter at the time but as the vital, sustaining bond that held society together. The foundation of all political organization, it permeated everyday discourse, education, social interaction, organization, and all matters of public commerce. Therefore new data-based queries rapidly escalated into controversies involving religion and the spiritual state of England, which in turn had the potential of disrupting the function of the state and established cultural relationships.

The clerics themselves stood disunited on the important religious issues of the day as they found themselves mired in bitter internecine disputes. In the sixteenth century, the general struggle between the Roman Catholics and the "Reformed" or Protestant churches had been resolved on the basis of a compromise under the Tudors.* The accession of Queen Elizabeth I to the throne of England in 1558 shattered this arrangement, marking the decisive victory for Protestantism [11].

However, the fabric of Protestant leadership threatened to become unraveled from new Puritan pressure. This new sect held that the work of Protestant reformation was incomplete and pushed for more changes that were unacceptable to new Protestant dogma. By the middle of the seventeenth century the Puritans were a large and broad-ranging group in English society, wielding profound influence within their local communities. With its strong patriotism and fierce anti-Catholic creed, Puritanism became a formidable force to be reckoned with in trade and commerce. Additionally, Puritans reached into the stratus of aristocracy, influencing the larger landowners and lawyers who populated the Houses of Parliament. However, at this point, the Puritans managed to divide themselves on matters of church organization.

---

* It was hoped that the compromise of declaring the monarch as the heard of national Anglican church, itself part Catholic (High Church) and part Protestant (Low Church) in structure, doctrine, and dogma, would provide a lasting solution.

The strong religious–culture link, in concert with inter-sectarian conflict, meant that changes in influence among the religious sects would be transmitted through the fabric of English culture. Thus, all intellectual work was interpreted in this religiously polarized environment, and the competing religious philosophies spilled over into contentious interpretations of the early demographers' work. Even John Graunt's reputation was besmirched by his conversion to Catholicism late in life [5].[*] It is easy to appreciate the irony in calling these early demographers not statisticians, but political arithmeticians.

However, the development of sample-based data collection continued. Throughout this period, the demographers' technical problem of estimation was taken up by the mathematicians Neumann, Halley, DeMoivre, Bernoulli, Euler, and other mathematicians throughout Europe. This work, further developed by Poisson and Laplace became the foundation of the laws of probability and the inception of the mathematical science of statistics.

Probability and the Return to Order

Probability, discounted as an alien effort by the deity-centric cultures of the Dark Ages developed its first real blooms in the 1600s. By the seventeenth century, as Graunt and others developed the concept of vital statistics, and games of chance continued to be the rave in England and France, gifted observers began to use the data from each of these endeavors. For the first time, this information was collected into datasets as these analysts explored the possibility of producing reliable predictions. The parallel development of mathematical notation sufficient to capture the reasoning process of these experts permitted important progress. A major advance was produced in the early 1600's by Abraham de Moivre, who developed the theory of the normal distribution as an approximation to the binomial distribution. His work, completed toward the end of the seventeenth century by Laplace, led to the conclusion that the mean of a small sample of data will approach a recognizable population mean in a predictable fashion.[†] This was the genesis of modern probability theory [5].

The cultural philosophy that had thus made no room for the role of randomness in the occurrences of life, and had previously dismissed attempts to predict the results of games of chance, had itself evolved. However, it continued to see the predictive, data-based calculations of gambling as disruptive. The DeMoivre–aplace theorem allayed this concern by demonstrating that random events followed their own laws; outcomes beyond the control of man were not unfathomable, but instead demonstrated an overarching order. This long-term view of random events revealed a stability that found a natural home in the religious–centric world.[‡]

---

[*] Graunt's work was criticized; he himself was subjected to the outrageous accusation that he was responsible for the great fire of London

[†] This was known as the DeMoivre–Laplace theorem, and is now recognized as the weak law of large numbers.

[‡] De Moivre, although impoverished his entire life and forced to make a living helping gamblers, was a very likable man and a good friend of Isaac Newton. De Moivre is believed to have died of somnolence, sleeping longer and longer each day in his old age until he finally did not wake up.

The drive to use mathematics to provide a clearer view of the world continued through Newton's work to the present day. However, the acceptability of the inclusion of probability in this quest was provided during the 17th century by DeMoivre and Laplace. Their results gave the process of studying random events an order, and therefore offered the world a lens though which it might gain an elevated perspective of the laws of the universe.

"Let Others Thrash It Out!"

As probability offered the world order by identifying how random events could be predicted, the issue of who would be the best interpreter of data continued to befuddle scholars of the time. The arguments took an interesting turn in the 1830 when a proposal was made to form a statistics section of the British Association for the Advancement of Science. Under the august leadership of Thomas Malthus, a sub-committee was created to answer the question, "Is statistics a branch of science?"

The distinguished committee readily agreed that the process by which the field of statistics collected, organized, and tabulated data was indeed a science. However the question, "Is the statistical interpretation of the results scientifically respectable?" produced vibrant polemics. The anti-inference sect won this debate. The decision to imbue the notion of inference with the respectability of science would have burdened statisticians with the responsibility for interpreting politically sensitive data accurately; this was a task beyond their abilities, since the science of inference had not yet been developed.

They repeated their victory a few years later in 1834 when the Statistical Society of London (later to become the Royal Statistical Society) was formed. Their victory was symbolized in the emblem chosen by the society — a fat, neatly bound sheaf of healthy wheat that represented the abundant data, neatly collected and tabulated. On the binding ribbon was the society's motto *Aliis exterendum*, which means "Let others thrash it out" [12].

Although this action appears out of step with current thinking, the decision provides insight into the prevalent perspective 200 years ago. At the time, statistics was not widely accepted as a science. Those working to correct this did not want to overwhelm the new discipline with politics. Permitting data interpretation to be incorporated as part of statistical science, with its social, economic, religious, and political undertones would provide the tendentious, nonscientific perspective the society hoped to avoid. Thus it was excluded. However, by 1840, the society began to push hard against this limitation.

Early Experimental Design

While the political arithmeticians developed and defended their work in the intellectual cauldrons of the urban environment, much of the development of eighteenth and nineteenth century experimental science took place in agricultural field studies. The parallel progress in experimental science did not rely on the advances of the probabilists and demographers/data analysts of the time. The agricultural science work was not a matter of the mere tabulation of data with associated inference, but of controlling the application of an intervention (e.g., a new seed). The process of designing the experiment to minimize any ambiguity of its conclusions did not draw on mathematics so much as it did on the powers of observation and deductive reasoning.

In 1627, Francis Bacon published an account of the effects of steeping wheat seeds in nine different "nutrient mixtures" on germination speed and the heartiness of growth [13].* One hundred fifty years later, a body of useful contributions to experimental design was constructed by a relatively unknown experimentalist.

Agricultural Articulations

In 1763, a young man, Arthur Young, inherited a farm in England. Within eight years, this agronomist had executed a large number of field experiments, publishing his conclusions in a three-volume book, *A Course of Experimental Agriculture* (1771). With clear insight, he articulated ideas that are the basis of current experimental methodology.

Young expressed the importance of surveying the available data, and each of his volumes began with a literature review. He paid particular attention to biases that were accepted as truth because they were expatiated by "authorities", frequently providing examples of authors who slanted the presented data to support their favored conclusion.

Additionally, Young stressed the importance of comparative experiments, insisting that, when comparing a new method and a standard method, both must be present in the experiment [14]. However, he recognized that, even in comparative experiments, many factors other then the experiment's tested intervention influence the final outcome. Soil fertility, drainage, and insects were just a few of the factors contributing to the yields of experimental plots. Because the overall impacts of these extraneous factors had a variable effect, increasing yields in some years while decreasing them in others, the results of a single experiment in one year could not be completely trusted. Young therefore concluded that experimental replication was critical in agricultural work, often replicating his experiments over each growing season for five years [14].

Additionally, Young was careful to measure the end result of the experiment accurately. When it was time to determine the experiment's outcome, all expenses that could be traced to the intervention being tested were recorded in pounds, shillings, pence, halfpennies, and farthings[14]. At harvest time, one sample of wheat from each of the control field and the treatment field was sent to market on the same day to determine the selling price.

Finally, he recognized the dangers of experimental result extrapolation, warning that his own conclusions about the influences of crop development and growth may not apply to a different farm with different soil and land management practices. By carefully noting that his results would not apply as a guide to long-term agricultural policy, he stressed the pitfalls of unjustified inference from a sample to a population [14].

These important principles of experimental design (review, control, reproducibility, and inference) focus more on the logical infrastructure of the experiment

---

* Bacon concluded that urine was the most effective "nutrient" mixture.

and not on the mathematical manipulation of the results. The work of Arthur Young helped solidify the foundation of experimental science, establishing the principle that the absence of a solid methodologic framework voids the mathematical results of a study.

James Johnson

Seventy-eight years later, James Johnson followed with his book *Experimental Agriculture* (1849), a treatise devoted to practical advice on agrarian experimental design [12].

One of the most important and unique articulations of this text is the consequence of the poorly conceived experiment. Johnson pointed out that a badly conceived experiment was not merely a waste of time and money, but perturbed future investigation. Results of the flawed experiment were incorporated into standard texts and accepted as truth by other experimenters. New and unproductive lines of research were commonly spawned by the false results, leading to wasted time as researchers, unable to understand the conclusions of these new experiments backtracked to find the original mistaken experiment. Additionally, money was lost as other farmers attempted to follow the precepts of the badly conceived experiment's results.

Johnson had other useful observations. Noting that plots of land near one another tended to give similar yields, he recommended that repetitions of the same treatment be spread across noncontiguous plots. The resulting balance of the common soil effect throughout the control and experimental plots reduced the role of soil in explaining the study's results. This presaged the use of randomization as a technique for balancing these influences. Johnson realized, however, that his own treatment-scattering maneuver to reduce the influence of variation was not enough, thereby recognizing his unfulfilled requirement for a quantitative theory of variation [12].

Fisher, Gosset, and Modern Experimental Design

Born in East Finchley, London, in 1890, Ronald Aylmer Fisher grew to be one of the giants in epidemiological thinking. Obtaining his schooling at Gonville and Caius College, in Cambridge, he started work in 1919 as a statistician at Rothamsted Experimental Station. He rapidly developed an interest in designing and analyzing agricultural experiments [7]. However, he realized, as Johnson had, that better methods were necessary to consider the natural variability of crop yields.

A major step forward in the theory of measuring effects in the presence of random variation had been taken while Fisher was still in training, the result appearing in the 1908 manuscript "The Probability Error of a Mean" [10]. Its author was William D. Gosset, using the pseudonym "Student." On leaving Oxford, Gosset went to work in 1899 as a brewer in Dublin for Guinness, a brewery whose owners preferred that their employees use pen names in their published papers[*].

---

[*] This requirement of a brewery that its employees use pen names when publishing always seemed odd to me. Apparently, the Guinness Brewery had given permission for the publication of the first scientific paper by one its employees on the condition that a pseudonym be

Gosset's work there exposed him to many measurement problems, where estimation was required from small samples. He was well aware of the problems of obtaining estimates from small samples of data, which had concerned Galton, another statistician — there just weren't enough observations in the sample to get a good sense for the distribution of the data. To estimate the variance in small samples was also difficult, for the same reason.

Gosset began by choosing the normal distribution for simplicity, stating "It appears probable that the deviation from normality must be severe to lead to serious error" [10]. He then showed that the sample mean and sample standard deviations from a normal distribution were uncorrelated and he correctly deduced that they were independent. The finding of independence simplified his next tasks immensely, leading to the identification of the distribution of the ratio

$$\left(x - \bar{x}\right)\Big/_{s}$$

as a t distribution (now known as Student's t–distribution). Thus, experimentalists could now identify the distribution of this normed difference even when the small sample size precluded a precise measure of the population variance. Agricultural scientists like Fisher could now incorporate the variance of the plot yield into a measure of the difference in plot yields and find the distribution of this normed difference, identifying extreme values. Building on this work, Fisher introduced the modern scientific era to the concept of significance testing and the p-value.

We will see in Chapter Five that acceptance of the p-value, especially in healthcare, has been doggedly resisted. However, the contention over the introduction of this tool demonstrated once again that the introduction of new mathematical concepts can take the scientific culture by surprise. The first reactions of astonishment produce firestorms of criticism that gradually recede as the new idea eventually finds its place in the panoply of available scientific tools.

However, some have argued that the p-value should never have had much of a place at all in healthcare research. To assess the validity of that perspective, we must examine the role of mathematics in generalizing sample results to populations in medical investigation.

References

1.   Stigler SM (1986) *The History of Statistics —The Measurement of Uncertainty Before 1900*. Cambridge, MA, and London: The Belknap Press of Harvard University Press, p. 4.
2.   Gerhard Rempel. Notes. Western New England College
3.   Hooker R: The European Englightenment
     http://www.wsu.edu/~dee/ENLIGHT/PRE.HTM.
4.   Holy Bible. New International Version. Luke 2:1.

used, possibly because competing companies might become knowledgable about ongoing work at Guinness[11].

5. Pearson K (1978) *The History of Statistics in the 17th & 18th Centuries* . London and High Wycombe: Charles Griffin .

6. Kendall, Sir Maurice, Plackett RL (1977) *Studies in the History of Statistics and Probability* (Volume 2) New York; Macmillan Publishing.

7. Hombas VC, Baloglou CP (2005) Gambling in Greek Antiquity. *Chance* **18**:49–50.

8. Sutherland I (1963) John Graunt: A tercentenary tribute. *Journal of the Royal Statistical Society* (A) **126**:537–556.

9. Gehan EA, Lemak NA (1994) *Statistics in Medical Research: Developments in Clinical Trials.* New York and London: Plenum Medical Book Company.

10. Kendall MG (1970) Where shall the history of statistics begin? From Pearson ES, Kendall MG *Studies in the History of Statistics and Probability*. Connecticut. Hafner Publishing Company.

11. Muhlberger S (1998) Notes. Nipissing University

12. Cochran WG (1976) Early development of techniques in comparative experimentation. From Owen D.B: *On the Hstory of Probability and Statistics*. New York and Basal Marcel Dekker, Inc.

13. Bacon Γ (1627) *Sylva sylvarum, or a Natural History*. London; William Rawley.

14. Young A (1771) *A Course of Experimental Agriculture*. Dublin; Exshaw et al.

1

The Basis of Statistical Reasoning in Medicine

1.1 What Is Statistical Reasoning?

"Well, do you believe the article, or not?" your impatient colleague demands yet again.

A 34-year-old woman is brought to the emergency room by her anxious husband. You're her doctor.

"She was fine until four hours ago!" her frightened husband blurts out. "She suddenly collapsed!"

You learn that your new patient, a cigarette smoker, didn't lost consciousness or convulse. She does use birth control pills. Your exam reveals a frightened but well-groomed adult female who is unable to communicate and can't control the right side of her body. Finishing your workup, you correctly diagnose an acute stroke and orchestrate her emergency care.

"Are you going to give her tPA[*] to help reduce the size of the stroke?" asks your colleague, who, observing the new case, wanders over to where you are now writing up the patient's record.

"No, " you reply. "Current protocols say to give tPA within three hours of symptom onset." Checking your watch, you add, "Its been almost four an a half hours now according to the husband. Giving it now would risk a major bleeding event."

"Hey!" your colleague retorts. "Didn't you see the article this month describing the latest research experience? It found that its safe to give tPA for more than three hours after the stroke. Actually," she adds, rummaging through a collection of papers, "I have it…right…Ah! Here it is." Your stomach squirms restlessly as she plops the manuscript on your desk right where you're writing the patient's orders.

"It's in a good journal," she persists. Turning to the relevant section, she says, "See? This is what I was talking about."

"I didn't see this," you confess thinking *Current tPA practice says that giving it now risks a major bleed. Yet if it could help…*

---

[*] Tissue plasminogen activator. This therapy is believed to reduce the magnitude of a stroke.

"Right here!" your colleague interjects, pointing to the abstract. "The study says the risk of a bleed is low and that patients do better with tPA administration even out to five hours after stroke symptoms."

Struggling to integrate the new material, you ask, "How many patients in the study?"

"A lot for a stroke trial," she responds at once. "It's a large subgroup analysis from a randomized, double-blind controlled clinical study with a combined primary endpoint and multiple secondaries. While the primary endpoint just missed stat significance, the secondary endpoint of reduced hospitalization…".

On and on your colleague goes, spewing out the study details. The clock is ticking as you struggle to decide if you believe the manuscript. *Is the analysis sound?* you wonder. *Does is apply to my patient? Can I believe the conclusion? Is it too late to apply it's results…*

"Doctor!" a nurse calls out, jolting you from your thoughts. "Just picked up a call from the paramedics. A motor vehicle accident with head trauma coming in. Any instructions?"

"Time's a'wastin, " your colleague reminds you.

Statistical reasoning in medicine is, at its heart, the process by which we determine if healthcare research results identified in one sample apply to others. For the emergency room physician in the previous example, the urgent question is whether the results can be generalized from the new manuscript to the stricken patient. Since this generalization is not automatic and commonly inappropriate, we must know when to generalize sample results versus when not to.

Before we delve into the statistical issues, we should first acknowledge that physicians have a built-in difficulty with these concepts. It's not our fault—we were engineered this way!

1.1.2 Physicians and the Patient Perspective

Physician training focuses on the individual patient to the exclusion of the population. We may call this the "single-patient perspective." The single patient perspective is inculcated in medical students from their first year introductory courses. The detailed instruction in anatomy, histology, biochemistry, and physiology we received was not so much to enhance our understanding of the constitution of the population, but to deepen our understanding of the structure of the individual. It was a discussion about facts. Exams were on facts, not on variability.

As medical students, we are trained to develop thorough and exhaustive differential diagnoses, compiling a complete list of possible explanations for the symptoms and signs the individual patient presented, with little thought given to the frequency of the disease in the population. In my medical education, a seemingly disproportionate emphasis was placed on rare diseases (e.g., Whipple's disease, or Tsushugamuchi fever). This exposure trained us to identify the one unexpected patient who might have that unusual disease. In essence we were taught to bring "the rare to bear" in developing a patient's diagnosis.

We remember the first time that we had responsibility for performing a history and physical.* Each of these experiences inculcates the "single-patient perspective"; i.e., our focus must be on the one patient before us.

Occasionally, during a short course in either epidemiology or biostatistics in the middle of medical school, we faced another point of view. General discussions about measuring effects in populations presented a perspective that suggested that there was a larger context for our work. However the concept was already a foreign one. After all, wasn't the best way to mend the health of a population to allow well-educated, individual physicians to treat individual patients, one at a time? Trained to place the patient in the position of pre-eminence, we found the new population-perspective was alien. Upon graduation, we took a patient-based, not a population-based, oath.

As house officers, we focused not on populations of patients, but on the few (although at the time it seemed like the many) patients on the wards, floors, and units that we covered. We attended lectures to learn how we might better help the patients directly under our care. Private practices were built one patient at a time, one family at a time. Every patient interaction offered a potential surprise or pitfall, and therefore required our complete attention. Since the most important patient that we would see is the one we were currently treating, all of our skills and energy had to be focused there.

1.1.2 Research and the Population Perspective

The patient-perspective remains preeminent for good and undeniable reasons. Examining, identifying, and treating the patient for his or her benefit alone is a tremendous responsibility for which we are disciplined and trained. We should not turn our faces from this challenge.

Yet the principles of research are different from those of medical practice. In fact, many physicians believe that in order to understand research tenets, they must embrace concepts that they have been specifically trained to shun.

One example of this disconnect between research and medical practice principles is the concept of the "average" patient. The average blood pressure produced by the active group in a clinical trial may be only 2–3 mm Hg. lower than in the control group, a finding heralded as an important advance by the research community. However, physicians treating patients in the community are not impressed with the change, asking how a 2-3 mm Hg reduction could possible matter in a patient where the daily stresses of work and family living generate changes in blood pressure that are more significant.

Another confusing message for the physicians laboring to understand research issues is the concept of variability. Treating physicians clearly understand that patients are very different from one another, unique in an infinite number of ways. We take this into account, adjusting the patient's visit schedule in accordance

---

* For me, it was an adult, deaf-mute male at North Shore Hospital on Long Island, New York, in March 1976.

with the patient's stability or our concerns.* We never think of modifying variability. Yet, researchers become experts at controlling, adjusting, or even removing
variability.

    The difference between the two groups of workers is perspective. Physi-
cian views develop from the patient-based perspective, while researchers are commonly population-based. Each perspective uses different tools because its goal's are
different.

1.1.3 The Need for Integration

The two examples cited above reflect the difficulties that complicate the physician's
attempt to integrate relevant research findings into their body of knowledge. The
different points of view between the population and patient perspective induce a
tension in physicians because their goals are different. Yet it is up to us to integrate
these disparate points of view, accepting the best of each while simultaneously understanding their limitations.

    We can begin this incorporation process by repudiating the idea that indi-
vidual patient preeminence is negotiable. In practice, the patient must come first —
subjugating our primary concern for the patient to any other perspective leads to
unethical, avoidable damage to patients and their families. However, embracing the
patient perspective blinds us to an objective view of the effect of our interventions.

    We as practicing physicians often cannot see the results of our own inter-
ventions in an objective light [1]. For example, if patients who respond well to our
treatments return to see us, while the poor responders drift away, we are lulled into
a false sense of confidence in the positive utility of the intervention. On the other
hand, if patients who are invigorated by our treatment do not return, while only the
dissatisfied come back to demonstrate the inadequacies of our therapeutic approach,
we may prematurely abandon an important and promising therapy. The fact is that
some patients improve (or deteriorate) regardless of what we do. By concentrating
on what we observe, to the exclusion of what should be considered but is unobserv-
able, we lose sight of an unbiased view of the intervention.

    Thus, while we require evidence-based medicine, the evidence we collect
from our daily practices is subjective and therefore suspect. The focus on the individual patient, while necessary, blinds our view of the true risks and benefits of the
therapy.

1.1.4 A Trap

An objective view of therapy begins with a balanced mindset, requiring that we
respond to our patients' trust in us by modulating our own belief in the therapies
that we advocate. We physicians as a group have become too easily enamored of
promising theories, e.g., the arrhythmia suppression hypothesis or the immunother-
apy/interferon hypothesis. These theories, well researched at the basic science level,
are replete with detail, holding out tremendous promise for our patients. This com-

---

* The simple, often mocked admonition "Call me in the morning", is a result of the fact that
the doctor, not knowing in precise detail what will happen to the patient, insists on being
provided with new information to determine if any unexpected event has occurred.

bination of innovation and hope can be hypnotic. Furthermore, initial findings in individual patients can lead to a domino effect of individual anecdotes, discussion groups, articles, and treatment recommendations. This set of theories can easily take on a life of their own.

Herein lies the trap. Well-developed and motivated theories are commonly wrong and unhelpful in medicine. Basing patient practice on an attractive but false theory has had and will continue to have devastating effects on patients, their families, and our communities. Accepting the conclusion before formally testing it is a wonderful principle in religion, but it is antipodal to science.

In order to keep our guard up, we must also remind ourselves, somewhat painfully, that professional and compassionate doctors who placed their patients first as we do, who were true to their oaths then as we are now, were often the source of destructive, barbaric treatments. For hundreds of years, compassionate physicians allowed infected wounds to fester because an ancient text declared authoritatively and erroneously that purulence was beneficial, and that cleanliness during surgery was unnecessary. More recently, we have learned that hormone replacement therapy for women as commonly administered for years is harmful.

The harmful actions of physicians based on our faith in false beliefs are the sad, natural consequences of accepting the patient-preeminence philosophy as an unbiased one. We must therefore recognize that, while the patient perspective is appropriate, we require additional tools to observe the effects of our therapies objectively. The population-perspective provides these tools. Thus, the population perspective does not represent a threatening viewpoint, but an additive one, and its consideration does not lead to philosophy replacement but perspective enlargement.

1.1.5 Clinical Versus Research Skills

Unquestionably, clinicians are professionals with important, even rare skill sets. While these capabilities include the capacity to diagnose patients and discuss complicated circumstances with patients and their families, one of our most important abilities is the capacity quickly to size up a particular clinical circumstance. The demands of medical school and residencies require us to size up a particular circumstance rapidly, identify the factors needed to make a decision, and then quickly select the right option. Doctors are taught not to be efficient, but to be hyper-efficient.

This skill is developed in training and becomes a natural habit pattern for physicians; it is perpetuated and taken advantage of in hospital wards and emergency rooms where rapid appraisal and assessment can be essential. In these circumstances, responding quickly, accurately, reflexively, and (of course) correctly becomes an admirable if not necessary adjunct to other clinical skill sets.

However, the fine clinical motivation for carrying out research can obstruct the conduct of that research. The impetus to use research to address an unmet medical need is closely aligned with an essential creed of modern medicine, to relieve pain and suffering. However, this can easily translate to the sense that great haste must be expended in the research effort. Left unchecked, this ideology can generate the belief that speed is everything, and that everything—discipline, standards, dialogue, methodology, quality, and good judgment — should be sacrificed for it. All of these principles add value to the scientific effort but unfortunately are shunned for the sake of rapid progress.

A fine counterexample to this is the practice of Dr. Stanley Cohen, the 1986 Nobel Laureate for Physiology and Medicine, Vanderbilt University School of Medicine. When asked about the caliber of his work that led to his award, he commented that, from the mid-1960s up to the present, technological advances permitted the automation of physiologic investigations; investigations that used to take days or weeks to carry out now took hours. Scientists found that they could execute experiments one after the other in rapid-fire succession [2].

Dr. Cohen, however, chose a different strategy. Rather than quickly execute a quickly excutable experiment, he would instead invest much of his time and best effort into pre-experimental thought, with attention focused on each of the possible outcomes of the experiment. Only when he was sure that each possible experimental result would teach him something that was both new and worth knowing would he proceed with the experiment. This was, in Dr. Cohen's view, the only noteworthy distinction between the character of his Nobel Prize–winning work and the efforts of his colleagues.

Dr. Cohen's experience emphasizes the importance of steady progress, as opposed to rapid progress. Science is not about speed. Other things — capitalism, politics, profit — are about speed. But not science.

1.2 Statistical Reasoning

The plenary session of a major medical meeting has just begun. A young, promising investigator steps to the podium. Assuredly, she begins her measured presentation illuminating a heretofore unexpected relationship between an exposure and the occurrence of disease. The well-rehearsed lecture goes smoothly as the scientist presents one slide after another with skill, poise, and aplomb. The audience listens to the presentation in rapt silence, anticipation building as the investigator reaches the apex of the 15 minute lecture with the demonstration of more disease among the exposed group of patients than among the unexposed group.

As the auditorium lights are raised at the conclusion of her concise presentation, the room erupts in questions. Is there a relationship between dose or duration of exposure and the disease frequency? What is the underlying biologic mechanism that explains the findings? Has anyone else demonstrated this relationship? The investigator responds clearly and honestly to these questions, and the entire room engages in one of the most satisfying experiences in science.

However, no one asks the simple question, "Do the results in your sample truly reflect the findings in the population from which your sample was drawn?" The question has nothing to do with the veracity of the investigator. She found what she claimed to find in her sample. But do her sample findings translate to the population from which the sample was obtained? Does the examination of the relationship between exposure and disease in her sample concisely and efficiently capture what one would find if they examined the entire population, or, alternatively, are the sample results merely due to a freak of chance, the vicissitudes of her inadvertent selection of the wrong, unrepresentative sample from the population. If the former is correct, than the whirlwind of scientific discussion is necessary and valid.

However, if the relationship is one that is seen only in the sample, and does not adequately depict a population finding, then the discussion is based on fantasy.

Discerning whether a sample's results applies to the population is the essence of statistical reasoning in medicine. Whether you believe in the use of p-values, confidence intervals, Bayes procedures, or alternatively, are unsure what to believe, you have to first decide if the sample results can be generalized.

1.2.1 The Great Compromise

A researcher studying a particular disease, e.g., congestive heart failure (CHF), would study every single patient with that disease everywhere if he could. He would identify the world population with CHF. Contacting each affected individual, the scientist would meet with him or her, taking a complete history and physical. Carrying out all requisite tests, the researcher would relentlessly record this data. He would do this not just at one time point, but periodically, over the course of the patient's life subsequent to their diagnosis.

This would be the definitive approach to the treatment of CHF. It is also hopelessly impossible. The financial, logistical, and ethical problems[*] remove it from serious consideration, and the researcher is blocked from access to the complete population (Figure 1.1).

Investigators

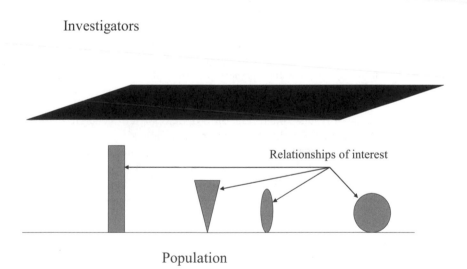

Population

Fig 1.1. The investigators are blocked from observing the relationship of interest in the entire population by financial, logistical, and ethical constraints.

---

[*] Even if our intrepid investigator managed to solve the Herculean financial, logistical, personnel, and travel issues, many patients might just refuse to be part of the study.

From Figure 1.1, we can see that the investigators are interested in examining the relationships in the population (denoted by the different geometric figures), but are obstructed because they do not have population data. In full recognition of this problem, the investigator compromises. He gives up the notion of studying every member of the population, replacing it with the concept of thoroughly studying only a sample of the entire population. Like every compromise, the sampling process provides something that the researcher needs, but it also requires that the investigator give up something of value. The heart of statistical reasoning in medicine is the implication of this compromise.

The sampling process provides executability for the researcher. While he is not in the position to study millions of subjects, he can pay for, obtain informed consent from, and thoroughly examine, 2,000 patients with CHF. The size of the study is now within his investigational scope, permitting him to learn of the experiences of this small cohort.

However, the investigator also gives up something of great value in this compromise — certainty. If the entire population is studied, the results of the population are known, and the answer to his scientific questions would be assured. However, studying only a small sample from a large population leaves most of the population unstudied. How then can the researcher have confidence in his answers when most of the population of interest remains unstudied?

In fact, many other independent samples can be drawn from the same population by equally diligent and capable investigators. Since these samples are composed of different patients with different life experiences, measurements on these patients will differ from measurements taken on patients in other independent samples. Results will vary from sample to sample.

The variability of the same measure across different samples, each generated by the same population, is *sampling error*. This variability is the new, important ingredient in the sampling approach that must be carefully examined and integrated into the research results' interpretation. Populations will generate many different samples. Since the price the investigator pays for taking one sample is the recognition that different samples, generated by different investigators, generate different results, why should one investigator's findings be believed over another?

Even a random sample, though it is planned, representative, and laudable, is, after all, just a single sample – it may not contain the truth about a population. Let's examine the effect of sampling error in a population.

1.2.2 Example of Sampling Error

To understand the different views a sample can provide of a population, let's carry out an artificial experiment. A population of 2,231 patients (all of the patients in the world with the disease) are at risk of death. A therapy will reduce the cumulative mortality rate for this population by 19% (producing a relative risk of 0.81). This is the "true state of nature" (Table 1.1).

Table 1.1. Effect of therapy on total mortality rate in a population of 2,231 patients

	Variable	Placebo	Active	Total	Rel Risk
		Patient Counts			
	Deaths	275	228	503	
Total	At Risk	1116	1115	2231	
Population	Total Mortality Rate	0.246	0.204	0.225	0.81

The population experienced a relative risk of 0.81, signifying a 19% reduction.

Now consider an investigator who does not know the true state of nature. The best that he can do is to take a random sample from this population and study the effect of the therapy. The investigator draws a sample of 216 patients from this population of 2,231, and observes the results (Table 1.2).

Table 1.2. Investigators' results from a random sample of 54 patients from the population of 2,231.

	Variable	Placebo	Active	Total	Rel Risk
		Patient Counts			
	Deaths	25	29	54	
Total	At Risk	109	107	216	
Population	Total Mortality Rate	0.229	0.271	0.250	1.21

Example of how a random sample can mislead. The relative risk of 1.21 is substantially different from the relative risk of 0.81 observed in the population.

This investigator's one sample reveals 25 deaths in the placebo group and 29 deaths in the active group, an excess of 4 deaths attributable to active therapy. The cumulative mortality rate for the placebo group is 0.229 (25/109) for the placebo group and 0.271 (29/107) for the active group, and the relative risk of therapy is 1.21. If the therapy were neutral, causing no more deaths in the active group than in the placebo group, the relative risk would be 1.00. The value of 1.21 suggests that therapy may be harmful, causing 21% increase in deaths in the treatment group than in the placebo group. This researcher might conclude that there is at least a trend toward excess mortality produced by the therapy.

To push this example a little harder, the promulgation of the investigator's one sample in the medical literature, at symposiums, at workshops, and conferences would suggest that the therapy is not helpful, and in fact may be harmful. Many researchers would labor to explain these surprising findings.[*] Some would theorize

---

[*] Possible explanations would be that the study explicitly excluded patients who would be helped by the medication, or that the causes of specific deaths should be examined to see if patients died of events not influenced by the therapy.

that perhaps the therapy itself did beneficially affect the course of the disease, but produced another unanticipated harmful effect that was fatal. Experienced academicians and researchers have watched this scenario play out in many circumstances. However, the role of sampling error is overwhelming, as portrayed by the display of other completely random samples from this same population of 2,231 patients (Table 1.3).

The sampling variability from Table 1.3 is stunning. In the population of 2,231 in which the therapy is in fact known to be effective, five of the ten small samples suggest a harmful effect. On the other hand, Sample 3 suggests a powerful beneficial therapy effect. Alternatively, sample 5 suggests a 43% increase in deaths. Imagine if these above ten samples reflected the results of each of ten investigators, one investigator to a sample. These investigators at a meeting would provide often long and sometimes loud commentary, laboring to justify their own findings. The "random" in random-sampling may not be chaotic, but this resulting situation surely is, and the confusion is solely due to sampling error.

This example demonstrates that, even with a perfectly random sample, it is possible that one clear relationship in the population will not be mirrored by the sample's result. In fact, we would have trouble identifying the true relationship between therapy and total mortality by looking at the ten sample results. This is why sampling variability is so dangerous to investigators. A clinician copes with the variability of a patient's response to a drug by using the traditional tools of clinical practice available to her. These tools include taking a family history, examining the patient's previous exposure to this class of drugs, and remaining vigilant for the occurrence of any adverse reaction. We need new tools to help us with sampling error so that we can assess the impact of the therapy in the community. Consider the plight of the investigators in the PRAISE investigations.

1.2.3 PRAISE I and II

In the 1980s, the use of calcium-channel blocking agents in patients with congestive heart failure (CHF) was problematic, as initial studies suggested that patients with CHF exposed to these drugs experienced had increased morbidity and mortality [3]. In the early 1990s, new calcium-channel-blocking agents appeared, with early data supporting their use in patients with heart failure. The Prospective Randomized Amlodipine Survival Evaluation (PRAISE) trial's long-term objective was the assessment of the channel blocker amlodipine's effect on morbidity and mortality in patients with advanced heart failure.

The primary measurement in PRAISE was the composite endpoint of all-cause mortality and/or hospitalization.[*] Patients with CHF (New York Heart Association (NYHA) functional class IIIb/IV and LVEF < 30%) were randomized to receive either amlodipine or placebo therapy beginning in 1992. Since the investigators suspected that the effect of amlodipine might depend on the cause of the patient's CHF, they balanced the use of therapy in each of two groups, (1) patients with ischemic cardiomyopathy and, (2) patients who had non-ischemic cardio-

---

[*] Hospitalization was defined as receiving in-hospital care for at least 24 hours for either acute pulmonary edema, severe hypo-perfusion, acute myocardial infarction, or sustained hemodynamically destabilizing ventricular tachycardia or fibrillation.

myopathy. By the end of the study, the PRAISE investigators randomized 1,153 patients, following them for a maximum of 33 months.

Table 1.3. Results of 10 random samples from a population of 2,231.

| Variable | Patient Counts | | | Rel Risk |
	Placebo	Active	Total	
Sample 1				
Deaths	25	29	54	
At Risk	109	107	216	
Total Mortality Rate	0.229	0.271	0.250	1.21
Sample 2				
Deaths	24	22	46	
At Risk	115	99	214	
Total Mortality Rate	0.209	0.222	0.215	1.13
Sample 3				
Deaths	35	15	50	
At Risk	122	92	214	
Total Mortality Rate	0.287	0.163	0.234	0.52
Sample 4				
Deaths	25	30	55	
At Risk	107	95	202	
Total Mortality Rate	0.234	0.316	0.272	1.43
Sample 5				
Deaths	31	17	48	
At Risk	112	96	208	
Total Mortality Rate	0.277	0.177	0.231	0.62
Sample 6				
Deaths	26	27	53	
At Risk	103	110	213	
Total Mortality Rate	0.252	0.245	0.249	1.02
Sample 7				
Deaths	27	24	51	
At Risk	104	106	210	
Total Mortality Rate	0.260	0.226	0.243	0.88
Sample 8				
Deaths	24	20	44	
At Risk	92	92	184	
Total Mortality Rate	0.261	0.217	0.239	0.82
Sample 9				
Deaths	31	20	51	
At Risk	110	99	209	
Total Mortality Rate	0.282	0.202	0.244	0.69
Sample 10				
Deaths	24	26	50	
At Risk	98	91	189	
Total Mortality Rate	0.245	0.286	0.265	1.01

Sampling error produces a wide range of relative risk for therapy from a population with a relative risk is 0.81.

At the conclusion of PRAISE, the investigators determined that in the overall cohort there was no significant difference in the occurrence of the primary endpoint or in total mortality between the amlodipine and placebo groups. However, there was a substantial reduction in all-cause mortality and/or hospitalization (58 fatal or nonfatal events in the amlodipine group and 78 in the placebo group), a 31% risk reduction (95% CI 2 to 51% reduction, $p = 0.04$) in patients with non-ischemic dilated cardiomyopathy. Further evaluation of these events revealed that there were only 45 deaths in the amlodipine group and 74 deaths in the placebo group, representing a 46% reduction in the mortality risk in the amlodipine group (95% CI 21 to 63% reduction, $p < 0.001$). Among the patients with ischemic heart disease, treatment with amlodipine did not affect the combined risk of morbidity and mortality or the risk of mortality from any cause. The effect of therapy appeared to be related to the classification of ischemic cardiomyopathy.

A second trial PRAISE-2 [4] was then conducted to verify the beneficial effect on mortality seen in the subgroup analysis of patients with heart failure of non-ischemic etiology in PRAISE-1. This trial, while focusing only on patients with heart failure of non-ischemic origin, was similar in design to PRAISE-1. The PRAISE-2 investigators randomized 1,650 patients to either amlodipine or placebo, following them for up to 4 years. However, unlike the first study, there was no difference in mortality between the two groups (33.7% in the amlodipine arm and 31.7% in the placebo arm; relative risk 1.09, $p = 0.28$) in PRAISE-2. Thus, the marked mortality benefit seen in the subgroup analysis in PRAISE-1 for amlodipine was not confirmed in PRAISE-2.

While several explanations have been suggested for the difference in the findings of the PRAISE studies, a possible explanation that cannot be excluded is simply that the patients in two essentially equivalent different samples responded differently, i.e., the results of the smaller subgroup analysis in PRAISE-1 were due to the vicissitudes of chance.* The issue of sampling error lies at the forefront of the interpretation of any sample-based research.

1.2.4 Fleas

Sampling error is the bane of the researcher's efforts. Research efforts that can include and study every single member of a small population of interest are more easily designed, more easily executed, more easily analyzed, and certainly more easily interpreted. However, what makes our sampling-based studies executable (i.e., the selection of a relatively small number of subjects from a larger population) is precisely what introduces sampling error and its implications into our effort. Consider the following passage from the novel *Arrowsmith* by Sinclair Lewis ([5] page 365). The quote is from Sondelius, an epidemiologist, dying from bubonic plague, for which the flea is a vector in the disease transmission.

> Gottlieb is right about these jests of God. Yeh! His best one is the tropics. God planned them so beautiful, flowers and sea and mountains. He made the fruit to grow so well that man need not work – and then He laughed,

---

* The problems of subgroup analysis will be discussed later in this text.

and stuck in volcanoes and snakes and damp heat and early senility and the plague and malaria. But the nastiest trick He ever played on man was inventing the flea.

Sampling error is the flea of our research tropics. We can't get rid of it, but we enjoy the "research tropics" too much to leave.

The principal use of statistics in research is to address the sampling error issue. The nonmathematical comprehension of this process is critical for the scientist who is interested in reaching useful conclusions about the population from which their research sample is drawn. Two important features of interpretable sample-based research are careful consideration of the sampling plan and careful execution of this prospectively declared plan. Since violation of either of these principles can render a sample-based research effort invalid, we will spend time discussing the necessary features of each of these two components.

1.3 Generalizations to Populations

When an investigator chooses a sample from a population, he has many selection schemes that he may follow. The investigator could select all males, for example, or restrict selection to only patients between 40 and 50 years of age. The selection criteria are arbitrary but the consequences can be profound. In order to choose the best criteria for selecting patients, we must remember that we rely on the sample to contain, reflect, and therefore reveal relationships that exist in the population.

The only purpose the sample serves, therefore, is to represent the population to which we would like to generalize the research result. The sample is our view of the population. If that view is blurred, bent, or otherwise distorted, we have difficulty discerning what is occurring in the population from what we see in our sample. We must choose our sample in the way that provides the clearest view of the population.

The clearest view of the population is provided if the sample is selected such that the sample resembles the population. However, typically small samples cannot look like the population in every detail. Populations are large, and have innumerable nuances and characteristics that overwhelm a small sample's ability to capture and reflect. However, samples can be generated that reproduce important features of the population.

1.3.1 Advantages of the Random Sample

To most people, the word "random" is associated with chaos. It refers to a thing that is unstructured, unplanned, directionless, and haphazard. Perhaps that is so for many events we deal with in the world, but it is not true for random-sampling schemes. One of the most useful sampling plans is the *simple random selection*. The simple random selection mechanism is that collection of procedures that draws subjects from the population in such a way that each subject in the population has the same, constant probability of being selected for the sample. This produces a sample that "appears like" the population. A sample that is selected using this mechanism is commonly known as a *simple random sample*.

This simple random-sampling approach is the best way to ensure that the selected sample represents the population at large, and that the findings in the sample can be generalized to the population from which the sample was obtained. If each population member has the same likelihood of being chosen for the sample, then no member is excluded a priori at the expense of another, and there are no built-in biases against any subject based on that subject's individual characteristics. This is one of the key requisites of the generalization process. Changes from the simple random-sampling plan must be carefully considered, since deviations impact the generalizability of the results.

Yet, although it is an admirable goal, the attainment of a simple random selection mechanism is commonly an unattainable goal in medical research. This is primarily due to its impracticability. Patients have the right to refuse participation in the study after being selected randomly. The influence of these individual decisions, in concert with the presence of specific patient inclusion and exclusion criteria, easily disables the random selection mechanism. Thus, this physician-researcher would have difficulty with any generalization because the inclusion and exclusion criteria necessary to make the study ethical can alter the sample so that it no longer represents the population. A well-designed study that examines the effect of therapy in one gender will commonly not be generalizable to people in the opposite sex.[*] Therefore, researchers and readers must take great care in correctly identifying the population to which a research sample can be appropriately generalized

1.3.2 Limitations of the Random Sample

There are two caveats that we must keep in mind when considering simple random samples. The first is that they can mislead. The second concern is that random samples are rarely achieved in clinical research, and almost never realized within the construct of a clinical trial. This is due to the operation of a set of inclusion and exclusion criteria. These exclusion criteria are required for logistical and ethical reasons. Sometimes they are used to identify a collection of individuals that are most likely to demonstrate the relationship that the research is designed to identify.[†] Since each exclusion restricts a patient from entering the study based on a characteristic of that patient, the body of exclusion criteria make the sample less representative of the general population. The inability of most clinical trials to achieve a sample that even approximates a simple random sample is an important limitation of this research tool.

A second caveat is the incomplete operation of the random chance mechanism in small samples. Since samples exclude most patients from the population,

---

[*] This was the case in the Physicians Health Study (Steering Committee of the Physicians' Health Study Research Group (1989) Final report on the aspirin component of the ongoing Physicians' Health Study. *New England Journal of Medicine* 321(3):129–35) that identified the cardio-protective effects of aspirin in male physicians. While few scientists had difficulty extending its results to male non-physicians, it was not clear whether the results should be extended to women.

[†] A fine example is clinical trials that exclude patients who are believed to be 1) unlikely to comply with the intervention if it is self-administered over a period of time or 2) unwilling to complete a rigid follow-up attendance schedule.

we would expect that a particular sample is not going to represent each of the innumerable descriptive facets of the population. A simple random sample of 1,000 patients from a population of 19 million diabetic patients will not provide representative age–ethnic-educational background combinations.[*] It is asking too much of the sampling mechanism to produce a relatively small sample that is representative of each and every property and trait of the individuals in the population. Thus, the sample must be shaped by the investigator so that it is representative of the population for the traits that are of greatest interest. This contouring process represents a compromise. Since the sample is created to be representative of some aspects of the population, it is not going to be representative of others. Thus, the resulting sample will have a spectrum of representation, accurately reflecting a relatively small number of traits of the population, and producing inaccurate depictions of others.

Investigators who are unaware of this spectrum, and who therefore, report every result from their study as though that result is valid and generalizable simply because it was produced by a random sample, can mislead the medical community. This is a dangerous trap for investigators because it is so easy to collect unrelated but "interesting" data from a study that was itself designed to evaluate a separate question.

1.3.3 Example: Salary Estimation

Consider, for example, a scientist interested in collecting and analyzing the annual salaries of all physicians who have been employed at their first post-training practice for five years or less. She is simply interested in identifying the mean average salary.

In this hypothetical study, she computes that she will need to collect this information from 1% of the population of physicians who have been in their position for less than five years. She selects her sample, sends all selected doctors a questionnaire, and subsequently constructs an answer to the salary question that they all answer.

However, suppose that before she send out her queries, she added questions about ethnicity and gender. Answers to these questions reveal that, of those who responded to the gender question, 40% were women and 60% were men. Carrying our further analyses, she finds that the mean salary of women is significantly greater than that of men. As this latter finding is the most provocative of her results, she focuses her conclusions on this surprising discovery. It was clear what the sample contained. Is it correct to generalize this finding to the population of physicians who are in their first post-training position for five years or less?

To evaluate this situation, we observe that the researcher carried out three analyses. The first is the assessment of the overall mean annual salary. The second is the evaluation of the gender composition of her sample. The third and most provocative result is the finding of higher salaries for female physicians. Of these three findings, the first is the most reliable. The additional findings cannot be assumed to

---

[*] For example if the proportion of subjects who are Mediterranean, between 30 and 45 years of age, and have a nursing degree is less than 1 in 1,000, then a sample of 1,000 patients is not likely to select any members of the population with these characteristics at all, and the sample will be unresponsive to any questions about this subgroup.

be representative and should be interpreted as crude and preliminary findings, requiring that a subsequent study be designed to answer these questions. The justifications for this narrow conclusion follows.

1.3.4 Difficulty 1: Sample Size and Missing Data

We begin our understanding of the researcher's three results by conceding the obvious. The researcher wishes to generalize the findings from her sample to the population at large. Specifically, she wishes to make a statement about the salaries of doctors, 99% of whom have never been queried. Ninety-nine out of one hundred physicians eligible for the sample had not taken part in the survey, had not had their data collected and tabulated, and had not provided information about their salaries to this research effort; yet the researcher wishes to draw conclusions about them. Describing people when you do not have data from them is potentially hazardous, certainly delicate, and can only be attempted after very careful consideration.

Methodology governs what generalization is acceptable. In this particular example, the sample was designed with the overall salary analysis in mind. It was constructed to be representative of the population and to have a sufficient number of members to identify the mean physician salary with precision. Specifically, the sample was obtained in order to reflect the annual post-training salary of starting physicians as a whole. The sample is therefore most representative of the location of the mean salary.[*]

However, the same cannot be said of the researcher's gender analysis. There is no doubt that the sample identified 40% of junior faculty as women. Since the sample was obtained randomly, does the random selection mechanism permit this finding to be worthy of consideration as "population truth also? No. The sample was identified and chosen to be representative of faculty salary, leading to its accurate and precise estimate. However, estimating the proportion of men and women with comparable precision of the salary estimate requires a different sample size. Thus, although her random sample provides accurate and precise estimates of the mean salary, the same sample does not, in general, provide precise and accurate estimates of gender.

A second complication with the gender assessment is that, while every subject in the sample contributed information about their annual salary (a requirement, since the goal of the sample was to obtain salary data), not every junior faculty member that was selected for inclusion in the sample supplied their gender. Thus, missing data about gender further distorts the estimates of the gender proportions in the population. Effectively, the missing data keeps the researcher from knowing the gender proportions in her sample, blunting her ability to estimate its relative size in the population. In this case, missing data on gender makes it impos-

---

[*] It must be pointed out that, even though the sample was selected to be representative of these salaries, it might nevertheless lead to the wrong conclusion about the amount of money earned on an annual basis by junior faculty. Despite her best efforts, the population might have produced a sample for the researcher that, just through the play of chance and the random aggregation of subjects within a sample, misleads her about the location of the population mean. The magnitude of these types of sampling errors (known as type I and type II errors) are what a good statistical analysis will identify.

sible for the researcher to know the gender distribution in her own sample, vitiating her ability to determine anything of value about the gender distribution in the larger population from which her sample was selected. This blocks her ability to carry out any gender analysis precisely, and obstructs the generalization of any of the gender-based results.

The problem that complicates the researcher's ability reliably to estimate gender proportions also obfuscates her attempts to draw conclusions from the comparisons of the mean salaries of men and women junior faculty. For example, she will observe that there were some subjects in her sample that responded to her query about salaries, but not about gender. What should the researcher do about this data in the gender-specific salary analysis? The missing gender information is critical in this gender–salary analysis but can be difficult if not impossible to collect when the research enters its analysis phase.

Each of the two variables (salary and gender) were obtained from the same random sample. However, a random sample cannot be representative of every variable that it measures. Sample-size requirements for each variable's analyses are different; in general the sample size for one analysis is inappropriate for the sample size of another evaluation. Additionally, variable-by-variable differences in missing data rates induce different levels of inaccuracy in the data analysis. And, since resources are finite, they cannot be applied uniformly across all variables measured in a sample. It follows that data quality, as well as precision of the estimates, suffers well.

Thus, while the sample is random, finite resources require that it be obtained with attention to one issue (i.e., the mean salary) to the exclusion of others. Thus, the random sample provides a clearer view of some aspects of the population than of others.

1.3.5 Sample Vision

Simple random samples are only representative of the aspect of the population that they were explicitly and overtly designed to measure. Observing a population through a sample is like viewing a complicated and intricately detailed landscape through glasses. It is impossible to grind the glass lens so that every object in the landscape can be viewed with the same sharp detail. If the lens is ground to view near objects, then the important features of the distant objects are distorted. On the other hand, if the lens is ground for the clear depiction of distant objects, then near objects are blurred beyond clear recognition (Figure 1.2). In this example, the research lens of the scientist was ground to provide a clear view of the overall mean salary of junior faculty. Her view of gender proportions using this same "research lens" is unclear and therefore unreliable. Commonly, the sample must be altered to gain a clear view of another relationship.

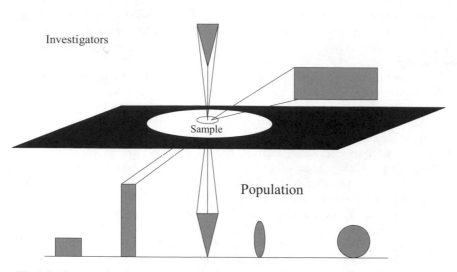

Fig 1.2. The sample allows a view of a relationship in the population (triangle). Note that the sample will not allow accurate views of all relationships (e.g., rectangle) for which it was not designed.

Therefore, since the research was not designed to evaluate gender, the 1) lack of statistical precision and (2) missing data combine to render the analysis of gender unreliable. If the goal of the research effort is different, the then optimal configuration of the sample must change (Figure 1.3).

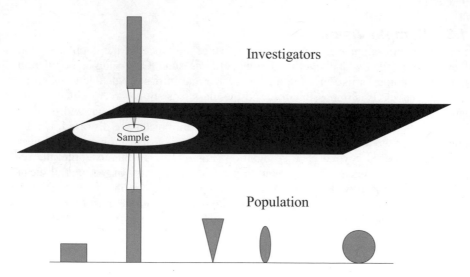

Fig 1.3. The optimal configuration of the sample must change in order to get the clearest view of other relationships in the sample.

However, in addition, there is yet one more difficulty with the gender–salary analysis, a difficulty that is both subtle and lethal. This will be the topic of Chapter Two.

References

1. Moore T (1995) *Deadly Medicine*. New York; Simon and Schuster.
2. Moyé L (2003) *Multiple Analyses in Clinical Trials. Fundamentals for Investigators*. New York; Springer.
3. Multicenter dilitiazem post infarction trial research group (1989) The effect of dilitiazem on mortality and reinfarction after myhocardial infarction. *New England Journal of Medicine* **319**:385–392.
4. Packer M (2000) Presentation of the results of the Prospective Randomized Amlodipine Survival Evaluation-2 Trial (PRAISE-2) at the American College of Cardiology Scientific Sessions, Anaheim, CA, March 15, 2000.
5. Lewis S (1953) *Arrowsmith*. New York; Harcourt, Brace, and World, Inc.

2

Search Versus Research

2.1 Introduction

As we saw in Chapter One, one of the difficulties of collecting a simple random sample was that it was not enough for the sample to be selected completely at random. In addition, the sample must be collected with a particular goal, or research question in mind. Just as one rarely has a successful vacation by simply packing up the car and leaving without knowing the destination, random-sampling without a research plan leaves most every desirable goal out of reach. And, just as leaving for one destination precludes seeing others, sampling that is designed to answer one question often makes it impossible to shed important light on other questions, even though they contain scientific interest of their own accord.

However, there is a second problem with carrying out an unplanned analysis suggested by the data. Like an iceberg, it is this second, submerged component that is commonly the most damaging when not recognized.

2.2 Catalina's Dilemma

Consider the following hypothetical example that is an illustration of a commonly occurring issue

2.2.1. Can Catalina Generalize?

An enthusiastic young researcher, Catalina, is interested in demonstrating the progressive deterioration in heart function observed in patients with mild CHF whose medical management is appropriate. She has designed a research program to examine the changes in left ventricular function over time, with specific attention to examining changes in end diastolic volume (EDV). During a six-month time period, Catalina recruits her sample randomly from the population of people with CHF seen at her hospital, and follows each patient for two years. For each patient, she measures heart function at baseline (i.e., when the patient agrees to enter the study) and again in 24 months. Every patient returns to have their heart function measured at the two-year time point. Although Catalina is focused on the change in EDV, the technology of the measuring tool permits her to obtain estimates of left ventricular ejection fraction (LVEF), end systolic volume (ESV), stroke volume (SV), and cardiac output (CO) as well.

Her colleagues who have contributed their own patients to Catalina's investigation are anxious to learn of the conclusions of her study. At the anticipated time, Catalina examines her data with great anticipation.[*] Comparing the baseline to 24 month change in EDV for each of her patients, she discovered to her surprise that the anticipated increase in EDV did not materialize. However although EDV has not increased, there has been a substantial increase in ESV. She therefore chooses to change the endpoint for the program from EDV to ESV. She presents her results in terms of the change ESV, saying little about the absence of a change in EDV.

2.2.2 Do Logistical Issues Block Generalization?

Admittedly, many researchers would have no problem with Catalina's last minute endpoint change. They would argue that since ESV and EDV reflect measurements of the same underlying pathophysiology and jointly measure the progress of CHF, they should be interchangeable as endpoints. In fact, they would applaud Catalina's doggedness in looking beyond the disappointing EDV finding, ferreting out the hidden change in ESV.

Others who have read Chapter One would argue that the analysis of ESV was inappropriate because the study was not designed to detect changes in ESV (even though that is exactly what the study did). These critics, drawing on the arguments demonstrated in Figures 1.1 and 1.2 would point out that a sample that was optimum for assessing the change in EDV might not be optimum in detecting the change in ESV. For example, a comparison of the standard deviation of the two measurements might lead to a different minimum sample size for the two analyses.

However Catalina, anticipating this argument, examines the data that led her to choose the sample size that she ultimately selected for the study. She finds that the sample size necessary for detecting the change in EDV would be sufficient for detecting changes in ESV. In fact, after a thorough examination of the design issues that would preface the analysis for each variable, she concludes that she would have made no change in design of the study if she had set out to detect changes in ESV rather than EDV. As it turns out, the sample was optimally selected to analyze either of these two variables. Does removal of the logistics argument now permit Catalina to generalize the ESV results?

2.2.3 Disturbed Estimators

Even though the logistical impediment to generalization has been removed, problems with the generalizability argument persists. There remains a critical difficulty with the statistical estimators that Catalina uses to measure the effect in ESV in her study — a difficulty that is induced by the change in endpoint from EDV to ESV.

---

[*] Since no intervention is being provided and she is not required to carry out any interim monitoring of her patients, Catalina can wait until the end of the two-year follow-up period to examine her data.

The decision to change the endpoint from EDV to ESV was based solely on the findings in the sample. Specifically it was not Catalina's foresight, but the data, that suggested ESV should be analyzed (because its results were positive) and not EDV. This data-based change introduces a new effect of sampling error, and the statistical estimators that we use (means, standard deviations, odds ratios, relative risks, confidence intervals, and p-values) are not designed to incorporate this effect. Specifically, her statistical estimators do a fine job of estimating the mean change when the variable is fixed and the data are random. However, when the variable itself is random (i.e., randomly chosen) these estimators no longer fulfill their functions well.

Did Catalina choose the ESV variable randomly? From her point of view, no. However, the sample chose it for her, and the sample contains random sample-to-sample variability.

To examine this issue further, let's say that another investigator (Susi) sampled from the same population as Catalina. Like Catalina, Susi chooses EDV for her endpoint. At the conclusion of Susi's study, her data reveal that, as was the case for Catalina, EDV did not change over time. However neither did ESV. For Susi's sample, it was the variable SV that changed over time. She therefore chooses to report the change in SV as the major endpoint in her study.

Finally, Al, a third investigator, sampling from the same population and like his two colleagues, focused on EDV as the variable of interest, finds that neither EDV, ESV, nor SV changed. For him, it was the change in CO that was positive. Thus, the three different researchers report their three different findings, (Catalina reports ESV, Susi reports SV, and Al reports CO). Nobody reports EDV, which was the prospectively identified endpoint chosen by each of these researchers. How can these results be interpreted?

Each investigator acts as though they can have complete confidence in their statistical estimators. However, for each there are now two sources of variability where there was only supposed to be one. The first source of variability is the variability of the measurements from subject to subject — easily anticipated and easily handled by the statistical estimators. These estimators incorporate this component well. The sample mean and standard deviation are accurate, a test statistic is computed, and the p-value nicely incorporates this subject-to-subject variability.

However, there is another source of variation that was never anticipated that is present in these research efforts — the variability of the endpoint selection. Each investigator selected, independent of the data, EDV as their endpoint. However, each investigator allowed the data to select another endpoint for them. Yet the selection mechanism was a random one, since each data set exhibits sample-to-sample variability.

Essentially, in the case of each of these investigators, the data have provided an enticing answer to a question that the researcher didn't think to ask. When the data determine the analysis, as in this case, our commonly used statistical estimators (i.e., means, standard deviations, confidence intervals, and p-values) do not function reliably. They were never designed to apply to this scenario, and the familiar formula for these quantities are no longer accurate. What has dismembered the formula is that there are now two sources of error, when they were designed to handle only one. This is the hallmark of *exploratory analyses*, or *random research*.

2.3 Exploratory Analysis and Random Research

Exploratory analysis is the process by which the investigator allows the data to answer specific questions that the investigator did not plan to use the data to address. There are two problems with exploratory or *hypothesis-generating research*. The first is that commonly, the sample is not an optimal one, since the investigator can only design a sample to answer questions that they knew to ask.

The second difficulty is a more pernicious one, requiring additional elaboration. We pointed out earlier that the careful selection of a sample to address the scientific question of interest does not prevent random-sampling error from generating the sample's answers. In order to measure the role of sampling error accurately, the investigator turns to the mathematical procedures supplied by statistics. From statistics, we find the computations that convert the sample's information (the data) into the best estimates of effect size (e.g., means or other measures of effect size, standard deviations, confidence intervals, and *p*-values). Researchers rely on the accuracy of these estimators to inform them about the population from which the sample was drawn

It is important to note that these estimators do not remove sampling error. Instead, they channel this sampling error into both the effect size estimates (e.g., means) and the variability of these estimates (e.g., standard deviations and confidence intervals). If the researcher is also interested in inference (i.e., statistical hypothesis testing), then statistical procedures will channel sampling error into *p*-values. Thus, when used correctly, statistical methodology will appropriately recognize and transmit sampling error into familiar quantities that researchers can interpret (Figure 2.1).

Unfortunately, these familiar estimators are corrupted when there is a source of random variability beyond that produced by sampling error. In the case of our investigator Catalina, the second source of variability is produced by random analysis selection.

Consider the simple example of the sample mean. If we select observations $x_1, x_2, x_3, \ldots x_n$, from a population, we commonly use

$$\overline{x} = \frac{\sum_{i=1}^{n} x_i}{n}$$

as an estimate of the population mean. We have come to accept its precision and reliability in many applications of research, and its ubiquity represents the confidence we have in this formula. It has taken statisticians a long time to figure out how to estimate from a sample [1].[*]

---

[*] The idea of repeating and combining observations made on the same quantity appears to have been introduced as a scientific method by Tycho Brae toward the end of the sixteenth century. He used the arithmetic mean to replace individual observations as a summary measurement. The demonstration that the sample mean was a more precise value than a single

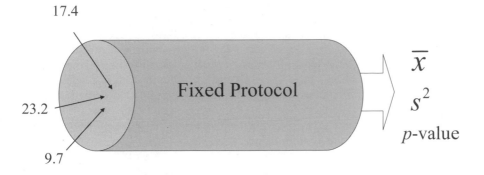

Fig. 2.1. A fixed, prospectively anchored protocol accepts random data and channels it into reliable, statistical estimators.

However, this formula was designed to work in a setting when there is only one source of error, sampling error. Specifically, it was created to work in the setting where the variable x is fixed, and then the sample of x's is selected randomly. While this is true in many circumstances, it is not the case with Catalina's EDV-ESV analysis. She did not choose the ESV analysis, but instead, allowed the ESV analysis to be selected for her by the data.[*] Thus, her original question has been supplanted by her observation that the ESV did change. This replacement was suggested to the investigator by the data. She would not have selected the ESV evaluation if the data didn't suggest that it deteriorated over time.

The sample data produced an answer to a question that the researcher had not asked, inducing the researcher to ask the question in a *post hoc* fashion. The effect of this data-driven choice is that the data contain sampling error. Therefore, as demonstrated with the experiences of Susi and Al, other datasets would produce

---

measurement did not appear until the end of the seventeenth century, and was based on the work by the astronomer Flamsten. At this point, the simultaneous organization of the formulation of discrete probability laws and the development of the differential calculus permitted an analytical examination of the probability distribution of the mean. In 1710, Simpson's work proved that the arithmetic mean has a smaller variance than a single observation.

[*] We can assert this claim because the investigator would never have highlighted the ESV analysis if its results did not stand out. The fact that she was drawn to the evaluation because of its magnitude and not because of any prospective plan to look at it is the mechanism of a data-driven analysis.

other intriguing results due to sampling error. Thus, different samples obtained from the same population would provide not just a different answer to the EDV deterioration over time, but, would also supply other "answers" to questions that had not been asked. Since the data are random and the data are proposing the research analyses, the analyses themselves are random.

In the random research environment, statistical estimators, e.g., the sample mean, lose their best properties of precision and reliability. They are constructed to operate best when 1) the analysis is chosen and fixed prospectively and 2) the resulting data are random. Their performance degrades when the analysis plan itself is random, distorting all measures of the magnitude and significance of the relationship. Operating like blind guides, they mislead us in the random research environment about what we would see in the population based on our observations in the sample (Figure 2.2). Therefore, since we do not have good estimators of the effect of interest in the population, the best that we can say is that these *post hoc* findings are exploratory, and require confirmation.

2.4 Gender–Salary Problem Revisited

Returning to the initial salary example, recall that this evaluation carried out by our researcher in Chapter One found that the salaries of female physicians were larger than the salaries of physicians who were men. We already understand that the impact of missing gender data can skew her analysis. The presence of this missing data means that we cannot even be sure what has happened in our sample, much less try to extend the sample result to the population.

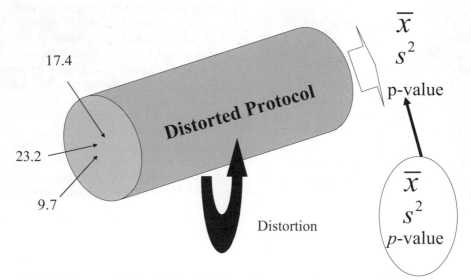

Fig. 2.2. A protocol, perturbed by a data-based, as opposed to a prospectively chosen-analysis plan, distorts the statistical estimators.

However, now assume that there is no missing gender data in the sample. Thus, the gender–salary analysis includes data from everyone in the sample. As we might anticipate from the previous discussion in this chapter, even though the sample database is complete, this gender–salary analysis is still likely to be misleading i.e., not at all representative of the population.

The unreliability of this sample-based result is rooted in the way in which the scientist's attention was drawn to the gender–salary relationship. Unlike with the overall salary evaluation that was designed a priori, the gender–salary analysis was unplanned. The researcher did not design the study to find this relationship. Instead she designed the study to obtain another measure, and was drawn to the gender salary relationship by its magnitude. In fact, the investigator was drawn to this finding by carrying out several non-prespecified evaluations, thereby discovering what the sample revealed about gender and salary. Since the source of this influence is sampling error, its presence generates misleading estimators (Figure 2.3).

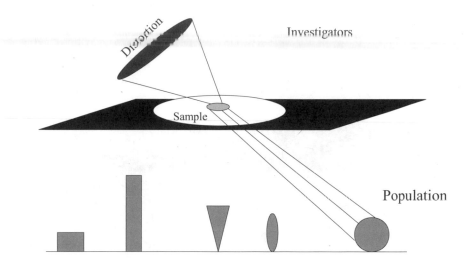

Fig 2.3. In the random research paradigm, a misdirected sampling scheme, in concert with untrustworthy estimators, misleads the investigators about the characteristics of the relationship. This is the hallmark of exploratory analyses.

As was the case with Catalina, this investigator did not choose the analysis. The data chose the gender–salary evaluation for her. Thus, her original question has been replaced by the question of the equality of salaries between men and women physicians. This replacement was suggested to the investigator by the data. Specifically, this means that the researcher would not have selected this question if the data did not suggest that the salaries of men and women were different.

As was the case with Catalina's cardiology research, the sample data produced an answer to a question that the researcher had not asked, persuading the researcher to ask the question in a *post hoc* fashion. She is not aware that other datasets will, due to the influence of sample-to-sample variability, generate other enticing results. For example a second data set might find no disparity at all between the salaries of male and female physicians but instead "find" a racial disparity, attracting the investigator's attention. A third sample may find neither of the previous two, but find a disparity in salary by zodiac sign. Thus, different samples obtained from the same population would provide not just a different answer to the gender–salary relationship question, but in addition, would supply other "answers" to questions that had not been asked. Since the data are random, and the data are proposing the research analyses, the analyses themselves are random. The estimators are derived to have the data selected randomly from sample to sample, not for the analysis plan itself to exhibit sample-to-sample variability.

A follow-up analysis designed to look at the gender–salary disparity would (1) choose the optimum sample (i.e., a sample with enough males and females), and (2) have the gender–salary question determined *a priori* (Figure 2.4).

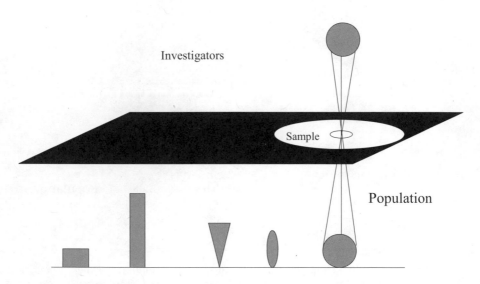

Fig 2.4. In the confirming analysis, the sample is specifically designed to focus on the aspect of the population of interest. The fixed analysis plan allows the statistical estimators to perform optimally. This is the hallmark of a confirmatory analysis.

2.5 Exploratory Versus Confirmatory

Both the hypothetical example from cardiology and the salary survey demonstrate the hallmark of exploratory analyses. By exploring, the investigator identifies relationships that were not anticipated but that the sample suggests are present. However, the presence of a relationship in the sample does not announce the presence of the relationship in the population. Additionally the statistical investigators were not designed to function when the analysis is random. They therefore add another level of distortion to the effect "identified" by the exploratory work.

The confirmatory evaluation provides the clearest measure of the magnitude of the effect of interest. Having its location determined by the exploratory analysis, the sample is optimally configured for the relationship that was suggested in the *post hoc* evaluation. Also, with the analysis fixed (i.e., the variable in which interest lies has been chosen prospectively and plans for its evaluation are already in place) the statistical estimators perform well, providing a reliable sense of effect magnitude and the degree to which that magnitude may vary from sample to sample. Generalization from the sample to the population is strongest when it rests on a confirmatory finding.

However, generalization should not be attempted when its basis is exploratory analysis. In the setting, the usual sample estimators are undermined because the assumption on which their accuracy is based is false. The two sources of variability wreck the capacity of our commonly used estimators to provide reliable estimates of the true population measures. This is the trait of exploratory estimators. Unfortunately, once the random research paradigm is in place, it can be very difficult to repair the exploratory analysis. While they can occasionally provide some light on the answer to a question the researcher did not ask, they require confirmation before we can accept the results.

2.5.1 Cloak of Confirmation

We will soon see how exploratory or hypothesis-generating research can be most useful. However, one area in which it is harmful is when it is represented as confirmatory research. This is what the salary researcher of Chapter One and Catalina of this chapter intended to do. Each believed that their research results were accurate and worthy of generalization to the population at large. However, further evaluations revealed that only a portion of the results (the mean salary for the entire sample for the salary researcher, and the EDV results for Catalina) can be generalized; the residual was exploratory or hypothesis-generating.

Exploratory analyses are dangerous when they are covered with the cloak of confirmation. This misrepresentation of exploratory analyses as confirmatory can be dangerous, misleading, and must be identified at once. The need for the research result can be overwhelming; yet, its correct identification (exploratory or confirmatory) requires vigilance, patience, and discipline. As Miles [2] points out "If the fishing expedition catches a boot, the fishermen should throw it back, not claim that they were fishing for boots."

As an example, consider the plight of a young parent who discovers that his child is sick. An emergency visit to the pediatrician reveals that the child suffers from an acute illness, but one that can be easily treated with the prompt use of a prescription medicine. Minutes later, the pharmacist reviews the prescription, telling the parent that the required medication is a combination of three compounds that can be quickly mixed and administered. The pharmacist returns with the preparation, and, anxious to follow the doctor's orders, the parent prepares to give the child the first teaspoon of medication right there in the pharmacy. However, just when the teaspoon is placed on the child's lips, the pharmacist rushes out, telling the parent that, although the medicine contains the right constituents, the proportions of those compounds are wrong because the device he used to mix them is defective.

The exploratory estimator, like the defective medication mixture, is a distorted and unusable concoction that should be avoided. Most parents would steel themselves, withdrawing the teaspoon containing the defective medication. Just as the bad medicine cannot be given, the researcher must exert discipline and avoid hasty interpretation of the exploratory estimator. It is the fortunately rare (and perhaps, rarely fortunate) parent who would insist on giving the defective compound to their child in the face of this news.

Now that the parent recognizes that the compound is faulty, what steps can be taken to correctly adjust the preparation at hand. Should it be diluted? If so, by how much? Should additional compounds be added? If so, in what quantities should they be added? Since the precise defect in the compound's formulation cannot be identified, the parent only knows that the medication is defective and that he cannot correct it. All he can do is ask the pharmacist to dispose of what he has in hand and then start the process again, this time using the required compounds in the right proportions.

Similarly, an exploratory estimator cannot be repaired. We only know that a critical assumption in the estimator's construction has been violated. Since we cannot rehabilitate the estimator, we can only ask that a study be carried out that does not violate the estimator's assumptions. Specifically, this means that the study is (1) designed to answer the prospectively asked question, and (2) the study is executed and its data analyzed as described in the protocol (concordant execution). In this paradigm, the estimators are trustworthy measures of population effects.

2.6 Exploration and MRFIT

A prime example of the harm that comes from exploratory analyses that are represented as confirmatory is one of the results from the Multiple Risk Factor Intervention Trial (MRFIT) [3] study. Published in 1982, it was designed to demonstrate that reductions in the risk factors associated with atherosclerotic cardiovascular disease would be translated into reduction in clinical events, e.g., myocardial infarction and stroke. Patients in the intervention group received treatment for elevated blood pressure, joined cigarette smoking cessation programs, reduced their weight, and lowered their serum lipid levels; patients in the control group followed their usual accepted standard of living. At the conclusion of the study, the investigators found and reported that there was no difference in clinical outcome between those patients who received risk factor intervention and those who did not.

These null findings were a disappointment to the risk factor interventionists, who then poured over the data to identify if any effect could be found in a fraction of the patients that might explain the null overall effect. They found one, and it was a bombshell. When the researches ignored the results in the entire randomized cohort (i.e., all randomized patients), and concentrated on men who were hypertensive and had resting electrocardiograph (ECG) abnormalities at baseline, they discovered that these patients had a worse outcome when randomized to anti-hypertensive therapy than those who received no such therapy.

This result was published, and had a major impact on the momentum to treat essential hypertension. At this time in clinical medicine, the importance of identification and treatment of hypertension galvanized physicians. Screening programs were well underway. New therapies (e.g., hydrochlorothiazide, alphamethyl-dopa, and clonidine) for the hypertensive patient became available. All of the necessary forces for a war on undiagnosed and untreated hypertension were maneuvering into position when the MRFIT analyses were released. This finding slowed the momentum for the treatment of hypertension by raising disturbing, and ultimately unhelpful, questions e.g., "Maybe not all hypertension was bad after all?", or "Maybe hypertensive disease itself was bad, but the treatment was worse?"

The real question however, was, "Is it just a distorted treatment effect?" For years after this finding, clinical trials in hypertension were forced to address this unusual result. None of the major studies ever found that hypertensive men with resting ECG abnormalities were better off when their hypertension remained unchecked. Nevertheless, an exploratory analysis, dressed as a confirmatory one, produced an important interruption in the treatment of a deadly cardiovascular disease.

2.7 Exploration in the ELITE Trials

Another, more recent example of the misdirection produced by exploratory analyses are the ELITE trials. There are many medications used to treat heart failure, one of which is angiotensin-converting enzyme inhibitor (ACE-i). This effective CHF medication's use dramatically increased in the 1980s. Unfortunately, many ACE-i treated patients experience undesirable side effects of this therapy; among the worst of these is renal insufficiency.

As a response to this undesirable side effect profile, angiotensin II type I receptor blockers were developed. In order to compare the relative safety of angiotensin type II type receptor blocker to ACE-i therapy, the Evaluation of Losartan in the Elderly Study (ELITE) was undertaken [4]. The primary analysis of ELITE was the comparison of the two drug's abilities to preserve renal function.

ELITE recruited 722 patients and followed them in for 48 weeks. At its conclusion, ELITE investigators determined that kidney function was equally preserved by the two medications. However, the investigators discovered that 17 deaths occurred in the losartan group and 32 deaths in the captopril group ($p = 0.035$). This finding received the principle emphasis in the discussion section of the manuscript. Although the need to repeat the trial was mentioned in the abstract, the balance of the discussion focused on the reduced mortality rate of losartan. According to the authors, "This study demonstrated that losartan reduced mortality compared with captopril; whether the apparent mortality advantage for losartan over captopril holds true for other ACE inhibitors requires further study." Others even went so far as to attempt to explain the mechanism for the reduction in sudden death observed in ELITE 1 [5, 6].

To the investigators' credit, ELITE II [7] was executed to confirm the superiority of losartan over captopril in improving survival in patients with heart failure. The primary endpoint in ELITE II was the effect of therapy on total mortality. This study required 3,152 patients (almost five times the number of patients recruited for the ELITE I) and also had to follow patients for 18 months (almost twice as long as the duration of follow-up in ELITE I). At the conclusion of ELITE II, the cumulative all-cause mortality rate was not significantly different between the losartan and captopril groups. The investigators conceded "More likely, the superiority of losartan to captopril in reducing mortality, mainly due to decreasing sudden cardiac death, seen in ELITE should be taken as a chance finding."

Although the finding in ELITE I may have been due to chance alone, the principle difficulty presented by the first study was that the statistical estimators commonly used to measure the mortality effect were inaccurate when applied to this surprise finding. However, since the sample was random (selected as one of millions of possible samples from patients with CHF), the selection mechanism for the analysis is random (since other samples would have produced other unanticipated findings). Specifically, by allowing their focus to be shifted to surprise mortality effect, the research paradigm became a random one (Figure 2.2). In this random analysis setting, the usual statistical estimators provide misleading information about the population effect from the observed findings in the sample. This is the hallmark of the random protocol. By letting the data decide the analysis, the analysis and the experiment becomes random, and the resulting statistical estimators become untrustworthy.

2.8 Necessity of Exploratory Analyses

Recognizing the importance of a guiding hypothesis is critical to the scientific thought process. This central hypothesis generates the finely tuned research design that, when executed per plan, permits a clear, defensible test of the core scientific hypothesis. This deliberative procedure stands in stark contrast to discovery or "exploration" whose use in sample-based research has limits as pointed out here and elsewhere [8,9].

Nevertheless, it is quite undeniable that discovery is important to science in general and in healthcare research in particular. Such findings can have important implications. The arrival of Christopher Columbus at the island of San Salvador led to the unanticipated "discovery" of the New World. Madam Curie "discovered" radiation. These researchers did not anticipate and were not looking for their discoveries. They stumbled upon them precisely because these discoveries were not in their view. However, as these prominent illustrations demonstrate, despite the weaknesses of the exploratory process, discovery has and will play an important role in healthcare research. This undeniable importance of this style of research is aptly demonstrated by the example of compound 2254RP.

2.8.1 Product 2254RP

During the height of World War II in France, Janbon and colleagues at the Infectious Disease Clinic of the Medical School in Montpellier quietly studied the effects of a compound that held out promise as an antibiotic.[*] An offshoot of the new class of sulfonamides, compound 2254RP was quite possibly a new treatment for typhoid fever. However the researchers were unable to maintain focus on the antimicrobial abilities of this agent because of its production of seizures. Even patients with no known medical history of epilepsy would commonly experience profound convulsions after the institution of 2254RP.

Further evaluation of these patients revealed that seizures were more likely to occur in patients who were malnourished. This unanticipated findings generated further queries, revealing that exposed patients were also rendered hypoglycemic by the compound.

Puzzled, Jabon transmitted these observation to a colleague, Auguste Loubatières who himself was engaged in research on the characteristics of seizure disorders in patients exposed to high concentrations of insulin. Loubatières hypothesized that both insulin and 2254RP produced hypoglycemia. After demonstrating the sequence of hypoglycemia followed by seizures in dogs treated with 2254RP, he verified the induction of hypoglycemia in three female patients by the compound. This collection of research efforts generated the development of the sulfonylureas as oral hypoglycemic agents in diabetes mellitus.

2.8.2 The Role of Discovery Versus Confirmation

Certainly, the production of hypoglycemia and seizure disorder was not part of the research protocol for Dr. Janbon and colleagues, and their unanticipated findings fell into the category of exploratory research. Janbon and colleagues would not be criticized for pursuing the surprise findings of their research efforts. The discovery that the antihypertensive agent minoxidil could unexpectedly reduce hair loss, and the finding that the antihypertensive, anti-anginal compound sidenafil can temporarily reverse erectile dysfunction are contemporary examples of the fruits of discovery.

Discovery must certainly play a major role in an environment where compounds have unanticipated and sometimes, even unimagined effects. The difficulty in sample-based research arises in separating true discovery from the misdirection of sampling error. What distinguished the "discovery" in MRFIT (that some hypertensive men should not be treated for their hypertension) from the discovery that the sulfonylureas had effects above and beyond antimicrobial abilities was confirmation. The MRFIT finding could not be confirmed. The 2254RP findings were. Therefore, discovery must be confirmed before it can be accepted as a trustworthy. Eccentricities of the discovery process e.g., faulty instrumentation, sample-to-sample variability, and outright mistakes in measurements and observations can each mislead honest researchers and their audience.

---

[*] This is taken from Chapter 6, Sulfonylurea Receptors, ATP-Sensitive Potassium Channels, and Insulin Secretion from LeRoith D, Taylor SI, Olefsky JM (2000). *Diabetes Mellitus: A Fundamental and Clinical Text. Second Edition.* Philadelphia: Lippincott Williams, and Wilkins.

This integration can be achieved by setting the discovery as the central *a priori* hypothesis for a new experiment that seeks to verify the discovery. For example, while it is true that Columbus discovered the new world, it is also true that he had to return three additional times before he was given credit for his discovery.[*]

Additionally, given that claims of discovery can commonly misdirect us, it is important to distinguish between an evaluation that uses a research effort to confirm a prospectively stated hypothesis, a process that we will define as *confirmatory analysis* (truly "*re*-searching") versus the identification of a finding for which the research effort was not specifically designed to reliably detect ("searching").

2.8.3 Tools of Exploration

While confirmatory analyses are prospectively designed, focused, and disciplined, hypothesis-generating analyses have other characteristics. Untethered by any early planning, they employ tools of elementary pattern recognition, requiring an open mind, and sometimes, a spark of imagination. Such analyses include, but are not limited to (1) changing a study's endpoint (i.e., exploring a new endpoint), (2) changing the analysis of an endpoint,[†] (3) subgroup analyses,[‡] and (4) data-based model building.[§] This type of investigational perspective is prevalent in healthcare research, is exciting to carry out, and is almost always interesting.

However, whenever the execution of a research effort is altered due to an unanticipated finding in the data as is the case with 1 4 above, the protocol becomes random, the research becomes discordant (i.e., its execution is no longer governed by the prospectively written protocol) and the analyses are hypothesis-generating. In these cases we must tightly bind the exploratory conclusions with the lock of caution until a subsequent confirmatory analysis can unlock and thereby generalize the result. To enforce this point, these exploratory, or hypothesis-generating results should be reported without *p*-values. *Z* scores would suffice very nicely here, since they provide a normed effect size, without mixing in the sampling error issue.

2.9 Prospective Plans and "Calling Your Shot"

It comes as no surprise that the advice from research methodologists is that exploratory or surprise findings do not carry persuasive weight primarily because they were not planned prospectively [10]. However, to many researchers, this requirement of "calling your shot," i.e., of identifying prospectively what analyses will have persuasive influence, seems much ado about nothing. After all, the data are, in the end, the data. To these critics, allowing the data to decide the result of the experiment can appear to be the fairest, least prejudicial evaluation of the message

---

[*] Columbus was essentially forced by Queen Isabelle of Spain to prove that he could find the New World when he was actually looking for it. Only when he did this three times (driving himself into poverty during the process) and other ship captains confirmed its location, was the New World finally accepted.

[†] For example, changing the evaluation of a 0-1 or dichotomous event to take into account the time until the event occurred (e.g., life table analysis).

[‡] Subgroup analyses is the subject of a later chapter.

[§] Regression analysis is discussed in Chapter Eleven.

they contain. When these debates involve patient well-being, the discussions can be explosive. Consider the case of carvedilol.

2.9.1 The US Carvedilol Program

In the late 1980s interest in the heart failure research community focused on the use of beta blockers. Considered anathema for the treatment of chronic CHF, re-investigation of the issue suggested that beta blockade could be useful in relieving the symptoms of heart failure. The US Carvedilol program [11] evaluated the medication carvedilol (previously approved for the treatment of essential hypertension) for the treatment of CHF.

In these research efforts 1,094 patients were selected for entry into one of four protocols, then randomized to either standard therapy plus placebo, or standard therapy plus carvedilol. There were 398 total patients randomized to placebo and 696 to carvedilol. At the conclusion of approximately one year of follow-up, 31 deaths had occurred in the placebo group and 22 in the active group (relative risk = 0.65, p-value = 0.001). The program's oversight committee recommended that the program be terminated in the face of this overwhelming mortality benefit. Both the investigators and the sponsor believed that since mortality effects were important, the beneficial effect of carvedilol on the total mortality rate should compel the federal Food and Drug Administration (FDA) to approve the compound as effective in reducing the incidence of total mortality in patients with heart failure.

However, FDA review of the program revealed some aspects of the carvedilol research effort that were not clearly elucidated in the *New England Journal of Medicine* manuscript. Although that paper correctly stated that patients were stratified into one of four treatment protocols [1, page 1350], the manuscript did not state the fact that each of these protocols had its own prospectively identified primary endpoint, nor did it acknowledge that the total mortality rate was neither a primary nor a secondary endpoint for any of the trials. Three of the trials had exercise tolerance as a primary endpoint and measures of morbidity from CHF as secondary endpoints. Furthermore, a protocol-by-protocol delineation of the primary endpoint results was not included in the manuscript.

Additional interrogation revealed that the finding for the prospectively defined primary endpoint in three of the studies were statistically insignificant ($p > 0.05$). The fourth study had as its primary endpoint hospitalization for heart failure (the statistical analysis for this primary endpoint was $p < 0.05$). Each of these four studies had secondary endpoints that assessed CHF morbidity, some of which were nominally significant ($p < 0.05$), others not. However, as pointed out by Fisher [12], total mortality was not an endpoint of any of the four studies in the program. Thus a research effort that at first glance appeared to be a single, cohesive trial with total mortality as its primary endpoint, was upon close inspection a *post hoc* combined analysis for a non-prospectively defined endpoint.

This observation, and subsequent arguments at the FDA advisory committee meeting produced a host of problems for the experiment's interpretation. The verbal debates that ensued at the Maser Auditorium in May 1996 between the Sponsor's representatives and the Advisory Committee were intense. The sponsor was taken aback by the unanticipated strong criticisms of its program with its strong mortality findings. Viewing the criticisms as small arguments over Lilliputian technicalities, the sponsor responded quickly and vehemently. The contentions spilled over from verbal debate into the literature, first as letters to the editor [13,14] and then as full manuscripts in their own right [12,15,16,17].

The proponents of carvedilol assembled a collection of compelling arguments both during and after the disputatious FDA debate. There was no question about the strength of the US Carvedilol's programs findings. Lives were prolonged for patients who had a disease that had no known definitive therapy and whose prevalence was rapidly rising. The Data Safety and Monitoring Committee[*] of the program had stated that, in the face of the large mortality benefit, it was unethical for the trial to continue merely to demonstrate an effect on its weaker endpoints. The FDA was reminded that the most compelling of all endpoints in clinical trials is total mortality, and the most laudable goal was prolonging life. There was no doubt that carvedilol had produced this precise result in the US Carvedilol Program.

In addition, the research community was asked to recall that at the outset of a research effort, investigators cannot be expected to identify the totality of the analyses that they will want to carry out at the study's conclusion. While scientists will certainly want to have a prospectively asked question that motivate the generation of the sample, the logistical efficiency of the research effort requires that they collect data extending above and beyond the prospectively declared analyses. When the manuscripts are submitted for publication, the authors must affirmatively reply to persistent journal reviewers and editors who may like to see additional analyses carried out so that the reader will have all relevant information required to make an independent judgment about the intervention's risk-benefit balance. To do anything else would open the investigators to the criticism of concealing critical information.

Finally, the sponsors were obligated to collect safety data. It was the FDA, the Advisory Committee was told, that required the US Carvedilol Program to collect mortality data in order to provide assurances that carvedilol did not shorten lives. Was the FDA, they asked, now to ignore the data they themselves demanded when the data demonstrated an unsuspected benefit of the drug? [†]

The US Carvedilol Program had complied with the requirements of the FDA in the design of the program and the studies' interim monitoring. From its advocates' point of view, scientists who criticized the US Carvedilol Program for not finding a statistically significant reduction in weaker endpoints e.g., exercise tolerance when carvedilol was found to prolong lives was tantamount criticizing a baseball player for not stealing any bases when all he did was hit home runs.

---

[*] The Data Safety and Monitoring Committee is a collection of distinquished scientists responsible for evaluating the interim results of the study to ensure the ethical treatment of its participants. Unblinded to therapy assignment, and privy to all of the data, this committee can recommend that the study be prematurely terminated if unanticipated harm or benefit has occurred.

[†] Certainly, if carvedilol had been shown to increase mortality, a clear hazard to patients, the sponsor's request for approval for a CHF indication would have been denied, regardless of the findings for the programs official panoply of primary morbidity endpoints. The asymmetry of safety findings is discussed in Chapter Eight.

However, critics of the program were equally vehement. There was no question about the findings of the US Carvedilol program. Lives had been saved. But, what did this collection of studies of just over 1,000 patients imply about the population of millions of patients with heart failure? Sample extrapolation is a dangerous process, and discipline, not hope should govern what sample results should be extended from the sample to the population. Samples are replete with "facts'; most of these facts apply only to the sample and not to the entire population. Healthcare has seen these kinds of failures of generalization before. Experience (e.g., that of MRFIT) suggested that the primary outcome analyses most likely represented the effects of carvedilol in the larger population.

Additionally, pre-specification of the anticipated analysis in the protocol of a trial has been an accepted standard among clinical trial workers [18] and certainly must be included in a manuscript describing that trial's results. In addition, the non-reporting of non-significant endpoints in clinical trials has been criticized [19]. Each of these principles was clearly violated in the manuscript published in *The New England Journal of Medicine*. The scientific community expects, and clinical trial workers require that analyses be provided for all prospectively stated endpoints. The fact that the results of a program claiming major benefit did not specifically define and report the analysis of the primary endpoint is a serious deficiency in the manuscript that purports to describe the effects of therapy.

Unfortunately, by violating these fundamental methodology tenets, the Carvedilol investigators open themselves to the criticism that they selected the total mortality analysis because of its favorable results, thus biasing the conclusions[*] and tainting the research effort. The mortality findings for the US Carvedilol were a surprise finding. They were an intriguing result, but the cardiology community was reminded that surprise "good findings are not uncommonly followed by surprise bad findings as the vesnarinone experience demonstrated.[†] Unanticipated surprise findings on non-primary endpoints weaken rather than strengthen the results of a clinical trial.

---

[*] This is a classic illustration of a random analysis.

[†]The contemporary reversal of the vesnarinone findings added more fuel to this raging fire. Vesnarinone was a positive inotropic agent that increased the pumping ability of the heart, holding out initial promise for improving the treatment of CHF. The first study, designed to randomize 150 patients to each of the three treatment arms, and follow them for 6 months, revealed a 62% reduction in all-cause mortality (95% CI 28 to 80; $p = 0.002$) which was not the primary endpoint of the trial (Feldman AM, Bristow MR, Parmley, WW et al. (1993). Effects of vesnarinone on morbidity and mortality in patients with heart failure. *New England Journal of Medicine* **329**:149–55.). However a second clinical trial reversed these findings to the confusion of the cardiology community. The vesnarinone investigators stated, "Examination of the patient populations in the two trials reveals no differences that could reasonably account for the opposite response to the daily administration of 60-mg of vesnarinone." (Cohn J, Goldstein SC, Feenheed S et al. (1998). A dose-dependent increase in mortality seen with vesnarinone among patients with severe heart failure. *New England Journal of Medicine* **339**:1810–16.)

2.9.2 Let the Data Decide!

Much of the discussion involving carvedilol revolved around the policy of disassembling the notion of a hierarchy of prospectively planned analysis, in favor of "letting the data decide." This latter point of view has a seductive, egalitarian sound. At first glance "letting the data decide" appears to liberate the interpretation of a study's results from the biases and preconceived notions of the investigator. It also frees the investigator from the responsibility of choosing arbitrary endpoint decisions during the planning stage of the experiment, selections that subsequently may be demonstrated by the data to be the "wrong choices." In fact, it can appear to be far better for the investigators to preserve some flexibility in their experiment's interpretation by saying little during the design of the experiment about either the endpoint selection or the analysis procedures. This would allow the data collected to choose the best analysis and endpoint as long as these selections are consistent with the goals of the experiment.

This "let the data decide" point of view may appear to be bolstered by the observation that researchers by and large understand and appreciate the importance of choosing the research sample with great care. Intelligent, well developed methodologies are required to choose the optimum sample size [20 — 24]. The sampling mechanism, i.e., the process by which patients are selected from the population requires careful attention to detail. Well-tested mechanisms by which patients are randomized to receive the intervention or the control therapy are put into place in order to avoid systematic biases that can produce destabilizing imbalances. In fact, the fundamental motivation for the execution of the simple random-sampling mechanism is to produce a sample that is representative of the population [25]. This effort can be an onerous, time consuming, and expensive process, but investigators have learned that it can pay off handsomely by producing a sample that "looks like" the population at large. Therefore, having invested the time and energy into producing a sample that is "as large and as random as possible," they would like the right to generalize any result "the data decides" from the sample.

Unfortunately, the utility of this approach as a confirmation instrument is undone by the wide range of sample-to-sample variability. The results from Table 1.3 demonstrate the wide variability in estimates of the mortality effect of an intervention. It is impossible to determine which sample provides the most accurate estimate of the effect in the population. In fact, from Table 1.3, we see that "letting the data decide" leads to a cacophony of disparate results from different samples. The data in fact doesn't decide anything, since the data vary so widely from sample to sample.

There are two additional problems with allowing the data to decide. The first is that the sample is commonly not drawn correctly to provide the best viewpoint to provide the answer. The appropriate sample size, as well as inclusion and exclusion criteria, can only be implemented if the research question is asked prospectively. Additionally, as discussed earlier, the statistical estimators in this approach do not perform optimally when *post hoc* analyses are carried out. This dangerous combination of suboptimal sampling frames and statistical estimators can misinform investigators. The delineated experiences of the MRFIT, Vesnarinone, ELITE, and PRAISE investigators requires us to distance ourselves from the alluring but ultimately misleading and disappointing approach of letting the data decide. While we must rely on data, the reliance pays its greatest dividend when the data are derived from a detailed, prospective plan.

The FDA refused the sponsor's application for the approval of Carvedilol for life prolongation in patients with CHF. However, six months later the compound was approved for CHF symptom amelioration. A more thorough evaluation of this second meeting is available [12,13], as well as an elaboration of the additional entanglements faced by clinical trials assessing the role of beta blockage in CHF [26]. Alternative points of view are available [12,14,17].

2.10 Tight Protocols

Well written protocols are the first good product of a well-designed research effort. The development of a tight protocol, immune to unplanned sampling error contamination, is a praiseworthy effort but takes a substantial amount of time and requires great patience. The investigators who are designing the study must have the patience to design the study appropriately. Its literature review is not just thorough and informative, but constructive, in that it guides the final assembly of a relevant research question.[*] They must take the time to understand the population from which they will sample, make a focused determination of the necessary endpoint measurements, and assess endpoint measures accurately and precisely. Occasionally, they should also have the patience to carry out a small pilot study, postponing the main trial until they have tested recruitment and data collection strategies. In the well written protocol, the methods section is elaborated in great detail. The source and numbers of research subjects or patients are provided. Data collection methods are elaborated. Statistical analysis tools are expounded. The specification of each endpoint's ascertainment, verification, and analysis is laid out in great detail.[†]

Those who make these efforts are rewarded with well-considered protocols that are executable, and have a clearly articulated analysis plan that is data independent. This is a heavy burden.[‡] This complete elaboration serves several useful purposes. A requirement of its development demands that the research effort itself be thoughtfully considered prospectively, a requisite for good research execution. In addition, the specifications in the protocol permit the conditions of the research to be fully illuminated, permitting other researchers to replicate the research design. Finally, a well-written protocol serves as an indispensable anchor for the study, keeping the analyses from being cast adrift in the eddies of the incoming data stream.

After the protocol is written and accepted, investigators must insist on nothing less than its rigorous execution. The protocol is the rule book of the trial,

---

[*] Arthur Young wrote of the necessity for a thorough review of the literature as a tool to create productive and useful research efforts. (Chapter One, page 12).

[†] In some cases, the protocol may discuss an analysis even though neither the endpoints of the analysis nor the details for the analysis are known during the design phase of the trial. An example is blood banking.

[‡] Investigators may profit from remembering the Quaker admonition "strength in this life, happiness in the next."

and all involved must strictly adhere to it. Information about a violation of the trial protocol must immediately raise concerns for the presence of study discordance with attendant alpha error corruption. As for midstream endpoint changes, consider the following true story.

> A 34 year-old automobile mechanic from Alamo, Michigan, was troubled by a noise coming from the truck he and his friend were driving. The mechanic insisted on finding the noise's source. Instructing his friend to continue driving so the noise would continue, the mechanic maneuvered outside of the truck and then, while the truck was still being driven, continued to squirm and maneuver until he was underneath the truck. While carrying out his investigation, his clothing caught on part of the undercarriage. Some miles later when his friend finally stopped the car and got out, he found his mechanic friend "wrapped in the drive shaft" – quite dead.

Avoid the temptation of changing a research program that is already underway, so you don't get "wrapped in drive shaft."

2.11 Design Manuscripts

Occasionally the investigators will choose to publish the protocol of their study as a "design manuscript." There are several advantages to this procedure. First, the appearance of the protocol in the peer-reviewed medical literature broadcasts to the research and the medical community that a research effort is being conducted to answer the posed scientific question. In addition, important assumptions underlying the sample size computation, aspects of the inclusion and exclusion criteria, and endpoint determinations are carefully elaborated, commonly to a greater degree than is permissible in the manuscript that will describe the study's final results.

Finally, a design manuscript is a message to the research community from the investigators that says "Here is the research question we wish to address. This is how we have decided to address it. Here are the rules of our trial. Be sure to hold us to them."[*] Examples of design manuscripts are available in several healthcare related fields [27 —32].

In addition, design manuscripts can be particularly useful for research efforts that examined disputed, sometimes litigious research questions in which strong, vocal, and influential forces have forcefully articulated their points of view before the research effort was conceived. At its conclusion, a well-designed, well executed research effort will be criticized because its results are at variance with the expectations of some, a level of criticism that is directly proportional to the controversial nature of the research question. Such criticism is inevitable and unavoidable.

---

[*] Design manuscripts have the additional advantages of (1) engaging the clinical trial investigators in the publishing process, an activity that can help to improve morale in a long trial, and (2) conserving space in the final manuscript that is published when the clinical trial has been completed by describing the trial's methodology in complete detail in the earlier appearing design manuscript.

However, one particularly sharp barb can be that the investigators sacrificed their objectivity by changing the research methodology to produce the desired answer. Like the unfortunate archeologist who was found with a hammer and chisel altering the length of one of the pyramids because it did not conform to his expectation, the researchers are commonly accused of warping their research (and their data) to get the desired answer. The appearance of a well-written design manuscript followed by the concordant execution of the protocol, like the apple of gold in the setting of silver, naturally fit together to blunt this especially visceral criticism.

2.12 Concordant Versus Discordant Research

As we have seen, the accuracy of statistical estimators in a sample-based research effort depend on the sources of variability. Define study *concordance* [33] as the execution of a research effort in accordance with a prespecified protocol and analysis plan. With study concordance, the analysis plan is prospectively fixed, sampling error only affects the values of the observations, and the estimators perform well. On the other hand, if the research plan is not chosen prospectively but is selected by the data, the influence of sampling error on the analysis selection perturbs the estimators. This circumstance is defined as study *discordance*. Since the random data have been allowed to transmit randomness to the analysis plan, and the research program's results, effect sizes, standard errors, confidence intervals, and *p*-values are unreliable since it is the result not just of random data, but of a random analysis plan.

However the notion of concordance or discordance is not one of absolutes. The unexpected affects every research effort, and some discordance is present in every research program.

2.12.1 Severe Discordance: Mortality Corruption

Severe study discordance describes the situation where the research execution has been so different from that prescribed in the prospectively written protocol that the sample provides a hopelessly blurred and distorted view of the population from which it was chosen. Estimators from these discordant studies are rendered meaningless and irrelevant to the medical community since the view of the population through the sample is smeared and distorted. This unfortunate state of affairs can be produced by the flawed execution of a well-written protocol. The situation can be so complicated that, in the case of a positive study, the estimators themselves cannot be incontrovertibly computed. Experiments that lead to this type of estimator corruption are essentially useless to the research community.

Consider the case of a clinical trial that will assign therapy to patients with advanced HIV infections. The study has two treatment arms, and patients are to be followed for four years. The endpoint of the study is the total mortality rate.

At the conclusion of the study, 15% of patients are lost to follow-up. What is the best interpretation of these results? The implications of this discordance are substantial, because the follow-up losses blur the investigator's view of the population. In essence, they obtained the sample to learn what would happen in the population, but now, with substantial follow-up losses, they never learned what really happened in their sample.

There are additional problems. How should the analysis be carried out? The problem here is not that statistical estimators are data-based (every statistical estimator uses data). The problem introduced by severe study discordance is that the very method of computing the estimators is data based. Should the computation assume that all patients who are lost to follow-up are dead? Should it assume that patients who are lost to follow-up in the active group are dead, and those who were lost to follow-up and in the placebo group are alive? Should it assume that an equal fraction of patients who are lost to follow-up are alive, regardless of the therapy group assignment? The best choice from among these possibilities is not dictated by the protocol. Instead, the choice of computation is based on belief and the data, which itself is full of sampling error.* Variability has wrenched control of the statistical estimator's computation from the protocol and complicates this study's interpretation.

The degree of discordance here depends on the magnitude of the statistical estimators. If the effect size and p-value remained below the threshold of significance in the most stringent of circumstances i.e., assuming that all lost patients assigned to the placebo group were alive at the trial's conclusion, but that all lost patients in the active group were dead, we must conclude the discordance is mild because the worst implications of the follow-up losses do not violate the results. However, if the p-value fluctuates wildly in this sensitivity analysis, the discordance is severe.

2.12.2 Severe Discordance: Medication Changes

Another example of severe study discordance is produced from a clinical trial designed to assess the effect of an intervention on patients who have established heart failure at the time of randomization. Patients are randomized to either control therapy or control therapy plus an active intervention. The prospectively specified primary analysis for the study is a change in the background medication for heart failure (e.g., increase in digoxin or diuretic use during the trial, or the addition of ACE-i during the trial), a change that would be triggered by deterioration of the patient's left ventricular function over time. The trial requires a sample size of 482 patients.

The trial protocol assumes that all patients will have an endpoint assessment. However, during the trial's execution, 40% of the patients have missing medical records precluding the determination of endpoint status, allowing endpoint computation on only the remaining 60%. Is this experiment interpretable? The investigators must carry out some post-hoc computation if the research effort is to convey useful information about the population to the research and regulatory community.

Clearly, the view is distorted if 40% of the sample has missing endpoint information. As before, there is disagreement on the computation of the trial's statistical estimators since different assumptions about the medication records for the

---

* Some of these computations will provide statistical estimators that support the investigators' ideas, while other computations provide antithetical measures of effect size, standard errors, confidence intervals, and p-values.

40% of patients with missing information would lead to different values of the effect size and confidence interval widths. For example should the *p*-values be computed assuming that the missing patients had no medication changes? Assuming only active patients had medication changes? Each assumption leads to a different effect size computation. Experimental discordance is potentially extreme, and if a sensitivity analysis reveals wide variation in effect size estimator based on the assumption about the 40% of patients with lost records, then the study will be uninformative about the effect of therapy on the CHF population.

2.12.3 Discordance and NSABP

As a final example of discordance, consider the findings of the National Surgical Adjuvant Breast Project (NSABP) [34] that examined the effect of different therapies for breast cancer reduction. After the study's results were analyzed and published, it was discovered that 99 ineligible patients were deliberately randomized with falsified data. Is this experiment hopelessly corrupted?

One way to resolve this dilemma was to examine whether the estimates of effect size, standard error, confidence intervals, or *p*-values were substantially altered in a sensitivity analysis by excluding the fraudulently entered 99 patients. This sensitivity analysis revealed no important change in the statistical estimators. However, a second relevant question of the interpretation of the trial had to be addressed since the presence of fraudulent data admitted the possibility of dishonest behavior elsewhere in the trial apparatus. To address this discordance issue, a full audit of the study data was carried out by Christian et. al. [35]. Since the protocol discrepancies identified were small in number and magnitude, the degree of discordance was assessed to be mild, and the conclusions of NSABP were allowed to stand.*

2.13 Conclusions

The supremacy of hypothesis-driven research does not eliminate surprises. Quite the contrary, we learn by surprises in science. The key features of our principle are (1) we cannot blindly take every finding in a sample and extend that finding to a much larger population and (2) the magnitude of the statistical estimators does not determine which finding should be extended to the population, and which should be left behind in the sample. The findings for which the experiment is designed are most likely to be the generalizable findings — those we take to the population with us. This applies to any sample-based research, from small observational studies to large, expensive state-of-the-art clinical trials.

During the design of a research effort, anticipate that there will be many more exploratory analyses than primary analyses. Investigators should be encouraged to triage their analysis plans [26], identifying a small number of primary analyses, followed by a greater number of secondary analysis, and even a larger number of exploratory analyses. This permits them to select a sample that focuses

---

* The controversy that swirled around this study involved several layers of investigation, including congressional inquiries. See Moyé L (2004) *Finding Your Way in Science: How You Can Combine Character, Compassion, and Productivity in Your Research Career.* Vancouver: Trafford.

on a small number of research questions for which they can provide confirmatory solutions. While the exploratory questions are interesting, the answers provided are only hypothesis-generating.

Similarly, reporting research results should follow a hierarchy as well. It is best to first report the findings that were the basis of prospective statements, on which some prior type I error has been allocated.* Once this has been completed, the researcher may announce other unexpected finding, but with the preamble that these are exploratory findings. These exploratory findings are disseminated to raise new questions — not to answer them.

Thus, research efforts are combinations of confirmatory and exploratory analyses. The sequence of events is typically that an interesting exploratory analysis is followed by a confirmatory one, the latter being used to confirm the former. This confirmatory analysis should not represent an attempt to reproduce slavishly the findings of exploratory analysis, as in the following humorous example:

> The chef at a hotel in Switzerland lost a finger in a meat cutting machine and, after a little hopping around, submitted a claim to his insurance company. The company, suspecting negligence, sent out one of its men to have a look for himself. He tried the machine out and lost a finger. The chef's claim was approved.

Exploratory analyses are commonly useful because they provide the first data-based view of the future. Thus, despite their limitations, exploratory analyses will continue to play an important role in research efforts. However, they should be reported at a level and tenor consistent with the inaccuracy of the estimators on which they are based.

On the other hand, the confirmatory work to reproduce the exploratory analysis should be designed to evoke and elaborate in detail the result of the exploratory analysis so that information about the mechanism that produced the exploratory relationship becomes clearer. The confirmatory analysis will, in all likelihood, require a different number of subjects, perhaps a more precise measure of the endpoint, and a different analysis than that presented in the exploratory study.

Ultimately, the value of the research depends on the generalizability of the research sample's results to larger populations. Well-designed research, well-chosen samples, and concordant execution are each required for this process to succeed.

References

1 .   Lehmann EL (1983) *Theory of Point Estimation.* New York; John Wiley. p 3.
2.   Miles JL (1993) Data torturing. *New England Journal of Medicine* **329**: 1196-1199.
3.   MRFIT Investigators (1982) Multiple risk factor intervention trial. *Journal of the American Medical Association* **248**:1465-77.

---

* Some uncomplicated advice on this allocation is provided in Chapter Eight.

4   Pitt B, Segal R, Martinez FA et al. on behalf of the ELITE Study Investigators (1997) Randomized trial of losartan versus captopril in patients over 65 with heart failure. *Lancet* **349**:747–52.
5   Jensen BV, Nielsen, SL (1997) Correspondence: Losartan versus captopril in elderly patients with heart failure. *Lancet* **349**:1473.
6   Fournier A, Achard JM, Fernandez LA (1997) Correspondence: Losartan versus captopril in elderly patients with heart failure. *Lancet* **349:**1473.
7.   Pitt B, Poole-Wilson PA., Segal R, et. al (2000) Effect of losartan compared with captopril on mortality in patients with symptomatic heart failure randomized trial–The losartan heart failure survival study. ELITE II. *Lancet.***355**:1582–87.
8.   Meinert CL (1986) *Clinical Trials: Design, Conduct, and Analysis*. New York. Oxford University Press.
9.   Friedman L, Furberg C, DeMets D (1996) *Fundamentals of Clinical Trials*. Third Edition. New York. Spinger.
10. Moyé LA (1998) *P*–value interpretation and alpha allocation in clinical trials. *Annals of Epidemiology.* **8**:351–357.
11. Packer M., Bristow MR Cohn JN et al (1996) The effect of carvedilol on morbidity and mortality in patients with chronic heart failure. *New England Journal of Medicine.* **334**:1349–55.
12   Fisher L (1999) Carvedilol and the FDA approval process: the FDA paradigm and reflections upon hypothses testing. *Controlled Clinical Trials* **20**:16–39.
13. Moyé LA, Abernethy D (1996) Carvedilol in Patients with Chronic Heart Failure (Letter) *New England Journal of Medicine.* **335**: 1318–1319.
14. Packer M, Cohn JN, Ccolucci WS (1996) Response to Moyé and Abernethy. *New England Journal of Medicine* 335:1318–1319.
15. Fisher LD, Moyé LA (1999) Carvedilol and the Food and Drug Administration Approval Process: An Introduction. *Controlled Clinical Trials.* **20**:1–15.
16. Moyé L.A (1999) *P* Value Interpretation in Clinical Trials. The Case for Discipline. *Controlled Clinical Trials* **20**:40–49.
17. Fisher LD (1999) Carvedilol and the Food and Drug Administration-Approval Process: A Brief Response to Professor Moyé's article. *Controlled Clinical Trials.* **20**:50–51.
18. Lewis JA (1995) Statistical issues in the regulation of medicines. *Statistics in Medicine.* **14:** 127–136.
19. Pocock SJ, Geller NL, Tsiatis AA (1987) The analysis of multiple endpoints in clinical trials. *Biometrics* **43**:487–498.
20. Lachim JM (1981) Introduction to sample size determinations and power analyses for clinical trials. *Controlled Clinical Trials* **2**:93–114.
21. Sahai H, Khurshid A (1996) Formulae and tables for determination of sample size and power in clinical trials for testing differences in proportions for the two sample design. *Statistics in Medicine* **15**:1–21.
22. Donner A (1984) Approach to sample size estimation in the design of clinical trials — a review. *Statistics in Medicine* **3**:199–214.

23. George SL, Desue, MM (1974) Planning the size and duration of a clinical trial studying the time to some critical event. *Journal of Chronic Disease* **27**:15–24.
24. Davy SJ and Graham OT (1991) Sample size estimation for comparing two or more treatment groups in clinical trials. *Statistics in Medicine* **10**:3–43.
25. Snedecor GW, Cochran WG (1980) *Statistical Methods, 7th Edition.* Iowa; Iowa State University Press.
26. Moyé LA (2003) *Multiple Analyses and Clinical Trials.* New York; Springer.
27. The SHEP Cooperative Research Group (1988) Rationale and design of a randomized clinical trial on prevention of stroke in isolated systolic hypertension. *Journal of Clinical Epidemiology* **41**:1197–1208.
28. Davis BR, Cutler JA, Gordon DJ, Furberg CD, Wright JT, Cushman WC, Grimm RH, LaRosa J, Whelton PK, Perry HM, Alderman MH, Ford CE, Oparil S, Francis C, Proschan M, Pressel S, Black HR, Hawkins CM for the ALLHAT Research Group (1996) Rationale and design for the antihypertensive and lipid lowering treatment to prevent heart attack trial (ALLHAT) *American Journal of Hypertension* **9**:342–360.
29. Moyé, LA for the SAVE Cooperative Group (1991) Rationale and design of a trial to assess patient survival and ventricular enlargement after myocardial infarction. *American Journal of Cardiology* **68**:70D–79D.
30. Pratt, CM, Mahmarian JJ, Morales-Ballejo H,Casareto R, Moyé, LA for the Transdermal Nitroglycerin Investigators Group (1998) The long–term effects of intermittent transdermal nitroglycerin on left ventircular remodeling after acute myocardial infaction. Design of a randomized, placebo controlled mulitcenter trial. *American Journal of Cardiology* **81**:719–724.
31. Moyé LA, Richardson MA, Post-White J, Justice, B (1995) Research Methodology in Psychoneuroimmunology: Rationale and design of the IMAGES–P (imagery and group emotional support study-pilot) clinical trial. *Alternative Therapy in Medicine* **1**:34–39.
32. Pfeffer MA, Sacks FM, Moyé LA et al. for the Cholesterol and Recurrent Events Clinical Trial Investigators (1995) Cholesterol and Recurrent Events (CARE) trial: A secondary prevention trial for normolipidemic patients. *American Journal of Cardiology* **76**: 98C–106C,
33. Moyé LA (1998) P value interpretation and alpha allocation in clinical trials. *Annals of Epidemiology.* **8**:351–357.
34. Fisher B, Bauer M, Margolese R. et al (1985) Eight year results of a randomized clinical trial comparing total mastectomy and segmental mastectomy with or without radiation in the treatment of breast cancer. *New England Journal of Medicine.***312**:665–73.
35. Christian MC, McCabe MS, Korn EL, Abrams JS, Kaplan RS, Friedman MA (1995) The National Cancer Institute audit of the national surgical adjuvant breast and bowel project protocol B-06. *New England Journal of Medicine.* **333**:1469–1474.

3

A Hypothesis-Testing Primer

3.1 Introduction

A critical compromise in research is the investigator's decision to study not the entire population of interest (which is, of course, impossible in most cases), but a small sample as a representation of that population. This decision permits researchers to carry out a thorough research effort on the sample that may be informative; however, he must give up certainty and confront the implications of sample-to-sample variability.

Accepting this compromise begs the question, Does the sample's answer to the research reveal a relationship embedded in the population or instead, is it a finding restricted to this one sample, with no broader applicability? The potentially disruptive presence of sample-to-sample variability undermines our efforts to try to explain the sample's findings. As physicians and investigators, we are anxious to learn from the data, and this motivation is manifested in our efforts to explain the study results in terms of underlying biology, pharmacology, or pathophysiology. However, before we attempt these incisive, evocative, and sometimes imaginative explications, the scientific community must come to grips with the sampling error issue. If sampling error is an explanation for the results, then there is little need to attempt a mechanistic or clinical explanation of the observed relationship.

The researchers can simplify the task of the community by recognizing the two influences sampling error can have. In the most pernicious circumstance, sampling error wrecks their research effort. Specifically, in the absence of a fixed protocol, the sample not only chooses the data but also chooses the analysis, suggesting the questions the investigators should have prospectively asked. Here, the sample is commonly chosen suboptimally, allowing only a poor view of the population's response. Additionally, the statistical estimators perform badly, creating inaccurate measures of effect sizes and standard errors, further distorting the sample's view of the population response. This research is commonly unreliable, must be viewed as exploratory, and requires confirmation.

However, in the presence of a sample that is tightly focused on a particular research question and is driven by a research protocol that is fixed prospectively, sampling error is well contained. The commonly used statistical estimators function remarkably well in providing accurate estimates. The researcher can simplify the interpretation of this research results by providing clear statements of their confirmatory analyses, followed by a summary of the exploratory analyses; these latter evaluations require their own confirmation in follow-up research efforts.

However, even in the circumstance of confirmatory analyses, the question still remains, Is the sample's answer to the research question generalizable to the population or it is a freak observation, applying only to the chance aggregation of individuals in a small sample? Even a confirmatory analysis will not answer this question with assurance. However, it does permit an answer with a corresponding measure of reliability.

3.2 The Rubric of Hypothesis Testing

There are of course important similarities between scientific and statistical hypothesis evaluations that allow statistical hypothesis testing to be very naturally and easily folded into the scientific method. Each procedure begins with a hypothesis, the veracity of which the investigator seeks to determine. In each case, the data must be the product of a well-designed and well-conducted research effort. Since the data are most commonly quantitative, both the scientific method and statistical hypothesis testing involve important mathematical computations. However, there is an important difference in the approach that is used by each that we must carefully examine.

The scientific method begins with a hypothesis or initial idea that the researcher hopes to demonstrate. Scientists have deductions they wish to prove. Columbus wished to prove that the earth was round. DeMoivre believed that comets were rogue entities with their own existence separate and apart from the planets. An oncologist may believe that a new cancer chemotherapy will lengthen the lives of her patients. These are affirmative beliefs of the scientist, and scientists possess powerful motivation to prove them.

However, statistical hypothesis testing does not start with the idea in which the scientist believes, but instead commonly begins with a hypothesis that the researcher hopes to disprove. Thus, its process is not one of confirmation, but of nullification. Yet, through the careful use of this negative proof, the researcher hopes to demonstrate that the only useful conclusion of the research is that their original, affirmative idea was correct.

A useful example to consider is that of obesity. The current cultural climate in the United States suggests that there is an epidemic of obesity in US men. Let's presume that a hypothetical investigator sets out to examine this issue for himself. Quantitatively, he seeks an estimate of how large US men are. However, his prior study and experience have generated his belief that male obesity is far more common a problem then is generally recognized. Thus, he enters this research project with a particular point of view.

There is nothing wrong with his *a priori* perspective. The researcher has some genuine interest in the problem and this level of interest is commonly and appropriately reflected in this opinion. However, the researcher must discipline himself to not let his belief or suspicion about the prevalence of male obesity spill over into the methodology of his research effort. He must differentiate between his *a priori* belief and his knowledge, that lags behind his belief and will be supplemented by the research effort.

However the statistical treatment of this commonly begins with a simplifying, useful, and surprising accurate assumption; the representative meaures of the underlying variable's distribution (e.g. the sample mean) follow a normal distribution.

3.3 The Normal Distribution and Its Estimators

Most of traditional hypothesis testing is based on the assertion that the variable of measurement is governed by the normal distribution. Although there are many probability distributions that have been discovered over the past 300 years, the one most frequently is the "bell-shaped curve" (Figure 3.1).

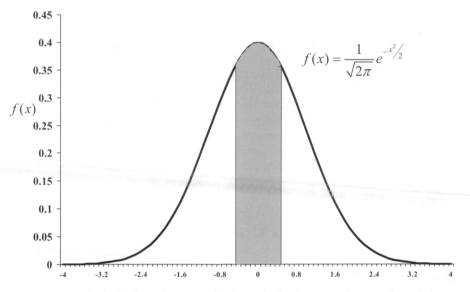

Fig. 3.1. The bell-shaped curve. The formula for the curve is complicated, but probability is measured as area under the curve, and provided in tables (Appendix A). The shaded area is the probability that a variable following this distribution lies between –0.50 and 0.50.

Formally known as the Gaussian distribution,[*] this probability distribution remains the most commonly used in statistical hypothesis testing. Its probabilities are for events on the real number line. The likelihood of any interval on that real line is the area under the curve depicted in Figure 3.1.

The formula for the curve is complicated. If z is a point on the real line then $f(z)$ is computed as

$$f(z) = \frac{1}{\sqrt{2\pi}} e^{-z^2/2}. \tag{3.1}$$

[*] Named for Karl Friedrich Gauss (1777–1855), a calculating prodigy who lived in the eighteenth century. His contributions to mathematics are numerous, including the development of the normal distribution, contributions to calculus theory, and the discovery of the "least squares" approach to statistical model building.

The complexity of this formula, ostensibly not directly related to healthcare variables, begs the question of how it could be so useful in clinical research. There are two reasons for its ubiquity.

The first is that, occasionally, an action is carried out whose outcomes have the precise probability that is the area under equation (3.1). Diffusion of gases and liquids is a prime example. However, the second, and most common, reason for its omnipresence has to do with the nature of the occurrences in general.

Outcomes are commonly the result of many influences, each exerting its effect separate and apart from others. For example, an individual's body mass index (BMI) is not the result of one force e.g., genetics. Instead, an individual's BMI results from a combination of effects that include but are not limited to genetics, activity, nutrition patterns early in life, and current dietary habits. Each of these major factors can be subdivided into smaller influences. However, although these individual influences are small, each has a specific direction i.e., some of them produce positive effects whereas others have negative ones. The mathematics of this process tell us that the distribution of the sum of this myriad collection of influences (in this case, the BMI) can be nicely approximated by the normal distribution.* This cumulative effect is seen time and again in healthcare research, hence the commonality of this probability distribution. In fact, the widespread use of this result is the motivation for the nickname of "normal distribution" for the bell-shaped curve.

3.4 Using the Normal Distribution

An important advantage in using the normal distribution is the relative ease of producing probabilities from it. Although the actual production of probabilities requires one to use a table (Appendix A)†, we need use only one table to produce probabilities for the many different normal distributions. This is due to the ease of transformation of normal random variables and the notion of symmetry.

3.4.1 Simplifying Transformations

The normal distribution is not just a single distribution, but is instead a family of them. In fact, there are an infinite number of normal distributions, each one characterized by its unique mean μ and variance σ^2. The mean provides the location of the distribution, and the variance characterizes the dispersion of the variable around that mean (Figure 3.2).

---

* The central limit theorem governs this use of the normal distribution.
† Spreadsheets and other calculating tools are available on personal computers as well.

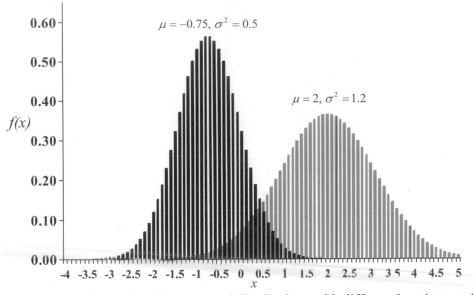

Fig. 3.2. Examples of two normal distributions with different locations and variances.

Figure 3.2 provides two members from the family of normal distributions. The central location of each is determined by the mean value μ, and its dispersal or spread is determined by and variance σ^2. The standard deviation σ is the square root of the variance.

The fact that the location and the shape of a normally distributed variable is governed by its mean and variance suggests that the investigator must incorporate these two parameters into any computation of the probabilities using these distributions. However, because there are an infinite number of combinations of these two parameters, a first impression is that an infinite number of tables are required. Fortunately, this complexity is bypassed by the fact that each member of the family of normal distributions can be related or transformed to another normal distribution. This observation produces the simplifying principle that any normal variable can be related or reduced to a single normal distribution. This single normal distribution has a mean of zero and a variance of one and is known as the *standard normal distribution*.

Therefore, if X follows a normal distribution with mean μ and variance σ^2, then X, and any event involving X can be transformed to a normally distributed variable with mean 0 and variance 1. Specifically, if X follows a normal distribution with mean μ and variance σ^2, then

$$\left(X-u\right)\big/_{\sigma}$$

follows a normal distribution with mean 0 and variance 1 (Figure 3.3).

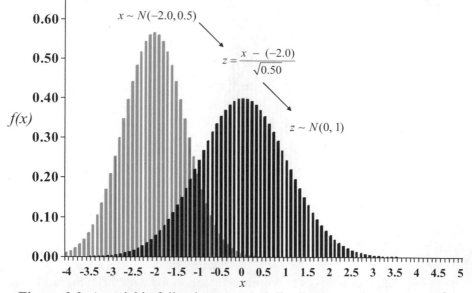

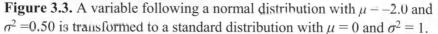

Figure 3.3. A variable following a normal distribution with $\mu = -2.0$ and $\sigma^2 = 0.50$ is transformed to a standard distribution with $\mu = 0$ and $\sigma^2 = 1$.

Thus, because every normally distributed random variable can be converted to a standard normal distribution, we require only a single set of tables that provide probabilities from the normal distribution.

For example, we can use this simplification to compute the probability that the normally distributed variables appearing in Figure 3.3 are less than −1.0. Since X follows a normal distribution with mean −2.0 and variance 0.50, we write

$$P[X \le -1.0] = P\left[\frac{X-(-2.0)}{\sqrt{0.50}} \le \frac{-1.0-(-2.0)}{\sqrt{0.50}}\right]$$

$$= P\left[Z \le \frac{-1.0-(-2.0)}{\sqrt{0.50}}\right] = P[Z \le 1.414].$$

Using Appendix A, we see that the probability that a variable that follows a standard normal random variable is less than 1.4 is 0.919, an approximate result sufficient for this example.

3.4.3 Symmetry

A second useful characteristic of the normal distribution is its property of symmetry. Examination of the curves in Figures 3.2 and 3.3 reveals that the shape of the

normal distribution is a mirror image of itself when divided at the mean. This produces some useful computation simplifications. Begin with a variable Z that follows
the normal distribution. $P[Z=0]=0$ from the concept of probability as area. We
also know from use of the property of symmetry of the standard normal distribution
that $P[Z<0]=[Z>0]$. Because the sum of these probabilities must equal one, we
see that $P[Z<0]=P[Z>0]=\frac{1}{2}$.

In fact, the use of symmetry produces the relationship that for any value z,
$P[Z<-z]=P[Z>z]$ (Figure 3.4).[*]

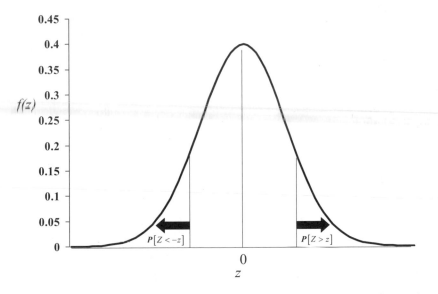

Fig. 3.4. Symmetry of the normal distribution. If Z follows a standard normal
distribution, then **P**[Z $<$ –z] = **P**[Z $>$ z].

This style of computation is frequently utilized. If we define
$F_Z(z)=P[Z\le z]$, then we know that $F_Z(-z)=1-F_Z(z)$. Let T be the test statistic
that is produced from a statistical hypothesis test, and $|TS|$ be its absolute value.
Then, if the TS follows a standard normal distribution,

$$P[Z\le-|TS|]+P[Z\ge|TS|]=2P[Z\le|TS|].$$

---

[*] For the normal distribution, the probability of a single value i.e., $P[Z=1]$ is zero.

We will have much more to say about this computation and its implications; but first we must return to our waiting investigator interested in assessing body mass index in a sample of patients.

3.5 The Null Hypothesis: State of the Science

Our investigator's plan to assess BMI in men is quite simple. He will draw a sample of subjects, compute each patient's BMI, and then draw a conclusion. However, while easily stated, this procedure requires some important preliminary steps.

First, he must determine just how many patients he will measure. Certainly, the larger the sample, the more the sample will resemble the population from which it was drawn. However, regardless of how large the sample will be, it is an insignificant fraction of the total population; since resources are restricted, he will need to be guided by a combination of fiscal restraint and scientific rigor.[*] Attention must also be paid to the process by which he draws his sample. If it is not drawn randomly, then the selection criteria that was used to draw subjects can hamper the generalization of the results to the population of interest.[†]

In addition, the investigator must plan what he will do with the sample once he draws it, with special attention to how he will interpret the results.

Assume the investigator recruits 100 subjects in his sample. From his point of view, there are two alternatives. One is that the current thinking in public health (i.e., the state of the science) is correct. The second, simply put, is that it is not. The use of classic statistical inference procedures reformulates the scientific hypothesis into two components; (1) the null hypothesis, and (2) the alternative hypothesis.

The null hypothesis is the hypothesis that the investigator does not believe, i.e., it affirms the current state of the science. In this case, the state of the science suggests that the mean BMI is 28. The investigator asserts this null hypothesis as

$$H_0: \mu = 28.$$

Since the investigator believes that the mean BMI is greater than 28, he thinks that his data will nullify H_0. However, he must proceed carefully if he is to persuade the medical community that the null hypothesis is false.

---

[*] Sample size computations will be discussed later in this text.
[†] This issue is commonly known as selection bias in epidemiology; while sometimes easily identified it can be difficult to assess. For example, an investigator who studies BMI in woman would quickly run into difficulty by generalizing the results to men, since the distribution of BMI is different in men. However, does a study executed in Europe that demonstrates the identification of a relationship between exposure to weight loss pill ingestion and primary pulmonary hypertension not apply to patients in the US simply because no US patients were included? In this case, the selection issue is clear (only European patients were selected). However, the central question is whether differences between the Europeans and Americans are so great that a relationship observed in one group does not automatically translate to a relationship in the other. In this case, even though there are important cultural differences between the two peoples, the mechanism of action of the diet drug, and the method of production of primary pulmonary hypertension are essentially the same. Therefore, the selection issue does not obstruct generalization of the European results the US.

If the null hypothesis is correct, then the researcher would expect that the BMI of all patients (and therefore the ones in his sample) will be normally distributed with a mean of 28 and a standard deviation of 5.5.

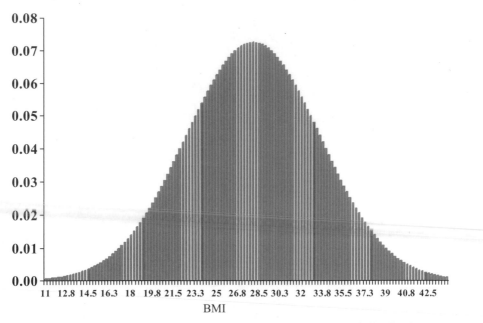

Fig. 3.3. Expected distribution of male BMI's assuming a normal distribution with mean 28 and standard deviation 5.5

Since the location of this normal distribution is what is in question, the investigator intends to focus on the sample mean, $\bar{x}$.

One advantage of the sample mean is that it is the best estimator of the central location of the population mean μ of a normal distribution. Another important characteristic of the sample mean is its smaller variability. Different samples will of course have different observations, but the sample means will not vary as widely from sample to sample as will the individual observations (Figure 3.4).[*]

---

[*] The distribution of the sample size for the mean comes from the following experiment. Choose 100 patients from the population. Compute the mean BMI from this sample and set it aside. Next, select another sample of 100 patients, and compute the mean BMI from this sample. As this experiment is repeated, a sample of the sample means is collected, and its distribution can be graphed.

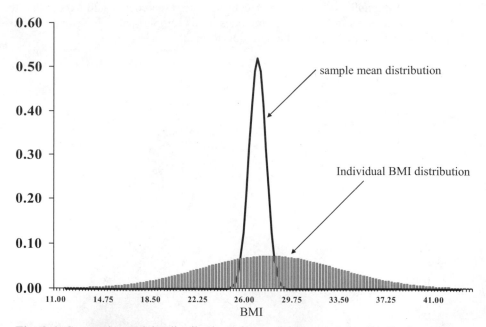

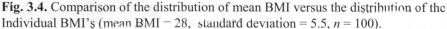

Fig. 3.4. Comparison of the distribution of mean BMI versus the distribution of the Individual BMI's (mean BMI ⁻ 28, standard deviation = 5.5, n = 100).

Thus while the sample mean will vary from sample to sample, its variability is not nearly as great as the variability of a single observation. This variability is reflected in its standard deviation. While the standard deviation of a single observation is 5.5, the standard deviation of the sample mean is $5.5/\sqrt{100} == 0.550$.

A comparison of the distribution of the individual BMI with that of the sample mean from Figure 3.4 reveals that the sample mean distribution provides more illumination about the location of the population mean μ then does the distribution of individual BMI's. Thus, the investigator chooses to compare the relative location of the mean $\bar{x}$ from his sample with the value of the mean under the null hypothesis. The closer they are to each other, the stronger the level of evidence the sample provides for the null hypothesis. The larger apart this difference, the less confident the investigator has in assuming that the population mean BMI for males is 28.

The investigator goes one step further by converting the distribution of the sample mean that, under the null hypothesis, has a sample mean of 28 and standard deviation of $5.5/\sqrt{100} == 0.550$. to a standard normal distribution (Figure 3.5).

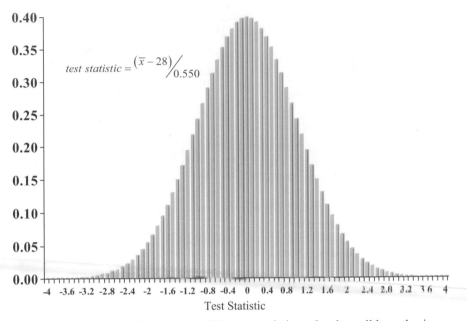

Figure 3.5. Sampling distribution of the test statistic under the null hypothesis that the mean BMI = 28.

Thus, the investigator focuses on the quantity

$$\frac{\overline{x} - 28}{5.5 \big/ \sqrt{100}} = \frac{\overline{x} - 28}{0.550}.$$

If the null hypothesis is correct, then the quantity $(\overline{x} - 28)/0.550$. will follow a standard normal distribution. This quantity is known as the *test statistic*. Evaluating the magnitude of the test statistic assesses the degree to which 1) the data support the null hypothesis and 2) the sampling error affects the decision process.

To see how this works, recall that there are two reasons that the investigator's sample mean would be different from the null hypothesis mean of 28. The first is that the null hypothesis is correct, but the process of sampling produced a value of $\overline{x}$ different from 28. The second reason is that the null hypothesis is wrong, in which case the best estimate of the population mean is not 28 but instead the value of $\overline{x}$. The sampling distribution of $(\overline{x} - 28)/0.550$ allows the investigator to take these different sources of variability into account by deciding what to do with extreme values (Figure 3.6).

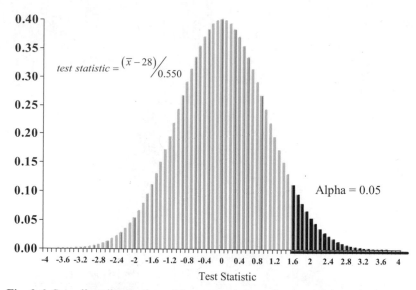

Fig. 3.6. Sampling distribution of the test statistic under the null hypothesis that the mean BMI = 28 with a one-sided (one-tailed) critical region (in black). Alpha is the area under the curve in the critical region.

Figure 3.6 contains the expected distribution of the test statistic. Examination of this distribution supports our intuition that if the null hypothesis was true and the sample mean is close to 28, then the value of the test statistic is likely to be close to zero. However, extreme values of the BMI undermine our confidence in the null hypothesis. In this case, the investigator has focused on values of the test statistic greater than 1.645 (the black bars of Figure 3.6). Values of the test statistic in these ranges are less likely under the null hypothesis and support the thesis that the mean BMI is greater than 28. The investigator decides to reject the null hypothesis if the values fall in either of these ranges. The range of values of the test statistic for which the investigator chooses to reject the null hypothesis is the *critical region*. In this example, he has chosen the critical region to be wholly on one side of the distribution of the test statistic.

Note that it is still possible that the null hypothesis is correct (and the population mean is 28) even if the test statistic falls within the critical region. Therefore, if the investigator decided to reject the null hypothesis based on this event, it is possible that he will be mistaken. The *type I error* is the probability that the decision to reject the null hypothesis based on an extreme value of the test statistic is wrong. This mistake is also known as the *alpha error*. Note that this error is strictly one of sampling i.e., it is the likelihood that a population governed by the null hypothesis generates an improbable sample that produces an extreme test statistic.

In this circumstance, the investigator is only interested in rejecting the null hypothesis if his sample mean is greater than 1.65. Thus, he only wants to reject the null hypothesis when the mean BMI is too large, and not too small. This is termed a *one-tailed* or *one-sided test hypothesis test*. In this one-tailed testing, the investigator is interested in rejecting the null hypothesis for the alternative hypothesis that the mean BMI is greater than 28. This is stated statistically as

$$H_0: \mu = 28 \text{ versus } H_a: \mu > 28.$$

where H_a refers to the alternative hypothesis. In this case, we can use the standard normal table to compute the probability that a type I error occurs is simply $P[N(0,1) \geq 1.645] = 0.05$. To avoid the complications of random research discussed in Chapter Two, the investigator chooses the critical region before the data is collected.

The investigator carries out his research effort, observing that $\bar{x} = 29.5$. He computes the test statistic as

$$\frac{\bar{x} - 28}{0.550} = \frac{29.5 - 28}{0.550} = 2.73.$$

This value falls in the critical region, and the investigator rejects the null hypothesis in favor of the alternative hypothesis. (Figure 3.7).

His best estimate of the mean BMI is now not 28 (that has been rejected), but 29.5. The *p*-value is the probability of a result at least this large under the null hypothesis, and may be computed as

$$P[N(0, 1) \geq 2.73] = 0.003.$$

Note that the *p*-value is less than the prospectively declared type I error rate of 0.05. The null hypothesis may still be true, but only three times in one thousand would a population with a mean BMI produce a sample with a mean at least as large as 29.5. Since this event is unlikely, the investigator rejects the null hypothesis. By prospectively stating the type I error rate at 0.05, the researcher declared that he would not reject the null hypothesis when the alpha error was greater than 0.05. Since the *p*-value is less than this *a priori* level, the investigator is comfortable rejecting the null hypothesis.

Note the difference between the alpha error rate and the *p*-value. The alpha error rate was set *a priori*, before the data was collected. It was part of the investigator's plan. However, the *p*-value was determined based on the data. It reflects one aspect of the researcher's results (Figure 3.7).

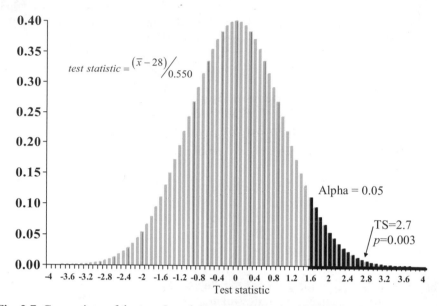

Fig. 3.7. Comparison of the type I or alpha error, determined before the data is obtained, with the *p*-value, the area under the curve to the right of the test statistic (TS).

This approach using statistical inference is one in which the investigator attempts to align his perspective with the state of the science. He first deduces what the distribution of this data should be if the state of the science is correct. If the state of the science is correct, then the observed data should nicely approximate this expected distribution. However, if the data do not match what is observed, then one of two things has happened: either (1) a sampling error has produced the aberrant result, or (2) the unanticipated finding negates the state of the science, and the current understanding should be replaced by the new finding.

However, there are other, somewhat less abstract implications for the alpha error. If a type I error occurs, then the investigator has erroneously concluded that the mean body mass index for men is larger than anticipated. This can lead to the initiation of well meant but erroneous public health warning that overestimate the magnitude of the obesity problem. The consequences of alpha errors in healthcare are commonly the institution of false and expensive programs that in the end serve no real public health benefit. Therefore, investigators choose lower levels of alpha, since the implications of their occurrence can be hazardous. However, we will moderate this conclusion after our discussion of power.

3.6 Type II Error and Power

In the previous section, the investigator observed a mean of 29.5, leading him to reject the null hypothesis in favor of the concept that the population mean BMI of males was greater than 28. However, what conclusions would the investigator have drawn if the result of their research revealed, not a BMI of 29.5, but instead, $\bar{x} = 28.5$? Would the investigator be comfortable not rejecting the null hypothesis?

Certainly, the test statistic would have been smaller. Its new value $(28.5 - 28)/\sqrt{0.550} = 0.674$ does not fall in the critical region. The p-value associated with this test statistic is $P[N(0, 1) \geq 0.674] = 0.250$, which is greater than the prespecified level of 0.05. Since the type I error is too large, the investigator would choose not to reject the null hypothesis.

However, this decision could also be a mistake; a mistake generated by sampling error. Specifically, it is possible that in the population, the mean BMI is actually 30, but the population has produced a sample with a mean much closer to the null hypothesis assumption of 28. This sampling error, where the population that demonstrates a difference produces a sample in which the state of the science (i.e., the null hypothesis) appears to be affirmed is a *beta error*, or a *type II error*. Just as with the alpha error, the beta error is strictly a phenomenon of sampling error.[*]

In addition, just as with the alpha error, the beta error is set *a priori*. In this setting, given the sample size of 100, the standard deviation of the mean, the type I error, and the value of the population mean under the alternative hypothesis (30), we can compute the probability of a type II error very easily.

We desire the probability that we do not reject the null hypothesis when the male population's mean BMI is 30. We reject the null hypothesis when the test statistic falls in the critical region, or $(\bar{x} - 28)/\sqrt{0.550} \geq 1.645$. This can be written as $\bar{x} \geq \sqrt{0.550}\ 1.645 + 28$. To find the probability of a type II error, we want the probability that the test statistic does not fall into the critical region, or $\bar{x} < \sqrt{0.550}\ 1.645 + 28$ (i.e., $\bar{x} \leq 29.22$) when the mean BMI is 30, i.e.,

$$P\left[\ \bar{x}\ <\ \sqrt{0.550}\ 1.645 + 28\ |\ \mu = 30\right]. \tag{3.2}$$

The solution is simple. We know that the distribution of $\bar{x}$ is not that of a standard normal distribution; however, the distribution of $(\bar{x} - 30)/\sqrt{0.550}$ is. We just convert the left hand side of the inequality to a standard normal random variable, carrying out the same operation on the right hand side to preserve the inequality. Thus,

$$P\left[\ \bar{x}\ <\ \sqrt{0.550}\ 1.645 + 28\ |\ \mu = 30\right]$$
$$= P\left[\ \frac{\bar{x} - 30}{\sqrt{0.550}}\ <\ \frac{\sqrt{0.550}\ 1.645 + 28 - 30}{\sqrt{0.550}}\ \right]$$
$$= P\left[\ N(0,1)\ <\ -1.052\right] = 0.146.$$

---

[*] If the sample size and the alpha error are selected, then the beta error is fixed. However, commonly the alpha and beta errors are selected *a priori*, and the sample size is derived from these selections. See Chapter Six for a full discussion, and Appendix B for the calculations.

Thus, one would expect the population with a mean BMI of 30 to produce a sample that supports the null hypothesis of the mean BMI = 28 almost 15% of the time.

The *power* of a study is simply the beta error subtracted from one. Power is a sampling phenomenon as well. It is the probability that the population whose mean value is proscribed by the alternative hypothesis produces a sample in which the alternative hypothesis is supported. Unlike alpha and beta, the power does not measure the probability of an error. Researchers wish to maximize power, and correspondingly, minimize beta.

Is the beta error low enough in the preceding example? For some researchers, a beta errors should be no larger than 5%. Others will accept a beta error as large as 20%, and would therefore be comfortable with not rejecting the null hypothesis in the preceding circumstances.

The relationship between alpha and beta errors can be easily demonstrated.

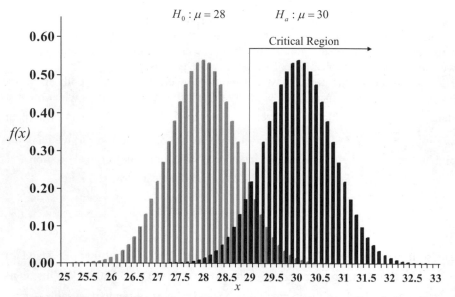

Fig. 3.8. Expected distribution of the sample mean under the null and alternative hypotheses. The critical region is delineated.

From Figure 3.8, we see that small values of the mean BMI (e.g., 27.8) are most likely under (and therefore most supportive of) the null hypothesis. For example, $\bar{x} = 31$ clearly favors the alternative hypothesis. However, the occurrence of values between the two means are the most problematic, since each of the null or alternative hypothesis are fairly likely to produce them. (Figures 3.9 and 3.10).

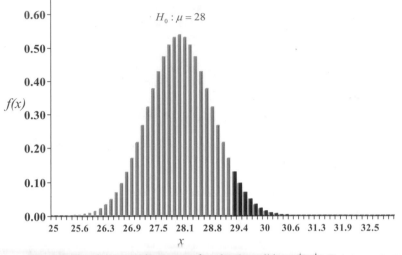

Fig. 3.9. The alpha error is computed under the null hypothesis.

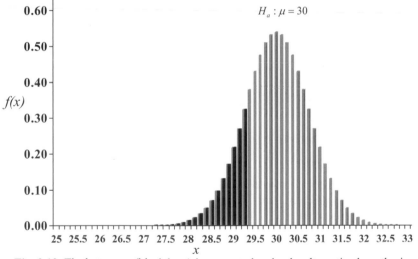

Fig. 3.10. The beta error (black bars) is computed under the alternative hypothesis.

3.7 Balancing Alpha and Beta

Recall the previous advice about selecting alpha errors. Early in this chapter, the case was made for keeping the type I error as low as possible to help reduce the number of false public health initiatives. However, the implication of a low alpha error or false-positive rate are clear from an inspection of Figures 3.9 and 3.10. By decreasing the type I error, moving the critical region further to the right, the likelihood of a beta error increases. This decrease in power means that the investigator is less likely to identify a true increase in the mean male BMI when in fact larger BMI's typify the population

Thus, decisions about type I and type II error rates must be jointly considered (Figure 3.11).

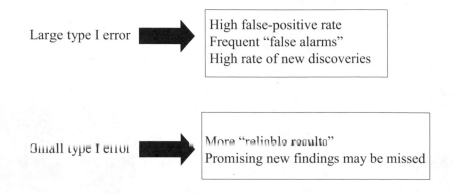

Fig. 3.11. Implications of large versus small type I error rates.

It can be quite reasonable for the researcher to consider an increase in the type I error rate to improve power. One way to calibrate the type I and type II error rates is for the researcher to consider the level of the medical community's satisfaction with the state of the science on the issue at hand. If the community is relatively comfortable with the standard for the issue, and changing that standard would lead to a costly intervention, then the likelihood of a type I error should be lowered and the identified effect size (in this case, a substantially larger mean BMI) must be provided to provide sufficient motivation for the scientific community to take action.

However, if there is a high level of dissatisfaction with the state of the science (e.g., a highly infective and lethal form of avian flu), then the medical community would be willing to accept a larger type I error rate in its search for an effective treatment. In this case, one would not wish to miss a promising therapy. The higher rate of type I error means the result has to be confirmed, but the investigator minimizes the risk of missing a promising therapy, even if some of the novel interventions are of no value in the long run.

By selecting a different alternative hypothesis, the investigator can alter the type II error level. For example, the selection of the alternative hypothesis H_a: μ =32 produces a smaller region of overlap of the distribution of sample mean under each of the null and alternative hypotheses (Figure 3.12).

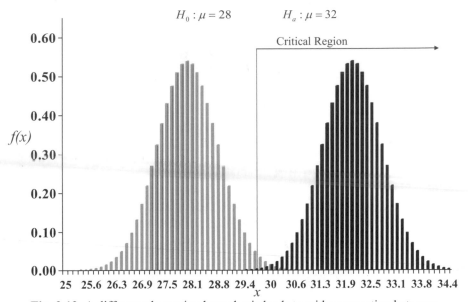

Fig. 3.12. A different alternative hypothesis leads to wider separation between the two distributions of the sample mean, decreasing the region of overlap and the magnitude of the type I and type II errors.

Thus, one mechanism that the investigator has at his disposal is to increase the distance between the mean value of the BMI under the null and alternative hypotheses. However, although the investigator has complete control over the selection of the mean values for the null and alternative hypotheses, his choices must be tempered by what is generally accepted by the medical community. Small distances between the null and alternative hypotheses tend to give statistical weight to unimportant findings. Alternatively, as we will see later, distances that are too widely separated lead to evidence that may clearly reflect an important clinical difference, but do not lead to rejection of the null hypothesis. Thus, the values of μ for each of the null and alternative hypotheses are best determined using clinical rather than statistical criteria.

3.8 Reducing Alpha and Beta: The Sample Size

One more level of control that the investigator has in this matter is the choice of the sample size. In the previous example, the investigator chose a sample size of 100 patients. Selection of a larger sample size would diminish the variability of the sample mean, thus diminishing the spread of two distributions under the null and alternative hypothesis (Figure 3.13).

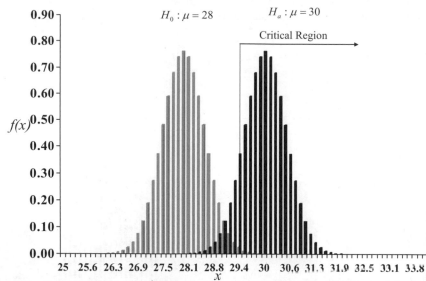

Fig. 3.13. Wider separation is produced between the distributions of the sample means when the sample size is increased from 100 to 400 subjects, decreasing the magnitude of the type I and type II errors. The critical region is delineated.

For Figure 3.13, we examine the distribution of the sample means under the original values of the null hypothesis H_0: $\mu = 28$ versus H_a: $\mu = 30$. However, now the sample size has been increased from 100 subjects to 400 subjects. By studying more patients, the precision of the mean increases.[*] Thus, by increasing the sample size, the variability of the sample mean decreases. Comparing the distribution in this figure to those in Figure 3.8, we see that the width of each of the two sampling distributions in Figure 3.13 is decreased. This concentration of probability in the center of the respective distributions decreases the area of overlap, making it easier to determine which distribution the sample mean is more likely to support.

Thus, the investigator has several means to reduce the influence of sampling error in his research effort. By increasing the distance between the values of the population means of the null and alternative hypotheses and increasing the number of subjects recruited in this research effort, the investigator can reduce the magnitude of the sampling error to any level. However, the investigator is also bound by (1) the expectations and demands of the medical community for a realistic choice of the alternative hypothesis, and (2) the logistics and costs of the additional

---

[*] Remember that the standard deviation of the mean of n observations, $\bar{x}$, $\sigma_{\bar{x}} = \sigma / \sqrt{n}$.

subjects on the other. These two important constraints require the investigator to choose a realistic value for the alternative hypothesis, and keep the sample size down to a practical number.

3.9 Two-Sided Testing

With the paradigm that we have constructed here, the p-value is relatively easy to understand and may be directly computed. The investigator has identified the critical region in which the test statistic falls. He now conducts the research effort as it was designed, collecting his sample of 100 observations. Assume that he observes a sample mean of 29. The researcher computes the test statistic of

$$\frac{(29-28)}{0.550} = 1.82.$$

Applying this calculation to Figure 3.6, we see that the test statistic does fall into the critical region. The p-value is computed based on this data.

Specifically, the p-value is the probability that the population in which the null hypothesis is true has misled the investigator. Specifically it misleads him by producing a result that was at least this extreme. The p-value, like alpha, assesses the sampling error. However, alpha is set in the absence of the data, during the design phase of the research. The p-value actually computes the sampling error rate based on 1) the critical region that was set up *a priori* and 2) the samples data that is now available.

Thus, in this case, the p-value is the probability that a standard normal distribution is at least as large as that observed in the data; this is easily computed to be $P[N(0,1) \geq 1.82] = 0.034$. Note that the p-value is computed based on the application of the test result to the prespecified critical region. This is an important combination to keep in mind as we now consider the critical region for a two-sided test.

Our BMI investigator believed that the mean BMI of males is greater than 28, and set up his test to reject the null hypothesis H_0: $\mu = 28$ for larger values of the mean BMI. He thinks that he has provided adequate protection for the possibility that his prior belief is wrong by allowing the data to demonstrate that the BMI may not be greater than 28. If his suspicion is incorrect, then he will simply not reject the null hypothesis. This is protection from a sampling error, it may not be adequate.

There remains the possibility that the researcher's intuition could be worse than he is willing to consider. Specifically, the distribution of male BMI's could be substantially less than 28. If this were the case, the critical region that he set up is inappropriate. While he can correctly assess sampling error for larger values of the mean male BMI, the investigator is unable to determine the role that sampling error would play when the sample mean BMI is lower than anticipated (Figure 3.14).

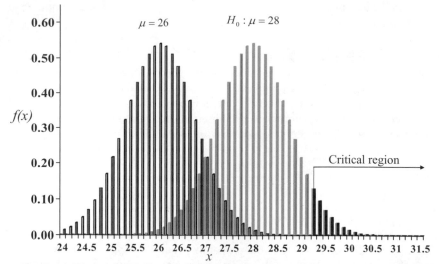

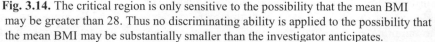

Fig. 3.14. The critical region is only sensitive to the possibility that the mean BMI may be greater than 28. Thus no discriminating ability is applied to the possibility that the mean BMI may be substantially smaller than the investigator anticipates.

Figure 3.14 reveals the potential problem that the investigator has in carrying out a test based on his own belief that the mean male BMI is greater than 28. Setting the location of the critical region only in one tail of the distribution does not permit him prospectively to identify departures from the null hypothesis in the other, lower tail of the distribution. Thus, although the investigator has laid out evaluations of positive excursions from the null hypothesis H_0: $\mu = 28$, he has given no thought at all to negative excursions.

This is understandable, however, because the research effort is based on his impression that the BMI was higher and not lower than 28. Since the researcher is well informed, understands the literature, and is bringing both his and the shared experience of his colleagues to this research effort, this hypothesis seems like an appropriate and defendable course of action. The investigator is of course not naturally prone to explore what his experience and intuition do not support. This is the common rationale for the one-tailed test.

However, this line of approach reveals a weakness; the researcher has foretold the direction of the result, and is using this prediction to sculpt the critical region. However, there are other possibilities that the investigator has not considered, specifically, that the mean male BMI may be substantially smaller than 28. Thus, while the investigator believes that the male BMI's will be larger than that suggested by the H_0, he does not know that result will occur. In the two-tailed test, the researcher provides additional protection for the occurrence of a type I error on the left side of the distribution even though a finding on this lower side of the distribution may be less likely.

Therefore, while the rationale for the one-sided test is understandable, it may also be wrong. Since reasonable deductions in medicine are commonly mistaken, prudent investigators build vigilance for the "reverse finding" into their protocols. Thus, in order to ensure that the investigator appropriately differentiates his belief (in this case, that the mean male BMI is greater than 28) from his knowledge (he actually doesn't know what the mean BMI is), he carries out a two-tailed evaluation (Figure 3.15).

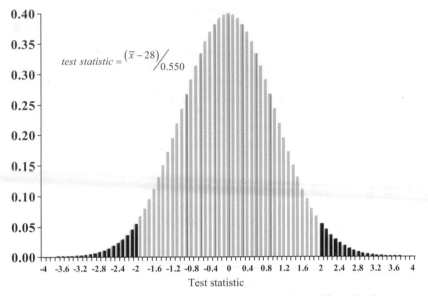

Fig. 3.15. Sampling distribution of the test statistic under the null hypothesis that the mean BMI = 28. The critical region (in black) is divided between the two tails.

The critical region from Figure 3.15 divides the type I error in the two tails of the distribution, leading to rejection of the null hypothesis when the mean male BMI is substantially lower than, as well as substantially larger than the null hypothesis mean value of 28.

The computation of the *p*-value in this setting is slightly more complicated than its calculation in the one tailed scenario. Recall earlier that when the investigator's data revealed a *p*-value of 1.82, he simply computed $P[N(0,1) \geq 1.82] = 0.034$. This was based on the fact that only large, extreme test statistics would fall in the critical region. However, for a two-sided test, test statistics could be more extreme and fall in the right tail of the distribution, or more negative and fall in the left tail of the distribution. The *p*-value must include this more extreme, reverse event as well. Thus, the *p*-value for the two-sided test is

$$P[N(0,1) \geq 1.82 \; or \; \leq -1.82] = P[N(0,1) \leq -1.82] + P[N(0,1) \geq 1.82]$$
$$= 0.034 + 0.034 = 0.068.$$

Thus the *p*-value for the traditional two-sided test is twice that calculated from the one-sided test.

To many investigators, the notion of a two-sided evaluation seems like "a lot of fuss over nothing." Suppose, in a one-sided test that the sample mean BMI was 27, producing a test statistic of $(27-28)/0.550 = -1.82$. Wouldn't this signify that the mean BMI was substantially less than expected, and therefore the null hypothesis should be rejected? One does not, it is argued, need formally to set a critical region to draw the correct reverse conclusion.

However, the absence of a critical region in this setting throws the researcher right into the waiting arms of random research. For his one-sided test, there was no *a priori* decision rule for the interpretation of this small sample mean. Thus, the surprise finding forces the investigator to redraw his critical region based on the unanticipated directionality of their finding. This is the hallmark of random research.

As we have seen, the random research paradigm makes any result difficult to interpret and generalize accurately.[*] In addition, the interpretation of the test statistic is not as clear cut as first anticipated. By dividing the type I error into two regions, the investigator must manage this division while still keeping the overall type I error level at 0.05. This means a contraction of each critical region. If the researcher wishes to divide the type one equally between the two tails, this division places a type I error of 0.025 in each tail, producing critical regions defined as: reject if the test statistic is less than -1.96 or greater than 1.96. In this setting, the investigators finding of a test statistic of -1.82 does not fall into the critical region at all.

By and large, two-sided testing is preferred in healthcare research efforts. Its uses and adaptations are examined in Chapter Eight.

3.10 Sampling Error Containment

A review of the ground that we have covered might be helpful. The occurrence of a type I error is solely a property of the sampling process. Since sampling is necessary for the research effort, the investigator understands that she cannot dismiss this possible explanation of these results. So, rather than try to remove it, an impossible task, she instead calculates the type I error, which is a measure of sampling error's effect on the degree to which the sample's results can be generalized to the population.

The investigator sets the maximum tolerable α error level as well as the largest β error (or alternatively, the minimum power = $1 - β$) at the beginning of the study. Since during the design phase of the study the researcher does not know whether the results will be positive or null, she must plan for each possibility; therefore each of these errors plays a role in the sample size computation.[†]

---

[*] As we will see later, when a research finding that falls in this unanticipated portion of the critical region produces clinical harm, the conclusions are ambiguous. The finding of harm cannot be ignored, but the measurement of the type I error rate is confused since the critical region was set up in a reactive, post hoc fashion.

[†] Sample size computations are discussed in Appendix B.

At the conclusion of the experiment, the investigator computes the *p*-value for the study's result. The *p*-value is the probability that a population in which there is no relationship between the treatment and the disease produces a sample that suggests such a relationship exists. Specifically, the *p*-value is the probability that we do not have a representative sample, i.e., that the sample-based evidence of a relationship is present just through the play of chance. The population misled us by producing an unrepresentative picture of itself. The *p*-value is the probability we have been misled in this fashion. That's all it is.

If the *p*-value is less than the α error rate that was prospectively identified, then researchers conclude that it is very unlikely that chance alone produced the findings of the study, and that the results of the study (be they clinically significant or clinically negligible) are truly reflective of what would occur in the larger population from which the sample was obtained.

Therefore, if (1) the systematic explanations for a spurious research finding are removed from the experiment by exceptional planning and good clinical trial execution, (2) the probability of a false finding just by chance alone is reduced to a small level (i.e., the *p*-value is less than the prospectively set α error rate), and (3) the magnitude of the findings are clinically important, then the medical and regulatory communities are assured that, to a reasonable degree of certainty, the positive results of the trial represent a true population finding.

3.11 Confidence Intervals

As we have seen, statistical inference summarizes a research result with one number. Its final product, the *p*-value, is an assessment of the role of sampling error in producing the research results.

However the point estimate can also be converted into another assessment of the role of sampling error. This second assessment yields not just a single measure and a *p*-value, but a range of estimates providing an understanding of how large an effect on the point estimate is caused by sampling error. The product of this effort is the *confidence interval*. The confidence interval provides an objective measure of the effect of sampling variability on the value of the point estimate itself. Confidence intervals are produced in different widths. The most commonly used confidence interval is the 95% confidence interval. It essentially examines the distribution of the point estimate and identifies that range of values that denote the center 95% area of the curve.

In an example, assume the investigator has computed that the mean BMI from 100 males is 30. Using what we know about the standard deviation, we understand that the estimate $\bar{x} = 30$ itself follows a normal distribution with a mean of 30 and a standard deviation of $5.5/\sqrt{100} = 0.550$. The probability distribution of this sample estimate is easily identified (Figure 3.16).

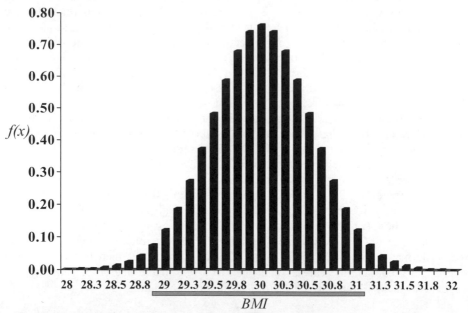

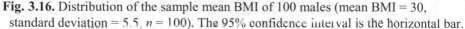

BMI

Fig. 3.16. Distribution of the sample mean BMI of 100 males (mean BMI = 30, standard deviation = 5.5, *n* = 100). The 95% confidence interval is the horizontal bar.

We can compute the 95% confidence interval easily. Since we know

$$P\left[Z_{0.025} \le \frac{30 - \mu}{0.550} \le Z_{0.975}\right] = 0.95.$$

Some algebra produces

$$30 + Z_{0.025}\left(0.550\right) \le \mu \le 30 + Z_{0.975}\left(0.550\right).$$

Remembering that $Z_{0.025} = -1.96$ and $Z_{0.975} = 1.96$, we compute,

$$30 - \left(1.96\right)\left(0.550\right) \le \mu \le 30 + \left(1.96\right)\left(0.550\right)$$
$$28.92 \le \mu \le 31.08.$$

Thus, the 95% confidence interval is for the mean male BMI is [28.92, 31.08]. The common interpretation of this confidence interval is that the user is 95% confident that the male mean BMI is between 28.92 and 31.08. However, the most accurate interpretation is that, if the research was carried out 100 times, each replicate producing a confidence interval, then the true population mean BMI for males would be contained in 95% (or 95) of them. We don't know whether the single confidence

interval contains this true mean value or not, just as, in the significance testing scenario, when the test statistic falls in the critical region, we don't know whether a
type I error has occurred.

Confidence intervals are more revealing about the variability of the estimate. Wide confidence intervals suggests that sampling error alone can generate
large changes in the point estimate, leading us to not be very "confident" about the
point estimate values. Alternatively, narrow confidence intervals suggest that the
point estimate is very precisely located and that other samples, generated from concordantly executed research, will produce a similar point estimate.

Confidence intervals have become quite popular among epidemiologists,
and this popularity has spread to the healthcare research community. Chapter Five
discusses the reason for the surge in their use.

3.12 Hypothesis Testing in Intervention Studies

In our previous BMI example, the researcher was interested in assessing whether
the mean body mass index of males was different then expected. He introduced no
intervention to reduce or otherwise influence the BMI's. He simply measured them,
comparing his results to what was expected. There was no intervention.

Healthcare research commonly involves an intervention. An intervention is
a maneuver that the investigator believes will affect the subjects in a manner worth
studying and reporting. The invention can be something that the investigator has no
control over (e.g. cellular phone use). Alternatively, it can represent a maneuver
that the investigators themselves deliver (e.g. cranial ultrasound therapy). The belief
is that the intervention will make an important difference.

The underlying thesis of intervention studies is simply that subjects treated
differently will differ more than subjects treated the same. Those who receive the
same treatment (be it the intervention or some control therapy) will differ from each
other due to the inherent and natural differences between them. However, a comparison of subjects who receive the intervention with those on control therapy introduces a new element. The natural, individual differences remain. However, there
is a new influence that is due solely to the intervention, and this new variability
element must be simultaneously considered.

Test statistics, constructed to identify and measure these two sources of
variability, are commonly ratios. The denominator is designed to contain and measure the variability of the subjects treated the same. This is the background variability. The numerator contains this variability plus the intervention effect. If this ratio
of these two quantities is large, we conclude that there is more variability among
those treated differently than those who received the same treatment. If the research
effort was well-designed and well executed, we attribute this excess variability to
the intervention. Converting the test statistic to a p-value helps to quantify the sampling error component of the process.

3.13 Community Responsibility

Chapter One outlined the second preeminent responsibility of physician scientists:
community protection. Every intervention has damaging side effects. Sometimes
these side effects are anticipated; other times they are new and surprising. Medica-

tions are prescribed by physicians because these physicians believe that the medicines, in balance, will do more good than harm. If the patients believe this as well, the side effects, with attention and treatment, will be tolerated. However, throughout this decision process, the physician must be assured that the medication is very likely to provide a benefit. Without this assurance, the patient is exposed to "medication" that is void of benefit, producing only side effects. This is the antithesis of "first do no harm," and the patient community requires protection from it.

This point is worthy of emphasis. Ineffective interventions in the medical community are not placebo; they are not harmless. Since medications have adverse effects, some of which can be severe, the physician must be convinced that substantial efficacy will be provided by the compound. The risk-benefit analysis that physicians internalize presumes that there will be benefit. The likelihood of a therapy benefit in the population can be quantified by physician investigators who fully accept their community responsibility.

The need for community protection is as critical as the need for patient protection. Physicians wisely use well established tools for patient protection. Among the first of these are a good history and physical exam. Should therapy be required after the diagnosis, we commonly begin with lower doses, gradually scaling the dose as needed. In addition, we monitor the patient frequently for evidence of side effects. These maneuvers are patient protective.

However, since the most objective view of a therapy's effect is population-based as we saw in the first chapter, we must learn to use tools that are not just patient protective, but provide community protection as well. Specifically, we must become adept at minimizing sample-based errors in the assessment of the likelihood that a therapy will be effective in a population.

The demonstration of efficacy comes from clinical testing in clinical research. Just as physicians must be vigilant against the use of ineffective medications in patients, physician-scientists who design, execute, and analyze research efforts must be especially watchful for the development of a therapy that lacks efficacy in the communities they study. In these research endeavors, adequate protection must be provided for the community in which the drug is to be used. One of the worst situations occurs with the adoption of a therapy for which the occurrence of adverse events is certain, but efficacy is absent. This is the consequence of a type I error. Since the occurrence of a type I error could lead to the wide use of a drug whose efficacy was demonstrated in the sample studied but has no efficacy in the community, the occurrence of a type I error in most cases must be minimized.

However the measure of sampling error has itself become controversial, as we will see in the next chapter.

4

Mistaken Identity: *P*-values in Epidemiology

4.1 Mistaken Identity

On the eve of one of his battle campaigns, the emperor Napoleon took the time to make an unannounced, personal inspection of his army. As he walked from unit to unit during his quiet evening examination, he came across a guard who had fallen asleep at his post. Shaking the dozing soldier awake, the emperor demanded to know his name. The guard replied smartly, "Sir, my name is Napoleon." The enraged emperor replied, "Either change your character or change your name!"

The *p*-value is a foot soldier mistaken for an emperor. It is falsely considered by many to be all that one needs to know about a research study's results. Perhaps this is because incorporated within the *p*-value are many of the measures that everyone agrees are necessary for a balanced interpretation of concordant research programs. The *p*-value's construction explicitly considers and includes sample size, effect size, effect size variability, and sampling error. Each of these components is important in the interpretation of a study. Since the *p*-value encapsulates these, it is easy to see why many could believe that the *p*-value is the sum (and perhaps greater than the sum) of its parts.

This "sum of its parts" philosophy has contributed to the *p*-value's preeminence in research. However, it is fallacious, and epidemiologists, quite vocal in their recognition of this problem of mistaken identity, have worked to topple the *p*-value from its position of dominance.

4.2 Detective Work

Epidemiology is the scientific discipline that applies clear powers of observation and careful deductive reasoning to identify the true nature of the exposure–disease relationship. This determination of whether a relationship is associative on the one hand, or causative, on the other, is a critical distinction that drives public health imperatives, and epidemiologists play a central role in these evaluations.

4.2.1 Association versus Causation

An *associative relationship* between a risk factor and a disease is one in which the two appear in the same patient through mere coincidence. The occurrence of the risk factor does not engender the appearance of the disease.

Causal relationships on the other hand are much stronger. A relationship is *causal* if the presence of the risk factor in an individual generates the disease. The causative risk factor *excites the production* of the disease. This causal relationship is tight, containing an embedded directionality in the relationship i.e., (1) the disease is absence in the patient, (2) the risk factor is introduced, and (3) the risk factor's presence produces the disease.

The declaration that a relationship is causal has a deeper meaning then the mere statement that a risk factor and disease are associated. This deeper meaning and its implications for healthcare require that the demonstration of a causal relationship rise to a higher standard than just the casual observation of the risk factor and disease's joint occurrence.

Often limited by logistics and the constraints imposed by ethical research, the epidemiologist commonly cannot carry out experiments that identify the true nature of the risk factor–disease relationship. They have therefore become experts in observational studies. Through skillful use of observational research methods and logical thought, epidemiologists assess the strength of the links between risk factors and disease.

4.3 Experimental Versus Observational Studies

The hallmark of an experiment is that the investigator controls the intervention, choosing which subjects will be exposed and which go unexposed. This critical research feature allows the investigator to deliver the exposure so that the effects produced by the research can be clearly attributed to the exposure.

We may divide experiments into two categories of experiments; randomized versus nonrandomized experiments. In randomized experiments, the selection of the intervention is not based on any characteristic of the subjects, insuring that the only difference between subjects who receive the intervention and those who do not is the intervention itself. Thus, when a difference in the endpoint measure between intervention groups is identified at the end of the study, that difference can be ascribed or attributed to the intervention.

4.3.1 The Role of Randomization

Randomization is the hallmark of modern experiments. Although its appropriateness in clinical experiments is still debated, it has had a major impact on the development of healthcare since the mid twentieth century.

Generally in clinical experiments, there are two levels of randomization. The first is the random selection of subjects from the population, and the second is the random allocation of the experimental intervention. Each has a different goal and follows a different procedure. It is desirable in clinical studies to utilize the random selection of subjects, and if an intervention is involved, to incorporate the random allocation of this intervention as well.

As we have discussed in Chapter One, the random selection of subjects from the population at large implies that not just every subject in the population has an opportunity to be accepted into the study, but that every subject has the same, constant probability of being selected. This simple random-sampling approach is the best way to ensure that the obtained sample represents the population at large, and that the findings in the sample can be generalized to the population from which the sample was obtained. Whenever random-sampling does not take place, generalizations from the sample to the population at large are often impossible.

In addition, this level of randomization creates in the sample the property of statistical independence, allowing the multiplication of probabilities so useful in the construction of both parameter estimators and test statistics.

4.3.1.2 Random Selection of Subjects from the Population

There is a second level of randomization, however, that is critical in many research efforts. The random allocation of therapy, when present, occurs within the selected sample itself. This procedure ensures that each subject in the sample has the same, constant probability of receiving the intervention, effectively prohibiting any link between the intervention and characteristics of the subjects themselves.

The presence of this level of randomization is crucial for the clearest attribution of effect to the intervention. In an experiment, the investigator wishes to attribute the effect to the intervention he has assigned. If the only difference between patients who received the intervention and those who received a control is the intervention (the percentage of males is the same across groups, the age distribution is the same across groups, the race distribution is the same across groups, etc.), then differences in the outcome measure of the experiment (e.g., mortality) can be ascribed to the intervention.

The absence of the random allocation of therapy in an experiment clouds the attribution of therapy effect. In an extreme case, if all patients who receive the active medication happened to be women and all who receive the control happened to be men, it is impossible to determine if the difference in outcome measure should be attributed to the intervention or to gender.[*] The random allocation of therapy is a design feature that, when embedded in an experiment, leads to the clearest attribution of that therapy's effect.

Large clinical trials attempt to take advantage of both of these levels of randomization. Undoubtedly, the researcher conducting the experiments have little difficulty incorporating the random allocation of the experimental intervention. Proven randomization algorithms are required to be in place at the trial's inception, assuring that every patient who is accepted into the trial must have their treatment randomly allocated. In addition, once researchers randomize patients, examinations of baseline characteristics in each of the randomized groups are thoroughly reviewed, ensuring that demographic characteristics, morbidity characteristics, and results of laboratory assays are distributed equally across the two groups. These procedures and safeguards work to guarantee that the only difference between subjects who receive the intervention and subjects who do not is the intervention itself. The treatment groups are the same with respect to all other characteristics, traits, and measures.

It is difficult to overestimate the importance of the random allocation of the intervention. Use of this tool not only protects the experiment from the influences of factors that are known to influence the outcome, but it also protects

---

[*] We say that the effect of therapy is confounded (or confused) with the effect of sex.

against influences not known to affect the occurrence of the endpoint, again because the random assignment of therapy does not depend on any characteristic of the individuals. When randomization fails to correct for a variable such as age, there are some techniques that can correct the analysis for differences caused by age. However, in randomized experiments, adjusted results will rarely differ markedly from unadjusted results.

However, clinical trials do not select subjects randomly from the population. It is true that large clinical experiments randomize patients from many different clinical centers. These centers represent different regions of a country, different countries on a continent, and sometimes different continents. This widespread recruitment effort is an attempt to be as inclusive as possible, and the investigators hope that it results in an acceptable approximation of this random selection mechanism.

One impediment to the random selection of subjects from the population in these large clinical studies is the use of exclusion criteria. Subjects who are in another study cannot be included, nor can patients who are intolerant of the intervention. Patients who have life-threatening illnesses are often excluded.[*] Subjects who are unlikely to be able to follow the compliance criteria of the experiment (patients who cannot take the intervention consistently or patients who refuse to adhere to a tight schedule of follow-up visits) are often excluded as well. These exclusion criteria are necessary for the successful execution of the trial, but they certainly weaken any argument that the experiment has followed a simple random-sampling plan. Thus, although large clinical trials successfully randomly allocate therapy, they are not so successful in the random selection of subjects from the population.

4.3.2 Observational Studies

Commonly the relationship between an exposure and the disease cannot be elucidated by an experiment. For example it is not feasible randomly to allocate subjects to either use cell phones and others to avoid them in order to determine if there is a causal relationship between these devises and brain cancer.[†] In these circumstances, the research must be observational. In *observational studies*, the investigators do not control the exposure. Instead, they observe the exposure–disease relationship already embedded in the population.[‡]

Observational studies are sometimes termed "epidemiologic studies." This is somewhat of a misnomer, since the interpretation of all research programs in healthcare (be they experiments or not) invoke epidemiologic princi-

---

[*] An unfortunate patient who has terminal pancreatic cancer with less than one year to live is unlikely to be randomized to a five-year trial assessing the role of cholesterol reduction therapy in reducing the number of heart attacks, even if he has met all other criteria for the trial.

[†] Subjects would find it difficult to avoid cell phone use in a society where these tools are so popular and convenient. Also, those who would be able to avoid their use would still be exposed to the electromagnetic radiation of people nearby who used these phones. Additionally, it is unethical deliberately to expose subjects to interventions when there is *prima facie* evidence suggesting that they will suffer harm that exceeds any benefit of the intervention.

[‡] As Yogi Berra said, "You can observe a lot just by watching." Taken from James N. Hyde's Tuft's University openware course entitled, "Epidemiology and Biostatistics 2004–2005."

ples. Nonrandomized, observational studies can sometimes do a better job than their counterpart clinical trials in randomly selecting subjects from the population. Although these observational studies are rarely able randomly to allocate exposure in their attempt to assess the relationship between exposure and disease, they nevertheless play a critical role in the development of public health.

Observational studies are often (but not always) less expensive and administratively easier than their randomized trial counterparts. However, they require great skill if the investigators are to draw the correct conclusions from them. The expert epidemiologist first selects the population in which the exposure–disease relationship exists. She knows that there are other relationships in the population as well (e.g., the effects of demographics, family history of disease, socioeconomic influences). These ancillary, confusing (or confounding) effects can generate biases, making it difficult to observe the direct effect of the exposure of interest. However, using a panoply of well-established research tools, the epidemiologist works to separate these other perturbing effects from the relationship of interest.

It is useful to think of epidemiologists as good detectives who get only the toughest cases to solve. Many important studies and landmark research efforts (e.g. the Framingham analyses) are observational. These studies have been, and will continue to be, critical. What is the relationship between the heavy metal content of tooth fillings and the occurrence of disease in later life? What is the relationship between silicone breast implants and autoimmune disorders? The relationship between magnetic field exposure and cancer in children? The relationship between prescription diet pills and valvular heart disease?

Unfortunately, in each of these circumstances, although it can be easier to select candidates randomly from the population at large, it is impossible to randomly allocate the exposure among subjects in the sample. Nevertheless, the answers to the exposure–disease relationship in each of these studies are critical. By and large, public health has advanced on the results of nonrandomized studies and the epidemiologists who design, execute, and analyze them. However, the inability to randomize exposure sharply circumscribes the conclusions drawn from these research tools.

It is useful to differentiate betweeen random and nonrandom observational studies. The term *random* here refers to selection of the control group. For example, in a study assessing the role of smoking and breast cancer, cases are identified from a hospital's cancer center. It is convenient to choose controls as nonsmokers who are also hospitalized. However, this inpatient control group can confuse the effect of smoking with the influence of being hospitalized. An alternative control group would be a random one, selecting its members at random from the community which the hospital serves. The criteria for inclusion in this control group is that subjects not have breast cancer and that they resemble the demographics of the cases.

4.4 Determining Causation

Just as justice is more than simply reciting from a book of laws, the determination that a risk factor–disease relationship is causal requires more than the blind application of artificial rules. Risk factor–disease relationships are unique and each require specific attention. For example, there are circumstances in which a strong risk factor–disease relationship first reported as suggestive of causation was subsequently shown to be non-causative and coincidental e.g., the relationship between coffee ingestion and pancreatic cancer. On the other hand, there are clear examples of risk factor–disease relationships identified by a single examination of a series of cases that are clearly causative.

The most important lesson one can take from this is that the determination of causality requires clear appreciation for the research methodology and careful consideration of the role of systematic biases and sampling error.

4.4.1 Causality Tenets

The fact that case reports are so useful in demonstrating the cause of a disease begs the question, What are the properties of a causal relationship?

In 1965, the epidemiologist Bradford Hill [1] described the nine criteria for causality arguments in healthcare. These nine rules or tenets are remarkably and refreshingly devoid of complex mathematical arguments, relying instead on natural intuition and common sense for the inquiry into the true nature of a risk factor–disease relationship. For example it is useful to identify the strength of the link between the exposure and the disease. Two questions that address this are, "Have there been more cases of the disease when the risk factor is present, and fewer disease cases when the risk factor is absent?" and Does a greater dose or duration of exposure produce a greater extent of disease?

Other questions asked by Hill explore the "believability" of the relationship. Some of these are; Is there a discernible mechanism by which the risk factor produces the disease? Have other researchers also shown this relationship? Are there other such relationships whose demonstration helps us to understand the current risk factor– disease relationship?

The nine Hill criteria are: (1) strength of association, (2) temporality, (3) biologic gradient, (4) biologic plausibility, (5) consistency, (6) coherency, (7) specificity, (8) experimental evidence, and (9) analogy.

> **1. Strength of association:** This tenet requires that a greater percentage of patients exposed to the risk factor develop the disease than those unexposed. This is commonly addressed by epidemiological studies that produce relative risks or odds ratios. The odds ratio is in general easy to compute. For example, if there are 30 patients exposed to an industrial solvent and cancer is subsequently seen in 5 of them, then the probability of cancer is $5/30 = 0.167$. The probability of no cancer is $1 - 0.167 = 0.833$. The odds of cancer is simply $0.167/0.833 = 0.200$. If there were 300 individuals unexposed to the solvent and seven had subsequent cancer, the odds are $(7/300)/(293/300) = 0.0239$. The odds ratio is simply the ratio of these odds, or $0.200/0.024 = 8.33$. Odds ratios can range from zero to infinity.[*] An odds ratio of one signifies that the odds of disease are the same in the exposed and unexposed groups, and there is no association between exposure and disease. The larger the odds ratio, the greater the strength of this association.

---

[*] Infinity is produced when all of the cases occur in the exposed patients and the unexposed patients are disease-free.

2. Temporal relationship: The directionality of causality requires that, if the exposure is to cause the disease, then it must be present before the disease. This is the proper temporal relationship that must be present in order to demonstrate causation convincingly. *Protopathic bias* (drawing a conclusion about causation when the disease process precedes the risk factor in occurrence) can result without appropriate attention to the research design. An evaluation of the relationship between seronin reuptake inhibitors (SSRI) and valular heart disease may demonstrate that these agents are associated with VHD. However, it is quite possible that the VHD was present (either congenitally or rheumatic in origin) well before the SSRI was implemented. Thus, a clearer assessment of the medication exposure-valular heart disease relationship requires that patients be screened for pre-exisiting VHD before they enter the study and those with a positive history be removed.

3. Biologic gradient (dose response): This assumes that the more intense the exposure, the greater the risk of disease. This intensity can be measured by dose, or by duration of exposure. Statistical measures can be of use here.

4. Biologic plausibility: There should be some basis in the underlying mechanism of disease production that supports an understanding of the relationship between the supposed "cause" and the effect. However, observations have been made in epidemiologic studies that were not considered biologically plausible at the time but subsequently were shown to be correct. An example is the relationship between rubella in the child's mother and subsequent birth defects in the child.

5. Consistency with other knowledge: Consistency requires that the findings of one study be replicated in other studies. Since research findings become more convincing when they are replicated in different populations and using different research methods and designs, different studies that examine the same exposure–disease relationship and find similar results add to the weight of the causal inference.

6. Biologic coherence: This implies that a cause–and–effect interpretation for an association does not conflict with what is known of the natural history and biology of the disease. Related to plausibility, this criteria focuses on the absence of a contradiction. For example, the observation that aspirin use does not prevent myocardial infarctions in patients born under Libra or Gemini is biologically incoherent.

7. Specificity: The specificity of a disease is directly related to the number of known causes of the disease. The greater the number of causes of a disease, the more nonspecific the disease is, and the more difficult it is to demonstrate a new causal agent is involved in the production of the disease. The presence of specificity is considered supportive but not necessary, and epidemiologists no longer require that the effect of exposure to an agent such as a drug be specific for a single disease. However, the more specific the disease, the more useful is the persuasive power of a case scries.

8. Experimental evidence: This includes in vitro studies, laboratory experiments on animals as well as human experiments. Experimental evidence also includes the results of the removal of a harmful exposure. These are termed *challenge–dechallenge–rechallenge experiments*

9. Analogy: This would include a similarity to some other known cause–effect association. For example, the relationship between thalidomide use and phecomelia is more clearly understood in the presence of the analogous example of rubella and congenital birth defects. The early demonstration of how a fetus's development could be influenced by the mother's exposure to a virus helped scientist to understand how the ingestion of thalidomide could have its damaging effects on the unborn child.

There are two noteworthy observations we may make in understanding how these criteria are applied. The first is that the firm establishment of a causal relationship does not require that all nine tenets be satisfied. Hill himself stated:

> None of my nine viewpoints can bring indisputable evidence for or against the cause–and–effect hypothesis, and none can be required as a *sine qua non*.

The second observation is that Hill did not require that any of his nine criteria be buttressed by statistical significance. There is not a single mention of *p*-values in his nine criteria.

4.5 Clinical Significance Without *P*-Values
Has there been an epidemiologic study that assessed causality in the absence of multiple studies with minimal reliance on *p*-values? Yes.

4.5.1 Thalidomide
The drug thalidomide has a long FDA history [2]. Thalidomide was hailed as a "wonder drug" that provided a "safe, sound sleep." It was a sedative that was found to be effective when given to pregnant women to combat many of the symptoms associated with morning sickness. No one suspected that the drug, whose name became synonymous with terrible adverse effects would cross over from the bloodstream of the mother to that of the unborn baby until it was too late.

Thalidomide was synthesized in West Germany in 1954 by Chemie Grünenthal and introduced to the market in the 1950s. It was approved in Europe in 1957, and marketed from 1958 to 1962, in approximately forty-six countries under many different brand names. A US marketing application for marketing thalidomide was reviewed by the F.D.A. for the United States in 1960 but was not approved because of concerns about peripheral neuropathy associated its use. While the agency was awaiting answers to these concerns, the link between thalidomide use and an epidemic of congenital malformations occurring in Europe exploded, and attributed to thalidomide in letters to the editor authored by Lenz and McBride [3].

When taken in the first trimester of pregnancy, thalidomide prevented the proper growth of the fetus, resulting in disfiguring birth defects and neonatal deaths. Any part of the fetus that was in development at the time of thalidomide ingestion could be affected. For those babies who survived, birth defects included deafness, blindness, disfigurement, cleft palate, many major internal disabilities, and the most common feature — phecomelia (shortening or absence of limbs). In addition, a percentage of the mothers who ingested thalidomide experienced peripheral neuritis.

The drug was withdrawn from the international market, and the tragedy played a part in the debate around the 1962 amendments to the Federal Food, Drug, and Cosmetic Act that resulted in specific effectiveness requirements for drugs.

The numbers vary from source to source, but it has been claimed that there were between 10,000 and 20,000 babies born disabled as a consequence of the drug thalidomide. Two thirds of those victims born alive are now dead. An English report suggests that adult survivors of thalidomide exposure have a greater incidence of children with birth defects of the limbs [6]. The extremely low prevalence of the conditions (particularly phecomelia) in the general population compounded with the marked rise in prevalence after exposure, obviates the need for multiple studies with accompanying p-values to infer causality.

4.5.2 The Radium Girls

"The doctors tell me I will die, but I mustn't. I have too much to live for—a husband who loves me and two children I adore. They say nothing can save me, nothing but a miracle." Ottawa native Catherine Donohue wrote those words and more from her bed to the Our Lady of Sorrows Roman Catholic Church in Chicago in the mid-1930s. She asked for a novena to bring her a miracle. She had to write the words, for she could not speak them. Her teeth and a large portion of her jawbone were gone. Cancer was eating away at her bone marrow. The doomed young mother weighed only 65 pounds [4].

Ms. Donohue was a charter member of The Society of the Living Dead, so called because its members had two things in common: all worked at the Radium Dial Company in Ottawa, Illinois, and all eventually suffered an agonizing death from radium poisoning.

Luminescent numbers on wristwatches designed for soldiers involved in the trench warfare of World War I became a consumer fad in the 1920s. Attracted by easy work and high wages, young women, mostly young and unmarried, were employed to paint the dials of watches with self-illuminating paint containing the relatively new element radium.

Besides the promise of decent work for decent pay, Clark writes, part of what must have made dial painting an attractive job was working with such a sensational product, glow-in-the-dark paint. The young workers were excited about their jobs. They were told that they would be working with products that would "put a glow in [their] cheeks." Assured that the radium-laced compound was completely safe, even digestible, they painted their clothing, fingernails, and even their teeth, "for a smile that glowed in the dark." When they went home from work, they thrilled their families and friends with glowing clothes, fingers, and hair.

Unfortunately, they were involved in a lethal activity. Dial painters were instructed in the technique of "lip pointing" to perform their finely detailed work. Mixing the dry, luminous paint powder with paste and thinner, the workers drew their small brush to a point with their lips before dipping it in the paint, and then meticulously filled in the numbers or other marks on clock faces or other equipment before repeating the process. The greatest exposure to radium was in the mouth and jaws, and 30 women contracted bone cancer.

Here again *p*-values played no role in the assignment of causation. When the finding of exposure is specific enough and the disease is extremely rare causality is easily established with careful observation and deductive reasoning.

This is not to say that statistical inference should be avoided. However, in some circumstances, the specificity of the disease, and the relationship between the occurrence of the disease and a new exposure, can call for a *p*-value-less conclusion. Waiting for an additional study before one puts the final nail in the causality argument is sometimes a luxury that the medical community cannot afford. Such is the nature of the mathematics–ethics tension in medical research.

While this is in general true, the historical examples of thalidomide exposure and birth defects, or toxic fish exposure and mercury poisoning, demonstrate that, in selected instances, complicated mathematics are not necessary to provide clear evidence of a relationship between exposure and disease.

4.6 Tools of the Epidemiologist

Practicing epidemiologists have many tools at their disposal as they attempt to illuminate the true nature of the exposure–disease relationship. Several of these are briefly discussed below.

4.6.1 Case Reports and Case Series

A case report is simply a summary of the findings of an exposure–disease combination in a single patient and the communication of those findings to the medical community. Many times that communication contains insufficient information. In other circumstances, the data from this report can be voluminous and complex. This material can consist of a complete medical history comprising all symptoms and signs the patient had experienced, in addition to information both about the patient's treatment and their ultimate disposition. A case series is a collection of case reports, linked together by a common thread (e.g., all of the patients were seen by the same doctor, or all patients were exposed to the same agent (e.g., cyclo-oxygenase [Cox-2] inhibitor therapy).

Case reports are somewhat paradoxical at the current stage of medical research and practice. Although the findings from case reports are commonly criticized by researchers, who utilize sophisticated mathematics and design methodology to examine exposure–disease relationships, carefully compiled case reports provide necessary observations from which clinicians and public health workers learn. Case reports remain the first data-based view of either a new disease or a potential cure for an established disease. Despite substantial criticism, it is undeniable that case reports and case series are among the most time-tested and useful tools epidemiologists have at their disposal to alert clinicians and the public to a possible health problem. For over 2000 years, the growth of medical knowledge has been fueled by the use and dissemination of case reports.

Like fire, when used constructively, case reports are the fuel that has historically propelled medical progress. A good case report is based on careful observation. It wasn't until the nineteenth and twentieth centuries, after 1800 years of the evolution of case reports, that modern statistical and epidemiological tools evolved to the point of providing a new, more useful perspective to healthcare research. However, even after the advent of these case control studies, new diseases, appearing in unusual settings, were successfully identified and their cause established using the method of case reporting. Examples of the more spectacular uses of case report methods to establish the cause of disease would be—

(1)   An outbreak of a very rare form of bone cancer in young women watch-dial painters in the Chicago area in the 1930s. It was established that radium used to paint the watch dial was the cause [4].

(2)   From the 1930s to the 1960s, a chemical company dumped tons of mercury into Mina Mata Bay in Japan. Thousands of people living around the bay developed methyl mercury poisoning through the consumption of contaminated fish. The victims suffered from severe neurological damage, that later became known as Mina Mata Disease. Symptoms of this disorder include tingling sensations, muscle weakness, unsteady gait, tunnel vision, slurred speech, hearing loss, and abnormal behavior such as sudden fits of laughter. The establishment that toxic fish ingestion was the cause of mercury poisoning in the Japanese fishing village of Mina Mata in the 1950s was established through the scientific examination of case reports [5].

(3)   The use of case reports in establishing the cause of a disease was the findings of Lenz [6] that thalidomide ingestion by pregnant women causes the birth defects phecomelia and achondroplasia.

(4)   The demonstration that the acute, debilitating pneumonia inflicting a collection of veterans attending an American Legion convention in Philadelphia, Pennsylvania in 1976 was due to a heretofore unknown bacterium, *Legionella pneumophila*. Although clinical trial methodology was well accepted as a research tool at this time, case report methodology accomplished the identification of the cause and cure of this disease.

(5)   The identification of the relationship between tick bites and Lyme disease. There are over 16,000 cases per year of Lyme disease, but its cause went unrecognized until the 1990s.

Case reports in combination with careful observation and deductive reasoning to this day continue to provide important insight into the cause of disease. A major reason they continue to be essential in the presence of more sophisticated research techniques is because at their root, well-documented case reports use the best skills of epidemiology and clinical medicine—skilled observation and careful deductive reasoning. In each of these circumstances, the use of case reports successively and accurately warned the medical community of an exposure that caused a debilitating disease or a birth defect. Even though modern epidemiological models were available, these advanced tools were unnecessary for a clear view of the exposure–disease relationships in the aforementioned circumstances. The argument that sophisticated epidemiological studies are always required to build a causal argument for disease is defeated by these forceful examples from history.

However, case reports must be reviewed critically. In general, there are three main categories of criticisms of case reports. The first is that case reports and case series do not provide quantitative measures of the relationship between an exposure and a disease.[*]

A second criticism of case reports is that they do not rule out other, competing causes of disease. The implication of this criticism is that case reports, because they reflect a finding in one individual, cannot possibly be known to have its implications extended to a larger population. One cannot deny that the best minds in cardiology, epidemiology, and biostatistics believe that large, clinical trials, despite the burden they place on healthcare resources, are required to evaluate the relationship between elevated cholesterol levels and myocardial infarctions. Why aren't case reports sufficient for a causality argument in this setting?

In fact, case reports lose their utility when the disease has many causes. We call a disease cause-specific if it has one cause, and cause-nonspecific (or just nonspecific) if it has multiple causes. Examples of cause-specific diseases are (1) the occurrence of fetal phecomelia with maternal thalidomide ingestion, (2) malignant pleural mesothelioma and asbestos exposure, and, (3) cinchonism that is unique to quinine exposure. In these circumstances, the identification of a disease that occurs only with the exposure defines the optimum utility of case reports. On the other hand, diseases such as atherosclerotic cardiovascular diseases have multiple contributing factors (genetics, obesity, cigarette smoking, diabetes, elevated lipid levels, and hypertension) requiring different data than that supplied in case reports to identify a new causative agent.

However, although it is clear that when a disease has many causes it can be difficult if not impossible to identify which cause was precisely the cause that excited the production of a disease in a given patient, one can often exclude other causes if there are only a few of them. Consider acute liver failure in the presence of diabetes. Acute liver failure does not occur as a well-known consequence of diabetes. If the common causes of acute liver failure can be removed as possibilities, the way is then open for establishing a new cause for the malady.

4.6.1.1 Do Case Reports Prove Causality?

A third and final criticism of case reports is the implication that by their very nature, case reports are unscientific. Consider the following quote from the Texas Supreme Court:

---

[*] While this is in general true, the historical examples of thalidomide exposure and birth defects, or toxic fish exposure and mercury poisoning, demonstrate that, in selected instances, complicated mathematics are not necessary to provide clear evidence of a relationship between exposure and disease.

The FDA has promulgated regulations that detail the requirements for clinical investigations of the safety and effectiveness of drugs. 21 C.F.R. §314.126 (1996). These regulations state that "isolated case reports, random experience, and reports lacking the details that permit scientific evaluation will not be considered." Id. §314.126(e). Courts should likewise reject such evidence because it is not scientifically reliable.

This has led to the unfortunate interpretation that all case reports are not scientifically reliable. In fact, when case reports are isolated, random, and lacking in scientific detail, they make no useful contribution to our fund of knowledge about the risk factor–disease relationship. However, case reports can be clustered, specific, and provide great attention to detail, thereby imparting useful information about the relationship between a risk factor and a disease. A fine example of such a case report is that of Monahan [7], who provided a clear measurement of the effect of the two drugs, Seldane and Ketoconazole, and the occurrence of dangerous heart rhythms. This case report was obtained in scientifically controlled conditions, clarifying the mechanism by which the Seldane–Ketoconazole relationship could cause sudden death.

Yet another example of the value of a case series was the identification of 24 patients in the upper Midwest United States by Heidi Connolly who had both exposure to the diet drug fenfluramine (fenphen) and heart value damage [8]. These case reports were not isolated but clustered.* Important detail was provided concerning the patients' medical history and exposure to the drugs. The patients underwent special studies of their hearts (echocardiography). In five cases, the heart valves themselves were recovered after the patients had undergone surgery and these heart valves were examined in a methodological, objective fashion. There was nothing unscientific about the evaluation of the patients in the Connolly case series. Although this study was followed by epidemiological studies, the findings of Connolly et al. and their implication that heart valve damage is caused by the fenfluramines have not been debunked.

Yet another example of the contribution of a scientific case control study was that of Douglas et al. [9], who demonstrated, again, under controlled, scientific settings, that the diet drug fenfluramine would consistently increase blood pressure in the pulmonary circulation of patients. This suggested that fenfluramine could be the cause of primary pulmonary hypertension. This study was followed by the case series of Brenot [10]. Although some have argued that this was not sufficient evidence for causality, the large epidemiological study that followed [11] validated the associations identified by the case report of Douglas or the case series of Brenot.

It is important to note that case reports have added value when they appear in the peer-reviewed literature. This is a sign that the study's methodology is consistent with the standard research procedures accepted by the scientific community. These articles must be given a greater priority than publications in non-peer-reviewed journals. Peer-reviewed journals also are superior to abstracts, which are themselves only brief, preliminary reports of non-peer-reviewed work.

---

* Examples of important information provided by clustered case reports are those of Lyme disease and of the illness caused by the Hanta virus.

The clear message from advances in scientific methodology is that good practice can produce useful results regardless of the methodology employed. While it is true that case reports, when shoddily documented or slovenly interpreted, will produce little of value, the criticisms are not specifically crafted for case reports but applicable as well to large epidemiological studies and placebo-controlled randomized clinical trials. Each of these scientific tools of investigation must be wielded carefully to be effective.

The utility of case reports and case series has taken on a new sense of urgency in the healthcare issues of today. Case reports are critical in quickly identifying the causes of disease. Today, citizens of New York City and the surrounding environs are not asked to await the results of a large-scale controlled clinical trial to provide conclusive evidence that the constellation of symptoms known as West Nile fever is caused by the West Nile virus, itself spread by a mosquito. The utilization of modern molecular techniques in concert with case-reporting systems identified the link between the mosquito and the outbreak of disease in the northeastern United States. In Texas, the scientific community has not been required to wait for an epidemiological study to determine if the annual appearance of fever, malaise, convulsions, and coma are due to St. Louis encephalitis virus, spread by the mosquito. Careful, patient work by epidemiologists has correctly obviated a requirement for large epidemiological trials in these critical public health areas.

4.6.2 Categories of Observational Studies

We have seen the criteria used to determine the presence of a cause–effect relationship. In order to demonstrate these tenets, epidemiologists have embedded structure into observational research design to demonstrate these tenets while maintaining the ability to efficiently work with data in several constructs. The result has been a collection of different research designs, each with the ability to satisfy some of the nine Bradford Hill causality tenets. An assessment of the strength of a causal argument comes from as evaluation of the entire body of knowledge, often times consisting of several observational studies of different designs. The job of the reviewer is to synthesize the total research effort, determining which of the causality tenets each of the research studies has satisfied.

Over the course of scientific research, several alternative nonrandomized investigative designs have evolved. It is useful to consider the nomenclature and the distinguishing features of these designs, keeping the focus on the correct interpretation of *p* values. As long as the *p*-value is relegated to a statement concerning sampling error, it is relevant in epidemiologic studies.

4.6.2.1 Directionality: Forward or Backward?

Directionality refers to the type of inference between the risk factor and disease in a research program's effort and determines the condition of the relationship between the risk factor and the disease. The program can either have a forward inference (risk factor presence implies disease prevalence) or a backward inference (disease status implies exposure). The concept of directionality is separate from the retrospective versus prospective concept that we will briefly describe momentarily.

To demonstrate the directionality characteristic in clinical research, let's consider two observational study designs evaluating the relationships between coffee ingestion and pancreatic cancer. The first investigator identifies patients with pancreatic cancer (cases), say, in a registry or in a review of hospital records. He then identifies patients who do not have pancreatic cancer (controls), derived from the same population as his cases. After this determination of cases and controls, the researcher looks into the history of these patients to determine their coffee ingestion history. The investigator then identifies the proportion of the cases who had exposure to coffee, and computes the proportion of the controls who had coffee exposure. The research question asked here is, given that a patient has pancreatic cancer, how much more likely is the patient to have ingested coffee? This is a backward inference, moving from case identification back through time to prior coffee exposure.

The second investigator starts by collecting not cases based on the presence of cancer, but cancer-free individuals who drink coffee. She identifies patients from the same population who do not ingest coffee, then follows her exposed and unexposed group forward through time, determining the incidence of pancreatic cancer. This would be a forward study, since first the exposure's presence is assessed, and then, for patients with the exposure and those without, the occurrence of the endpoint is measured. The research question is, How much more likely is pancreatic cancer in those who drink coffee than in those who do not? This is a forward inference and can be easier for the non-epidemiologist to understand.

Both of these designs address the coffee ingestion–pancreatic cancer issue, but from different directions. The first (backward approach) moves from the case identification to the exposure. This is commonly known as a *case-control study*. The second (forward approach) begins with the exposure and moves to identify disease. This is called a *prospective cohort* study, since the cohort or group of patients entered into the study is identified prospectively before the endpoint has occurred and followed forward in time. Determining the criteria on which the cohort is assembled is the hallmark of directionality. If identified by exposure status, the design is forward; if identified by case status, the design is backward. Alternatively, a study that examines a cohort of patients at a single point in time, assessing for each patient both a history of coffee ingestion and the presence of pancreatic cancer, is known as a *cross-sectional study*. Cross sectional studies are neither forward nor backward.

Typically, when the case prevalence is rare, forward direction studies will require many more patients than backward studies, since the forward study must identify a large number of exposed and unexposed patients to collect an adequate number of cases. For the backward study, since the cohort is selected first based on cases, attention is focused on first identifying an adequate number of cases matching them to controls, and ascertaining exposure on this relatively small cohort.

4.6.2.2 Retrospective Versus Prospective

Timing can be retrospective, or prospective. Unlike directionality which addresses the characteristic on which the cohort was chosen, timing addresses whether the information was collected in the past or will be collected in the future. When did the risk factor and disease onset occur? If these occurred before the research was undertaken, and we must gather this information reflecting only past events, our research is completely retrospective. If the exposure ascertainment will occur in the future, and the disease onset occurs in the future, we have a completely prospective design.

In a retrospective study, the researcher uses information that has been collected from the patient in the past. Thus, the investigator is compelled to review records about the patients' past experiences. The investigator identifies the information about exposure from subject recall, previous medical records, and even from autopsy and postmortem toxicology information. To identify disease status, he again identifies the past occurrence of disease and is totally dependent on what information was available in the past. Thus, in retrospective studies, the design is held captive by the abundance or dearth of this historical data.

Prospective designs allow the researcher more flexibility. Not being limited to past information, the researchers can tailor the collection process to the research program, fortifying the ability of their effort to identify the risk factor–disease relationship. In a prospective design, the researcher has the opportunity to collect the information about the patient's current condition directly from the patient with little reliance on recall. The investigator can choose the level of information detail, rather than settling for what is available in a retrospective research program. Thus, in a prospective program the data can be collected to address more subtle issues in the exposure– disease relationship, often making the research program more convincing. For example, the researcher can choose to measure different levels of exposure that would allow an examination of the dose-response relationship in the research program. Also, if randomization of exposure cannot be implemented, the researcher can collect information that is known to be correlated with either exposure or case prevalence, allowing a more convincing covariate-adjusted analysis.[*]

4.6.2.3 Case Control Studies

Subjects are identified as having an event (e.g., a stroke). Patients who do not have the event (controls) are then chosen. The history of each case and control subject is then searched to determine if the patient has the risk factor (e.g., hypertension). In a sense, the passage of time is backward, i.e., first identify cases and controls, then go back to see if the patient had the risk factor. For these reasons, classic case control studies have a backward directionality. The investigator hopes to show that patients with stroke are more likely to have hypertension than are patients without stroke, i.e., hypertension is more prevalent in stroke patients. However, this is not equivalent to demonstrating that patients with hypertension are more likely to have a stroke than are patients without hypertension.

4.6.2.4 Cross-Sectional Studies

In these studies, both exposure and disease status are measured simultaneously. Thus, these research programs are non-directional; they involve no passage of time. However, since this design provides no sense of time, the timing criteria of the tenets of causality cannot be assessed. For example, a cross-sectional study can identify the prevalence of cardiac arrhythmias in patients on antiarrhythmic

---

[*] This will be discussed in Chapter Eleven.

agents, but it cannot determine if those agents change the occurrence of these heart rhythms.

4.6.2.5 Prospective Cohort Studies

These studies can be very persuasive, since they first identify the risk factor, then follow the patients forward (prospectively) to determine if the endpoints (e.g., heart attacks) occur. However, they are not experimental since the investigator does not assign the risk factor, and therefore the attribution of effect can be problematic. Consider a research program designed to measure the relationship between homocysteine levels and the occurrence of heart attacks. Researchers measure patients' homocysteine levels and then follow them for three years to assess the incidence rate of myocardial infarction (heart attack). It is possible to link the incidence of myocardial infarction to the presence of levels of homocysteine. However, since there may be many of the differences between patients with low and high homocysteine levels that may not be known and therefore cannot be adjusted for, this study cannot successfully attribute differences in myocardial infarction to differences in homocysteine levels.

4.6.2.5 Historical Cohort Studies

The historical cohort study is an example of a retrospective, forward-directional design. It is related to a prospective cohort study, but it is "run in the past." For example, in the homocysteine level–heart attack study described as a prospective, cohort study, the investigators observe homocysteine levels now, then follow patients into the future to determine which of them sustain heart attacks. Suppose instead that this study was carried out in an established, complete database. The investigator first looks back into the early segment of the database to determine each patient's homocysteine level, and then looks forward in the database to determine the occurrence of heart attacks. This is like a cohort study embedded in retrospectively collected data. Since it is retrospective, it contains the additional problem of being unable to correct for differences in the groups not already measured and available in the database.

4.6.3 Variable Adjustments

We have pointed out that, in observational studies, there is no random allocation of exposure, with consequent difficulty in effect attribution. Regression analysis is sometimes used to correct observational studies by adjusting for differences between the exposed and unexposed groups.[*]

Many persuasively argue that this adjustment is more important in observational studies, since in these studies there is no random allocation of the risk factor of interest, and that there are differences between exposed and unexposed patients that confound our ability to ascribe an effect to the risk factor of interest. These adjustments may go a long way in reducing the problem with effect attribution in observational studies. By reducing the influence of known confounders on the exposure–disease relationship, the attribution of effect becomes clearer.

In general, adjustments are not as useful in randomized studies. Nor can *post hoc* adjustment be accepted as an adequate substitute for randomization.

---

[*] Regression analysis and *p*-value interpretation are discussed in Chapter Eleven.

One can correct an observational study for the effect of age using regression analysis, but that correction does not remove all of the imbalances between the risk factor and non- risk factor groups. In fact, an investigator can correct for all known differences between the risk factor and non-risk-factor groups through the use of regression analysis. However, because the investigator can correct only for known risk factors (assuming he has the values of these risk factors in the dataset) and unknown factors may be determining the differences between the two groups, he will never fully get the exposed groups and unexposed groups statistically equivalent. In the random design, however, the use of the random allocation assures the investigator of equivalence between the intervention and nonintervention groups.* Adjusted analyses are very useful, but cannot replace the random allocation of exposure.

The use of the procedure of adjustments through regression analysis can help to clarify the attribution of effect. However, the light shed by the *p*-value remains the same. It illuminates only sampling error. Even in adjusted analyses, *p* values must be interpreted jointly with sample size, effect size, and effect size variability.

4.7 Fenfluramines

The utility of modern observational studies is illustrated by the diet drug fenfluramine.[†] The chronologic examination of the relationship between exposure to the fenfluramines and primary pulmonary hypertension (PPH) is a fine example of the evolution of scientific thought from observation to hypothesis generation to hypothesis confirmation.

Primary pulmonary hypertension is serious disorder in which the pulmonary vascular tree, normally a low-pressure environment, is exposed to sustained high pressures in the pulmonary arterioles. PPH is progressive, commonly producing death within a few years of diagnosis. The background rate of PPH is approximately 1 – 2 patients per million per year.

The fenfluramines were approved in the United States as appetite suppressants in 1972. Widely used worldwide, their use in the US exploded in the 1990s when fenfluramine was combined with phentermine, producing the popular "fenphen" craze.

From 1968 to 1972, a sudden rise in the incidence of PPH was observed among pulmonologists and epidemiologists in Austria, Germany and Switzerland. Careful examination of these cases revealed that the common link among the patients was use of the new drug aminorex, an amphetamine derivative that had become popular as a weight loss aid. The epidemic first appeared several months after aminorex was introduced in these three countries. Once the PPH cases were linked to the diet drug and aminorex was removed from the European market, and the PPH epidemic abated shortly thereafter [12].

These reports were followed by observations describing PPH in young women taking fenfluramine for weight reduction [13]. With the increased consumption of dexfenfluramine (a derivative of the original fenfluramine molecule) in Europe, case reports also appeared linking it to PPH as well [14,15,16].

---

* The use of randomization may fail for an isolated variable, but once the adjustment is made using regression analysis, the groups are equivalent since the randomization procedure all but assures equivalence on all other risk factors.
[†] The author is a paid expert for plaintifs in the fenfluramine litigation.

In 1993, Brenot and coworkers in 1993 [10] provided the first retrospective analysis that linked PPH with fenfluramine use. These researchers showed that 20% of their patients with PPH had taken fenfluramine; these patients' survival times were as poor as those who have PPH without exposure to these drugs.

Finally, prospectively designed research effort was executed to assess the relationship between the fenfluramines and PPH. The International Primary Pulmonary Hypertension Study's (IPPHS) [11], carried out in Europe, was a case-control study. This study included 95 patients with PPH matched to 355 controls, Dexfenfluramine and fenfluramine constituted 90% of all anorexigens used by the PPH patients. The IPPHS study concluded that the risk of PPH was 6.3 times higher in patients who were exposed to anorexigens (primarily fenfluramine and dexfenfluramine) for all definite users of these anorexigens compared to non-anorexigen users. This study, in concert with previous published work, provides important evidence that there is a causal link between fenfluramine and dexfenfluramine and PPH.

4.8 Design Considerations

The goal of research efforts is often to examine the relationship between a possible risk factor for a disease and the occurrence of the disease. We have seen here that scientists have a range of study designs at their command to investigate this question. Each of these types of study designs provides important information. However, there is a relationship between the cost (financial cost, logistical cost, patient cost) and ethical considerations of that study, and the type of information each study provides about the risk factor – disease relationship

Many consider prospectively designed, double-blind clinical trials to be the state-of-the-art investigational tool of clinical investigators. The (approximate) random selection of subjects from the population and random allocation of therapy allow for the clear attribution of therapy effect. However, the cost of selecting a large number of patients from the population at large, controlling the intervention and following patients prospectively for years is often prohibitively expensive. The retrospective case-control study is an alternative design that provides important data on the relationship between a risk factor and a disease. Because they involve carefully choosing the level of exposure to observe and methodologically measure the occurrence of the disease, these prevalence studies provide important information on the relationship between the risk factor and disease. These studies not only conserve financial resources—they conserve patient and administrative resources as well.

However, the price one must sometimes pay for these cost-effective retrospective studies is the potential distortion of the risk factor–disease prevalence relationship through the operation of biases (e.g., selection bias, recall bias, and ascertainment bias, to name just a few). Thus, researchers must balance the relatively weaker causality arguments developed from the cost-effective retrospective studies against the stronger causality evidence from the prohibitively expensive prospective randomized trials.

In weighing the relative advantages and disadvantages of these different designs, scientists have reached a consensus. Like a tool in a tool kit, each design has a set of circumstances to which it is uniquely suited. In the first investigation of a rare disorder, there often are not the financial resources or the groundswell of support from the public health community for a large-scale, prospective clinical experiment. In this circumstance, the researcher will reach for the retrospective, observational study. Easily designed and relatively inexpensive, it will efficiently capture and quantify the magnitude of the relationship between the risk factor and the disease. If the strength of the relationship (the signal) is strong enough to overcome the methodological biases that can sometimes blur or distort this signal, enthusiasm grows for carrying out more expensive experiments.

The causality tenets are the filter through which each of the research efforts is poured. This filter traps the limits and weaknesses of the designs, and executions. What is left is the strength of evidence for a causal relationship between exposure and the disease. When applying the causality tenets, one would like to identify a growing body of evidence that contributes to the strength of association. For example, in the investigation of the relationship between cholesterol levels and ischemic heart disease, the first observations of cases were followed by case control studies, and then by studies that examined the effects of cholesterol levels on a population (ecological studies). These were then followed by case studies that demonstrated the reduction in the incidence of heart attacks by cholesterol reducing therapy, again through case studies, and then by observational studies [17]. These studies were followed by randomized controlled clinical trials e.g., WOSCOPS [18], 4S [19], and CARE [20] LIPID references).

Regardless of which research design is implored, the *p*-value must have a tightly circumscribed sampling error interpretation. In concordant, observational studies where effect attribution can be difficult, as well as in concordant clinical trials that employ the random allocation of therapy, the study interpretation must include explicit consideration of each of the *p*-value, sample size, effect size, and effect size variability as well as the quality of the research design and execution.

4.9 Solid Structures from Imperfect Bricks

The demonstration of a causal relationship between a risk factor and a disease is complex. The assessment of this relationship cannot and must not be viewed solely from the perspective of a randomized controlled clinical trial, and the point of view that randomized controlled clinical trials are necessary for causality must be shunned.

There has been no randomized clinical trial to demonstrate the asbestos exposure-pulmonary disease link, yet advocates of clinical trials have not called for a trial that randomizes (i.e., chooses at random) patients to receive a deliberate heavy asbestos exposure in order to demonstrate the harm asbestos can cause. There has been no randomized clinical trial to demonstrate the hazards of ingesting foul, soiled water, yet the hazard has been made amply clear, justifying important community standards for fresh, healthy water. There have been no randomized clinical trials to demonstrate the hazards of smoking (any attempt would be correctly seen as flagrantly unethical) yet the hazards of smoking are amply apparent. Clearly, randomized clinical trials are not necessary to demonstrate causation.

Observational studies are not randomized, yet they can be so well-designed and executed that they become the kernel around which a persuasive body of knowledge for a cause and effect relationship crystallizes. In 1998, the federal Food and Drug Administration (FDA) removed terfenadine (Seldane) from the market due to evidence of an undesirable effect of the combined used of seldane and some antibiotics. This decision was made not based on a clinical trial, but based instead on compelling data from case report information and from observational studies. Mebifridil (Posicor) was removed from the market-place by the FDA in 1998 in the presence of compelling information from case series reports despite equivocal evidence from a clinical trial. In each case, the information for causality was satisfied by information from nonrandomized re-search efforts. Clearly, there is ample precedent for deciding causality in the absence of a randomized controlled clinical trial.

4.10 Drawing Inferences in Epidemiology

The collection of such studies, each of which examines the risk factor – disease relationship must be considered as the body of evidence. No study, not even the gold standard, randomized clinical trial is perfect. Nevertheless, buildings of sound and solid constitution can be constructed from imperfect bricks. In the end, it is the final edifice that must be judged.

It cannot be overstated that, although the p-value must be carefully evalu-ated in nonrandomized studies, these studies can still be designed and executed skillfully to provide important, unambiguous evidence for causality. Epidemi-ologists recognize that the nonrandom nature of the most commonly used de-signs does not preclude them from building a strong argument for effect size in the population. Epidemiologists build inferential arguments by following these guidelines:

> 1. **Choose the sample with care**. Epidemiologists would pre-fer random samples from the population. This can rarely be achieved. However, a nonrandom sample does not mean a careless sample. If the epidemiologists are choosing cases and controls, they must ensure that patients who are cases and con-trols come from the same population. If they are choosing ex-posed patients and unexposed patients, they must ensure that these exposed and unexposed patients come from the same population.

> 2. **Use the tool of matching judiciously**. Matching ensures that an effect size in the end cannot be due to the matched variable (e.g., sex or treating physician), since the distribution of the matched variable is the same between cases and con-trols. It is a useful tool in clarifying effect attribution.

> 3. **Execute the effort concordantly.** Although it is a maxim that well-designed research is prospectively designed research, a necessary corollary is that the research must be well exe-cuted, minimizing protocol deviations. This concordant execu-tion allows a clear separation between prospectively planned analyses, and exploratory

> 4. **Report sample size, effect size, confidence intervals and p-value.** Each of sample size, effect size, confidence intervals

and *p*-value provides important information. The information from each of these sources is not independent. Sample size information is incorporated into effect size measures, and sample size, effect size, and effect size variability are incorporated into the *p*-value. Consideration of the information from all four sources provides the clearest assessment of the strength of association between exposure and disease.

5. Rely on adjusted analyses. Regression analysis is a necessary procedure in observational studies, since they have no random allocation of the risk factor of interest, and there are differences between the group with the risk factor and the group without. This adjustment is carried out by first isolating, and then identifying the relationship between first, the covariate and exposure, and second, between the covariate and the disease occurrence.[*] These relationships are removed before the assessment is made. These corrections, provided as adjusted odds ratios or adjusted relative risks, are important ingredients of epidemiologic studies, that attempt to clarify the attribution of the effect to the risk factor. Such adjustments are not essential when exposure can be randomly allocated, but, in observational studies, adjustments ensure that the results can not be explained by differences in known risk factors for the disease, and add greatly to the clarity of effect attribution. Adjusted analyses, although they do not replace the random allocation of therapy, are a very useful tool in epidemiology.

4.11 Study counting: The *ceteris paribus* fallacy

Study counting is simply counting the number of studies that address a risk – factor disease relationship and deciding if there are enough studies to support the notion that the risk factor causes the disease. Some who are involved in study counting argue that there must be more than one study. Others say that the number of positive studies must outnumber the number of negative studies. Only the fortunately rare and rarely fortunate epidemiologist reduces the argument of causality to "study counting." Instead, the scientific reasoning process assesses in detail each of the available studies, carefully dissecting the methodology, sifting through the patient characteristics, and methodically considering the conclusions. Study counting represents the wholesale abandonment of the intellectual principles of careful consideration. In a word, study counting is scientific thoughtlessness and should be rejected as a tool of inquiry.

This point requires a more detailed examination. The specific problem with "study counting" is the implicit *ceteris paribus* (all other things being equal) assumption, i.e., that all of the studies that are being included in the count are equal in methodology, equal in the thoroughness of their design, equal in the rigor of their execution, and equal in the discipline of their analyses and interpretation. This fallacious assumption is far from the truth of scientific discovery. Studies have different strengths and different weaknesses. Different investiga-

---

[*] There is a more complete discussion of adjusted analysis in Chapter Eleven.

tors with their own nonuniform standards of discipline execute the research efforts. Some studies give precise results, while others are rife with imprecision. The studies are known not for their homogeneity but for the heterogeneity of their designs and interpretations.

We must distinguish between the appearance of an *isolated* study, i.e., one study whose finding was contrary to a large body of knowledge available in the literature, and the occurrence of a sole study. There is ample epidemiologic evidence that single studies, when well-designed and well executed can be used to prove causality (e.g., the thalidomide investigation). What determines the robustness of a research conclusion is not the number of studies but the strength and standing of the available studies, however many there are. Science, like the courts, does not *count* evidence — it *weighs* evidence. This is a critical and germane distinction. Study counting turns a blind eye to study heterogeneity. Our business in science is to think — not to codify thoughtlessness.

4.12 Critiquing Experimental Designs

A valuable skill of healthcare workers who review research efforts is critically reviewing the design, execution, and analysis of a research effort. This ability is essential to sifting through the weight of evidence for or against a scientific point of view, and this comes only with practice.

To start, begin with the realization that the successful critique of an experiment does not end, but rather begins with, a list of that research effort's strengths and weaknesses. The best critiques (you should not begin a critique unless it is going to be a good one; a poor one is a waste of your time) converts the catalogue of strengths and weaknesses into an argument for accepting or rejecting the findings of the research.

A useful approach to the critique of a research effort is as follows. Start with a review of the hypothesis and goals of the research effort. Then, before proceeding with the actual methodology, turn away from the manuscript and begin to construct for yourself how you would address the hypothesis. Assume in your plan that you have unlimited financial resources, unlimited personnel resources, and unlimited patient resources. Think carefully and compose the best research design, the design that builds the most objective platform from which to view the results. Only after you have assembled this design yourself should you return to read the methodology, the results, and the actual interpretation of the research effort that was executed.

Having constructed your own "virtual" state-of-the-art design, you can easily see the differences between your design and the one that was actually executed by the researchers. After identifying these differences, ask yourself whether and how the compromises made by the researchers limit the findings of the research effort. It they pose no limitations when compared to your design, the researchers did a fine job by your standards. If the researchers have substantial limitations, then the analysis and its generalizability may be crippled. The researchers may have had understandable reasons for the limitations, but these limitations can nevertheless undermine the strength of their findings.

4.13 Conclusions

Epidemiologic studies have been the cornerstone of the development of public health research programs and continue to make important scientific contributions to public health understanding and policy. Unfortunately, the nature of these programs often precludes the random allocation of exposure.

P-values have a rich history of use in observational studies, and although, at one time they were embraced, *p*-values have fallen into some disrepute. The difficulty with *p*-values in these important, nonrandomized efforts is that they have erroneously but commonly been interpreted as binding up the truth of the trial—sample size, effect size, sample variability and effect attribution—into one number. Workers who interpret *p*-values in any research study, imbuing them with interpretative powers beyond an assessment of sampling variability, unfortunately do so at their own risk. The situation is more acute in nonrandomized studies due to the absence of the random allocation of exposure in the sample chosen from the population. *P*-values can play a useful role in the causality debate if the researchers are clear that *p*-values were not designed to measure sample size, effect size or effect attribution, only sampling error.

References

1. Hill B (1953) Observation and experiment. *New England Journal of Medicine* **248**:995–1001.
2. Times Newspaper Ltd., *The Sunday Times of London* (1979) Suffer the Children:the Story of Thalidomide.
3. Lentz W (1962) Thalidomide and congenital abnormalites (letter to the editor)*The Lancet*:**45**
4. Clark C (1997) *Radium Girls: Women and Industrial Health Reform, 1910-1935*. University of North Carolina Press, Chapel Hill, NC.
5. Pepall J (1997) Methyl mercury poisoning: the Minamata Bay disaster. Copyright © International Development Research Centre, Ottawa, Canada .
6. Lenz W (1962) Thalidomide and congenital abnormalities. *Lancet* **1**:45.
7. Monahan BP, Ferguson CL, Killeavy ES, Lloyd BK, Troy J, Cantilena LR Jr (1990) Torsades de pointes occurring in association with terfenadine use. *Journal of the American Medical Association* **264**:2788–90.
8. Connolly, HM, Crary JL, McGoon, MD, et al (1997) Valvular heart disease associated with fenfluramine–phentermine [see comments] [published erratum appears in *New England Journal of Medicine* **337**:1783.
9. Douglas JG, et al. (1981) Pulmonary hypertension and fenfluramine. *British Medical Journal* **283**:881–3.
10. Brenot F, et al. (1993) Primary pulmonary hypertension and fenfluramine use [see comments]. *British Heart Journal* **70**:537–41
11. Abenhaim, L., et al.(1996) Appetite–suppressant drugs and the risk of primary pulmonary hypertension. International Primary Pulmonary Hypertension Study Group [see comments]. *New England Journal of Medicine* **335**:609–16.
12. Gurtner HP (1979) Pulmonary hypertension, plexogenic pulmonary arteriopathy and the appetite depressant drug aminorex. Post or propter? *Buletin of European Physiopathology and Respiration* **15**:897–923.
13. McMurray J, Bloomfield P, Miller HC (1986) Irreversible pulmonary hypertension after treatment with fenfluramine. *British Medical Journal Med J (Clin Res Ed)* **292**:239–40.

14. Atanassoff PG, et al. (1992) Pulmonary hypertension and dexfenfluramine [letter]. *Lancet* **339**:436.
15. Roche N et al.(1992) Pulmonary hypertension and dexfenfluramine [letter]. *Lancet* **339** 436–7.
16. Cacoub P, et al. (1995) Pulmonary hypertension and dexfenfluramine [letter]. *European Journal of Clinical Pharmacology* **48**:81–3.
17. Gordon T, Castelli WP, Hjortland MC, Kannel WB, Dawber TR (1977) High-density lipoprotein as a protective factor against coronary heart disease: The Framingham Study. *American Journal of Medicine* **62**:707–714.
18. Shepherd J, Cobbe SM, Ford I, et al. (1995) Prevention of coronary heart disease with pravastatin in men with hypercholesterolemia *New England Journal of Medicine* **333**:1301–7.
19. Scandinavian Simvastatin Survival Study Group (1994) Randomized trial of cholesterol lowering in 4444 patients with coronary heart disease. *Lancet* **344**:138–89.
20. Sacks FM, Pfeffer MA, Moyé LA, Rouleau JL, Rutherford JD, Cole TG, Brown L, Warnica JW, Arnold JMO, Wun CC, Davis BR, Braunwald E for the Cholestrol and Recurrent Events Trial Investigators (1996) The effect of pravastain on coronary events after myocardial infarction in patients with average cholesterol levels. *New England Journal of Medicine* **335**:1001–9.

5

Shrine Worship

5.1 Introduction

Chapter Three discussed how statistical hypothesis tests generate p-values. Designed to assist both the investigator and the medical community in assessing the role of sampling error in research results, they have become omnipresent in healthcare research efforts. In fact it is difficult to get away from p-values in medical investigations. Manuscripts produce p-values by the dozens, and sometimes by the hundreds.

However, although available for over 70 years, inference testing and its p-value products have been continuously embroiled in a controversy from which they have yet to emerge. While p-values can be useful tool, reliance on them to exclusion of other considerations can be fraught with danger.

5.2 The Nightmare

Here is one variation on a common nightmare for contemporary investigators.

> After years of practice and careful observation, a distinguished physician developed a theory for the treatment of a disease. A time of arduous work followed, during which he convinced his colleagues of the truth of his thesis. He worked patiently to build a funding base and assembled a cadre of capable investigators. Finally, he was in a position to put his clinical hypothesis to the definitive test through a formal, randomized, double-blind, placebo-controlled clinical trial.
>
> Several more years of diligent and patient work elapsed as the trial was executed, during which time our scientist could only watch from the sidelines. Finally, after many seasons, the trial concluded and its results were revealed. The therapy produced the desired beneficial effect; however, the p-value was 0.06. As the implications of this statistically insignificant finding broke through to this investigator, he, in absolute frustration and despair exclaimed, "Why must we worship at the shrine of 0.05?" [*]

---

[*] From a story related by Dr. Eugene Braunwald.

It is the goal of this chapter to provide sound advice to this investigator. But first, let's feel his pain.

5.3 *P*-value Bashing

Thinking physicians, statisticians, readers, editors, and regulators have, at one point or another, grappled with the rigidity of *p*-values. As physicians we learn to expect variability in our patients, and have developed a fine tool to deal with it — flexibility. We adjust treatment regimens if patients don't respond as anticipated. We alter testing schedules, increasing or decreasing the frequency of laboratory evaluations accordingly. We ask our colleagues to see our patients and we listen to their sometimes surprising advice. Flexibility serves us well in reacting to patient variability in our practices.

However, it seems that statisticians replace flexibility with staggering hyperrigidity: $p = 0.05$. One either meets this threshold or one does not. Period. If the *p*-value is greater than 0.05, then, "You missed it. What a shame. You worked so hard." Alternatively, if your *p* value is less than 0.05, then, "Congratulations. Outstanding work. When will you publish?" Is it unfair to an investigator to permit all of the work invested in a research program, all of the variability in investigators and in patients, all of the toil in collecting thousands of case report forms, and hundreds of thousands of bits of information to be supercondensed into one number? Is it appropriate to reduce this effort down to a single entity that dispenses judgment on research programs without feeling or adaptability, dispassionately granting publication acceptance, grant awards, academic progress, and regulatory approval? These *p*-values seem to make or break careers and spirits, and the investigator may be forgiven for believing that he are at their mercy.

Given that the *p*-value has so much influence, it is perhaps only natural that investigators would attempt to reverse the tables by influencing them. Significance testing can be easily described as flexible and adaptable, with a plethora of hypothesis testing tools (e.g., adjusted analyses, unadjusted analyses, analyses with missing values imputed to name just a few). There are many such adaptations, and their presence offers false hope to the investigator who, with $p > 0.05$ in hand, believes that he only need select the tool that reduces his *p*-value below the threshold 0.05 level. These desperate attempts have pulled the *p*-value farther from its intent and true meaning, sapping it of its true statistical intent, leaving behind only the chimera of utility.

Let's take a few minutes to figure out how we got here, before we decide where to go.

5.4 Epidemiology and Biostatistics

The *p*-value battle has commonly been typified as a clash between biostatisticians, typecast as champions of *p*-value implementation, and epidemiologists, accused of viewing its use with scorn. There is a basis of truth in this, but the conflict is, at its heart, more about the correct role of mathematics in healthcare research. Specifically, should mathematics be supportive or ascendant?

5.4.1 The Link Between Epidemiology and Statistics

Epidemiologists and biostatisticians have much in common. In healthcare, they both focus on identifying the true nature of a relationship. However the tools used to get at the heart of this relationship are different. It is this difference in which the controversy about the role of mathematics and p-values in particular, first took root.

5.4.2. Exposure–Disease Relationships

Both epidemiology and biostatistics pay important attention to the true nature of the exposure disease relationship. Given an exposure and a disease (or perhaps, amelioration of the disease), it is possible that the exposure caused the disease. Alternatively, the exposure's presence may merely be coincidental. The question of causality can be a complicated one, and the distinction between a relationship based on association and one based on causation is critical. In the "association" circumstance, the risk factor and the disease just happen to occur together, appearing jointly.

However, a causal relationship is much different. A risk factor causes a disease if that risk factor excites the production of the disease. There is a clear directionality in the risk factor–disease causal connection that is absent in a serendipitous risk factor–disease association. The time sequence embedded in the causal relationship is that (1) the disease is absent, (2) the risk factor is introduced, and (3) the risk factor working in ways known and unknown produces the disease.

The classification of a relationship as associative or causal can be a public health urgency. However, this classification can also be a complex, time consuming task, since multiple risk factors and diseases can congregate. This complex coexistence can make it difficult to separate the causal risk factors from the associative ones. Both epidemiologists and biostatisticians are called upon to help disentangle the risk factor–disease connection, and have historically emphasized the use of different research tools. These different emphases, like forces on the opposite sides of a rope, have pulled the p-value at varying times too then away from respectability.

5.4.2.1 Epidemiology and the Power of Observation

As we saw in Chapter Four, epidemiologists rely on powers of careful observation and deductive reasoning. Using the Bradford Hill tenets of causality as the metric, they measure the strength of evidence for a causal relationship between the exposure and the disease. An example of the successful implementation of this approach is the identification of the bacteria *Legionella pneumophilia* as a cause of a new and unrecognized pneumonia at a Veterans' meeting in Philadelphia [1].

This research style requires great sensitivity, sharp powers of observation, and clear reasoning skills. In short, epidemiology is a thinking person's business. However, to the classical epidemiologist, the role of mathematics is merely supportive, and not transcendent in understanding the exposure–disease relationship. This perspective has pitted these workers against the philosophical approach used by biostatisticians.

5.4.2.2. Modeling Sampling Error in Biostatistics

While one of the goals of biostatisticians is the same as that of epidemiologists, namely, the classification of the exposure–disease relationship as associative or causal, the emphasis of the biostatistician is mathematical. Since research in healthcare often begins with the selection of a sample from a large population or universe of patients, statisticians use quantitative tools to examine the effect this sampling process can have on the results of the research effort.

Specifically, biostatisticians focus on identifying why some groups of patients have results that are more disparate (i.e., have greater variability) than others. While one explanation might be that patients have different exposure histories, a second is that the results are simply due to the random aggregation of this collection of subjects in the sample.

This perspective on how samples can produce variability permits biostatisticians to model, partition, separate, examine, and compare the variability of subjects with different levels of exposure to that of subjects with the same. This comparison permits them to quantify the likelihood that the research results were driven by the exposure rather than generated by the random play of chance.

This is a mathematical process, leading the biostatistician to lean on sophisticated mathematical modeling techniques. *T*-testing, logistic regression analysis, Cox proportional hazard modeling, and Bayes procedures are all tools that essentially do the same thing – separate the error variability or "noise" introduced by the sampling process from the directional variability produced by the exposure–disease relationship.

Thus, the traditional epidemiologist is an expert observer, and the classic biostatistician is an expert mathematical modeler.[*] This distinction created the charged grid on which the polarizing debates about *p*-value occurred.

5.5 The Initial Schism

Since epidemiologists and biostatisticians have the same goal, i.e. the identification of the causes of disease and their treatments, it is not surprising that they would work together. Perhaps the more famous early case of this joint effort was in the identification of the effectiveness of smallpox vaccinations.[†]

Epidemiology was ascendant at the dawn of the twentieth century. Its contributions to understanding disease at that point were undeniable, and the creation of criteria (e.g. Koch's postulates) promised that medicine would now have objective assessment criteria as it awakened to the possible role of microorganisms as the cause of human disease. The observation that the single most effective way to reduce surgical infection is for clean surgeons to use clean instruments with clean hands (the *primum movens* for the hyperclean surgical

---

[*] This is not to say that epidemiologists do not use mathematical tools (or that biostatisticians do not use deductive reasoning). Because workers in biostatistics often observe carefully, and epidemiologists readily use some modeling tools, there has been an important overlap in experienced workers in these fields.

[†] To demonstrate the effectiveness of the Jenner "variolation procedure," the statistician (Daniel Bernoulli) produced a computation of the expected number of deaths, and the epidemiologists, in concert, collected the "observed" number of deaths. Inspection of this data led leading scientists to conclude that the Jenner procedure was effective.

suites of today)[*] was demonstrated using the basic observational principles of epidemiology. There was a strong feeling that modern medicine would be propelled forward by the thrust of diligent, observational epidemiologists.

However, an unexpected theoretical impediment was innocently dropped directly in the path of this progress by the physicist Albert Einstein, who, working in isolation on his days off from the Patent Office, produced a remarkable observation of his own. While many of his observations were about what would occur at relativistic speeds (i.e., speeds close to the speed of light),[†] his theories about Earth-bound observation were directly apropos to the science of the time.

Einstein, in 1905, and again during World War I, said that observational scientists maintained an unjustified reliance on the power of observation. Two observers could watch an event and come to different conclusions; according to Einstein both would be right. The difference in these observations resided in the characteristics of the observation point, not the observational prowess of the observers. According to the new laws, physical findings and measurements could no longer be trusted. Concepts easily understood and taken for granted for centuries were found to be inconstant—merely a function of the observation point of the viewer.

Einstein's work implied the only appropriate substitute would be mathematics. Additionally, Einstein's demonstration that advanced mathematics revealed findings in the real world that scientists trained to observe had missed, suggested that mathematics was superior to observational science in its ability to reveal the truth of our surroundings and mankind's interrelationship with them.[‡]

The observational disciplines, poised for a period of dramatic progress into the new twentieth century, were now stricken with insecurity. Their scientists were now forced to question the reliability of their own tools; the seeds of doubt sown by advanced, impenetrable, but irrefutable mathematics.

The discovery that (1) all observations are inherently biased, and (2) events in nature can be predicted from cloistered mathematical work, shook epidemiologists, forcing them to question and sometimes stridently defend their point of view against a correct but abstract argument. No one questioned the veracity of their findings in the past. It was the implications for that discipline's future that placed the core themes of epidemiology in jeopardy.

---

[*] The work of Holmes (1809–94; Boston, 1843) and Semmelweis (1818–65; Vienna, 1858) proved that the doctors and midwives carried infection, and that by simply washing their hands could reduce death rates dramatically.

[†] In Einstein's new world, space could no longer be seen as an empty stage on which objects moved and performed, but instead had its own properties that changed when mass was present. In the absence of mass, space can appear alien. Geometry is no longer Euclidean. Parallel lines do not exist. The angles of a triangle no longer have a sum of 180 degrees nor do perpendiculars to the same line converge.

[‡] Not only epidemiologists but, in addition, traditional probabilists, were threatened by this inexorably progressing logic. The findings of the Russian mathematician Kolmogorov revealed that all of probability— with its rich history of observations based on natural phenomena, stock market predictions, and games of chance—was only a subarea of the larger mathematical field of real analysis. Advanced mathematical analysis, functional analysis, and the complicated area of measure theory now jointly subsumed probability, reducing the latter to a mere application. Once again mathematics seemed to be driving out, pushing aside, and supplanting observation-based research.

Fisher's findings were released into this new threatening environment. His conclusions represented the match that was struck in an intellectual powder keg of controversy, igniting explosions that still reverberate today.

5.6 Appearance of Statistical Significance

Born in East Finchley, London, in 1890, Ronald Aylmer Fisher was one of the giants of twentieth century statistical thinking. Upon finishing his schooling at Gonville and Caius College in Cambridge, he started work in 1919 as a statistician at Rothamsted Experimental Station. He rapidly developed an interest in designing and analyzing agricultural experiments. As he concentrated on the design and analysis of these experiments, he recognized as James Johnson had in the previous century, that better methods were necessary to consider the natural variability of crop yields.*

5.6.1 Introducing the 0.05 Level

Fisher's earliest writing on the general strategy in field experimentation appeared in the first edition of his 1925 book *Statistical Methods for Research Workers* [2], and in a short 1926 paper entitled, "The arrangement of field experiments" [3]. This brief paper contained many of Fisher's principal ideas on the planning of experiments, including the idea of significance testing. It is in this paper that the notion of a five% level of significance first appeared.

Fisher's example to motivate the use of significance testing was the assessment of manure's influence on crop yield. In this circumstance, the yields of two neighboring acres of land, one treated with manure and the other without were to be compared.

Fisher observed that the manure-treated plot produced a 10% greater crop yield than that of the non-treated plot. This result suggested a benefit attributable to the manure, yet Fisher grappled with how one could decide that the greater yield was due to the manure and not to the random play of chance. In this case the role of chance exerted its influence in the random aggregation of factors that affect crop yield, e.g., soil moisture, seed quality, and insect presence. The question came down to how likely would one expect to see a 10% increase in crop yield in the absence of the manure by chance alone?

Fisher concluded that if there was only a one in twenty chance that the play of chance would produce a 10% difference in crop yield, then

> ...the evidence would have reached a point which may be called the verge of significance; for it is convenient to draw the line at about the level at which we can say "Either there is something in the treatment or a coincidence has occurred such as does not occur more than once in twenty trials." This level, which we may call the 5 per cent level point, would be indicated, though very roughly, by the greatest chance deviation observed in twenty successive trials [3].

---

* See the Prologue for a discussion of James Johnson's ideas of research design.

This appears to be the first mention of the 5% level of significance level. Note that its underlying philosophy is rooted in what might have been expected to occur naturally, i.e., under the influence of only random variation.[*]

Fisher went on, justifying the 0.05 level of significance in his own work, adding

> If one in twenty does not seem high enough odds, we may, if we prefer it, draw the line at one in fifty (the 2 per cent point) or one in a hundred (the 1 per cent point). Personally, the writer prefers to set the low standard of significance at the 5 per cent point, and ignore entirely all results which fail to reach this level) [3].

He continued to say that if he had the actual yields from earlier years, and could compute the variability of the yields, then he might use Student's t-tables to compute the 5% significance level. These were the building blocks of the test statistic.[†] The significance level of 0.05 was born from these rather casual remarks [4]. It cannot be overemphasized that there is no deep mathematical theory that points to 0.05 as the optimum type I error level — only Fisher's arbitrary decision.

It is useful to note that Fisher himself was not wedded to the 0.05 level as the only level of statistical significance. In his text *Statistical Methods for Research Workers*, he makes the following assertion about the chi-square goodness-of-fit test, in which the investigator focuses on whether the discrepancy between observed and expected proportions is important, suggesting other thresholds maybe useful:

> If P is between 0.10 and 0.90 there is certainly no reason to suspect the hypothesis being tested. If it is below 0.02 it is strongly indicated that the hypothesis fails to account for the whole of the facts…A value of χ^2 exceeding the 5 per cent point is seldom to be disregarded. [page 80]

Here he suggests a range of significance levels, with 0.02 providing strong repudiation of the null hypothesis, and 0.05 level reflecting a more tepid

---

[*] The use of the occurrence of naturally occurring events as a surrogate for random variability is remarkably similar to the thinking of the eighteenth-century physician, Dr. John Arbuthnot. In 1710 he noticed that for the past 82 years, London consistently produced a higher ratio of male to female births. Understanding that this tendency might be due to chance alone, Arbuthnot deduced that its probability should be relatively high. However, when he computed the probability that in each of 82 successive years there were more male than female births as $(\frac{1}{2})^{82}$, an exceedingly small number, he concluded that there was some other systematic influence driving the relatively high number of male births. This was perhaps the earliest use of a formal probability calculation for a purpose in statistical inference [15]. One hundred years later, the idea of using probability to assess the likelihood of a chance occurrence in a research setting was adopted by Laplace, who in 1812 used statistical measurements to confirm astronomical findings.

[†] Fisher went on to develop the notion of the use of randomization of the intervention in the agricultural experiment, the factorial design (analysis of variance).

finding, setting the stage for equating the p-value magnitude with "strength of evidence".

5.6.2 "Dangerous Nonsense"

Fisher's work introduced a new quantitative tool for scientists involved in studying results from samples. The notion of sample-to-sample variability had been known to investigators for years. Finally, here was a way to deal with the chronic problem of sample-based research using objective mathematics.

But, perhaps, even more importantly, Fisher's innovations strengthened the field of statistical inference. For over 150 years, the field of statistics had struggled with its correct role in data interpretation and generalizing sample results to larger populations.[*] At last, a method was emerging that would provide formal and reproducible mathematical structure to the inference process.

Yet, Fisher's point of view on experimental design became the flash point of a new controversy. Many observationalists in science believed that the significance testing scenario was counterintuitive, representing the unhelpful type of thinking that was likely to be produced by mathematical workers who did not spend sufficient time in the observationalists' world of data collection and deductive reasoning. Epidemiology, already bruised by the two decade-old assault on its philosophical opinions by physicists and mathematical theorists[†], reacted quickly. They had to take the irrefutable arguments of Einstein. They did not have to sit still while Fisher lectured them on the scientific method. The field responded vehemently, with comments that reverberate to this day.

To epidemiologists, Fisher's approach was the reverse of the scientific method. Specifically, this new, upside-down paradigm of statistical significance appeared to deny the scientist the ability to prove the hypothesis he believed was correct. Instead, the scientist would be required to replace the strong assertion of his own affirmative scientific hypothesis with the tepid alternative of disproving

---

[*] See the Prologue.

[†] Over time, epidemiologists have successfully defended their time-tested methodologic perspective. Of course, the flaw in all of the criticisms regarding the use of observation as a foundation method of epidemiology lies in the difficulty in translating findings that are germane in one field (physics) to that of another (life sciences). While the findings of the relativity laws are in general true, they are most useful in physics. The theoretical physicist may be correct in asserting that every observer is biased and that there is no absolute truth about the nature and magnitude of the risk factor–disease relationship. However, this does not imply that all platforms are equally biased. Epidemiologists never stopped striving to find the most objective position possible. Certainly, if bias cannot be removed, it should be minimized. The fact that bias may not be excluded completely does not excuse its unnecessary inclusion.

Second, while mathematicians are capable of predicting results in physics, they have not been able to predict disease in any important or useful fashion. No mathematical models warned obstetricians or their pregnant patients of the impending thalidomide–birth defect link. Similarly, mathematical models did not predict the birth defects that mercury poisoning produced in Japan. While physics often studies processes in which mathematics can reign supreme, real life and its disease processes have proven to be painful, messy, and chaotic affairs. The substantial role of epidemiology is incontrovertible in the development of the most important new healthcare research tool of the twentieth century—the clinical trial. The time-tested tools of epidemiology continue to prove their utility in the present day.

a hypothesis that he did not believe. To traditional observationists, Fisher's significance testing appeared to be just the type of indecipherable, mathematical, reverse logic that had already shaken the foundations of early twentieth-century epidemiology. It therefore comes as no surprise that the epidemiologists' reaction to Fisher were profoundly negative. One said,

> What used to be called judgment is now called prejudice, and what used to be called prejudice is now called a null hypothesis ... it is dangerous nonsense ... [5]

However, there was also real enthusiasm for the notion of significance testing. In the 1930s, Egon Pearson and Jerzy Neyman developed the formal theory of testing statistical hypotheses [6]. In this paradigm, the investigator must choose between two hypotheses. The first is what we now know as the null hypothesis, aptly named because it is the hypothesis that is to be nullified by the data. The alternative hypothesis is commonly what the investigator believes represents the true state of nature. From this emerged the notion of alpha errors (identified then as the error of the first kind), beta errors, and power[*]. These workers also developed the foundation for the confidence interval [7 9]

The advances and resulting codification of Fisher's innovative approach into a theory based collection of procedures did little to reduce the severity of criticisms leveled at statistical inference. Joseph Berkson was especially critical. Karl Pearson's maxim of — "After all, the higher statistics are only common sense reduced to numerical appreciation" — was widely accepted by the world of observationalists. This tenet, he argued was violated by Fisher's seemingly reverse-logic significance. Published papers by Berkson [10,11] and Fisher [12] provide some feel for the repartee between these two researchers as they struggled to understand the complex implications of the hypothesis testing scenarios. Much of the criticism Berkson leveled at Fisher was in the interpretation of the extreme findings (i.e., findings associated with small p-values). Returning to Fisher's manure example at the 5% level, Berkson contended that, just because the 10% yield produced on the field treated with manure would not be anticipated in 20 such experiments does not preclude its occurrence by chance. He argued that, if we accept the notion that it is relatively rare for a human who is between 20 and 30 years of age to die, a statistician would conclude, confronted with a dead person in his twenties, that the dead person was not human! This was amusingly refuted (although the refutation was not always amusingly received) by Fisher, who said that "It is not my purpose to make Dr. Berkson seem ridiculous nor of course for me to prevent him from providing innocent entertainment" [12].

The difficulty was that many workers believed Fisher was equating small p-values with a causality argument (i.e., a small p-value was the sin qua non of a causal relationship), yet all Fisher claimed to provide was an assessment of the likelihood that the larger crop yield was due to chance alone. Critics of the putative link between significance testing and causality assessment would find ample targets for these cogent arguments 60 years later.

---

[*] Discussed in Chapter Two.

5.7 The *P*-value Love Affair in Healthcare

Despite these deep–seated, articulate criticisms expressed by devoted experimentalists, exploration and acceptance of the notion of significance testing continued. Neyman and Pearson helped codify the notion of significance testing by its formalization, leading to the first early sample size computations. Now, researchers had a formal, objective way to compute the size of their research effort, helping to protect adequately against both type I and type II errors. They themselves stated [8],

> But we may look at the purpose of tests from another viewpoint. Without hoping to know whether each separate hypothesis is true or false, we may search for rules to govern our behavior with regard to them, in following which we ensure that, in the long run of experience, we not often be wrong.

In addition, the intense quantification of healthcare research, starting in the 1930's was an important new trend, boosting the utility of inference testing and *p*-value implementation. World War II, with its requirement for new, improved medicine and delivery of healthcare services to both soldiers and refugee populations, produced a surge in healthcare research. Research teams, including such renowned groups as the Medical Research Council (MRC) of England, were assembled to develop not just new medications, but new research methodology as well.[*] These efforts explored, and in many cases embraced, the use of statistical hypothesis testing.

This explosive growth in healthcare research had predictable consequences—the population of new investigators generated a demand for new and higher levels of research findings. The product of these new research efforts required an outlet in the peer reviewed medical literature, a field of journalism that in the 1940s was a small, cloistered industry controlled by a handful of powerful editors. Harried grant administrators together with overworked journal workers were overwhelmed by the demand for their diminished resources, and each struggled with how to separate "the wheat from the chaff" in the myriad submitted grant applications and manuscript drafts.

This was not malicious. The grant administrators and journal editors wished to fund and ultimately publish the best research. The difficulty was that there was no objective way to separate reliably the strength of evidence provided by the investigators from the authors' persuasive claims, sometimes buttressed by imaginative calculations. These powerful oversight groups decided that their decisions could be improved by the inclusion of a mathematical, objective measure of a research effort's results. This would allow the data to speak for itself in a structured fashion, free of the bias that an investigator would bring to the research paradigm.

This influential group concluded that *p*-values were the needed objective measures of research result. The *p*-value, being data-based, was a readily available, easily computed tool that was entirely mathematical, incorporating the

---

[*] The MRC engaged the help of Sir Bradford Hill in carrying out the first modern clinical trial — an investigation of the risks and benefits of streptomycin in the treatment of tuberculosis.

concerns for sampling error. It also was devoid of investigator subjectivity. Thus, not only would the p-value be the basis of grant awards and manuscript publication, but it would also be the best basis for therapeutic options and determining government health policy. A more thorough discussion of this complex process is available [13].

Moving on this conclusion, these administrators quickly required that research grants and manuscripts should include formal statistical hypothesis testing in general, and p-values in particular, in order receive active consideration for funding or publication. The embrace of p-values by granting agents and academia was followed by their wholesale acceptance by the regulatory industry and consequently, the pharmaceutical industry.

The technique of significance testing itself was to undergo a refinement into its present form. The threshold significance level (type I error probability level) was utilized by Neyman and Pearson as a criterion that should be determined in connection with the type II error level. Thus, the null hypothesis was rejected if the p-value fell below a threshold. The exact value was not reported, only whether the null hypothesis was rejected or not.

It is interesting to note that Fisher was opposed to the interpretation of the type I error rate as a rejection rate. Instead, he emphasized the significance reflected by the actual p-value (i.e., the smaller the p-value, the greater the strength of evidence that the relationship identified in the sample is not due to chance alone). Thus, as the use of significance testing grew, the belief that this estimate of the level of significance should be sharpened was encouraged. Also, the availability of more extensive tabulations of probabilities eased the computation for the exact value of this quantity. Thus, it became the custom to report the exact p-value ($p = 0.021$) and not just the inequality ($p < 0.05$). This is how p-values are currently reported.

The p-value genie was now out of the bottle.

5.8 Use and Abuse of *P*-values

It is not tragic that the use of p-values accelerated; however, it is unfortunate that they began to take on a new, subsuming, and inappropriate meaning in the medical research community. Medical journals, at first willing merely to accept p-values, now not only demanded them but also required that they fall below Fisher's 0.05 threshold level for acceptance. Thus, inadvertently, the stage on which p-values would be the major player was set.

This situation degenerated when p-values stampeded over the well-established epidemiologic tenets of causality. Elaborated by Sir Austin Bradford Hill [14], these tenets served as the basis of epidemiologic causal thinking in the mid-twentieth century. Free of complicated mathematics, these hallmarks of a causal relationship have twin bases in common sense and disciplined observation. The nine precise Bradford Hill criteria are (1) strength of association, (2) temporality, (3) dose–response relationship, (4) biologic plausibility, (5) consistency, (6) coherency, (7) specificity, (8) experimentation, and (9) analogy. These are well elaborated in the literature [15].

These criteria acknowledge that a greater number of disease cases in the presence of the risk factor than in its absence raise a causal suspicion. In addition, determining that greater exposure (either by dose or duration) to the risk factor produces a greater extent of disease changes our perception that the exposure is controlling the disease's occurrence and/or severity. These two features are important characteristics of a cause–effect relationship.

Other questions posed by Hill permit us to explore the "believability" of the relationship. Is there a discernible mechanism by which the risk factor produces the disease? Have other researchers also shown this relationship? Are there other examples that help us to understand the current exposure–disease relationship? These are all incorporated in Hill's criteria. Statistical criteria are not.

However, Hill's thoughtful, accepted approach was beginning to be supplanted by the following style of reasoning:

> Since the study found a statistically significant relative risk …
> the causal relationship was considered established [16].

While this type of comment was not typical, it did demonstrate the extreme conclusions that were beginning to be based solely on the p-value. What had been offered by Fisher as an objective sense of the strength of evidence of research result was now being transmogrified into a popular but inadequate substitute for good, causal thinking.

Workers, accepting the important new role of the p-value in promulgating their research results, were now replacing their own thoughtful, critical review of a research effort with the simple evaluation of the p-value. In some studies, highly statistically significant effects (i.e., small p-values) are produced from small, inconsequential effect sizes. In others, the p-values themselves were meaningless regardless of their size since the assumptions on which they had been computed were violated. Finally, there was the paradox that statistical significance may not indicate true biologic significance.

It was inevitable that some scientist would actively resist this degradation in the scientific thought process. In healthcare, the common abuse of significance testing was driving its critics to conclude that significance testing was replacing well reasoned, thoughtful consideration of research results. Some in this camp argued against the use of significance testing altogether.

The dispute broke out into the open again in 1987, when the prestigious and well-respected *American Journal of Public Health* solicited an editorial arguing that significance testing be purged from articles submitted for review and publication. Subsequently, the epidemiologist Alexander Walker debated with the statistician T.W. Fleiss over the use of significance testing [17–21], with Fleiss, supporting the use of this statistical procedure.

Fleiss conceded, however, that there had been abuse of statistical inference procedures in healthcare. He was particularly concerned about a new confusion between the concepts of statistical versus clinical significance. Specifically, he feared that many workers now assumed that a finding of statistical significance was synonymous with clinical significance.[*]

In addition, Fleiss pointed out the other side of the coin. Healthcare research efforts could and commonly did produce p-values greater than 0.05, i.e., statistically insignificant; however, many readers equated a statistically insignificant finding with the conclusion that the definitive demonstration that there

---

[*] This is discussed in detail in Moyé L (2003) *Multiple Analyses in Clinical Trials: Fundamentals for Investigators*. New York: Springer. pp. 327–331.

was no effect. By doing so, the mis-interpreter missed two important points. The first is that the research effort must be appropriately designed to reach either a positive or a null conclusion. For example, a study that is designed to demonstrate the effect of an intervention but uses a homeopathic dose of the intervention will produce a small treatment effect and in all likelihood, a larger p-value. However, this doesn't mean that the therapy, when appropriately administered at the correct dose, is worthless.

Secondly, in the presence of a large p-value (reflecting a test statistic that did not fall into the critical region) the reader must focus on the power of the study. Recall from Chapter Three that when the researcher claims the study findings are null (i.e., there is no effect of therapy), the sampling error of greatest concern to the reader is that produced by a type II error. If this error rate is high, suggesting that there was a treatment effect in the population at large but the play of chance produced a sample in which this effect could not be observed, the null results of the sample must be set aside. Thus, null findings from underpowered studies are simply uninformative.

However, Fleiss defended significance testing, saying that it keeps us from coming to our own conclusions about the results of an experiment. He claimed that we need safeguards against diversity of interpretation, imaginative theorizations, and the possibility that "my substantive difference may be your trivial difference."

However, the theme that p-values were inappropriately substituting for a detailed, well-considered review of research results hit a responsive chord. Charles Poole [22] pointed out that the mechanical, reflexive acceptance of p-values at the 0.05 level (or any other arbitrary decision rule) is the nonscientific, easy way out of critical discussion in science. Under the guise of "intellectual economy" scientists were being encouraged by the advocates of statistical inference to give up their ability to come to their own conclusions. These workers were to substitute independent thought and consideration of a research effort's meaning with the simple observation of whether the p-value was above or below 0.05.

This criticism of p-values lead to the rise of the confidence interval as its replacement.

5.8.1 Confidence Intervals as False Substitution

In the frustration with the problems introduced by significance testing, many workers have argued that confidence intervals can replace p-values as a summary measure of an research effort's results. In fact, the *American Journal of Public Health*, and *Epidemiology* have each proposed that this substitution be made.

Certainly, the use of confidence intervals betrays a dimension of the effect that p-values do not. Recall from Chapter Three that a confidence interval reveals information not just about the magnitude of the effect size, but in addition provides a perspective on the variability of that magnitude. It, like the p-value provides useful information about the influence of sampling error on the effect size. However, while the p-value internally incorporates this dimension, the confidence interval converts this sampling error into a range of values for the parameter estimate.

However, there is a natural correspondence between the p-value and the confidence interval that permit the abuse of both. Since each can be derived from the other, they both address the issue of whether the research data supports the null hypothesis. Specifically, if the p-value is less than 0.05, signifying the null hypothesis has been rejected, then the 95% confidence interval for the point estimate does not include its value under the null hypothesis. Alternatively, a p-value > 0.05 ensures that the confidence interval will contain the value of the point estimate under the null hypothesis.

This one-to-one correspondence between p-value and confidence interval interpretation creates a potential trap for the investigator. The researcher, accepting the notion that significance testing has important flaws, may choose to eschew p-values for confidence intervals. However, if this investigator chooses to judge the significance of his work by assessing whether the confidence interval contains the value of the point estimate under the null hypothesis, then he is essentially constructing his own p-value from the confidence interval.

This "back-door significance testing" offers no real advantage over the p-value assessment. Any thoughtless approach, whether it involves p-values or confidence intervals, is inadequate if it substitutes mathematics for careful judicious thought.

Additionally, Chapter Two pointed out the difficulty in interpreting research efforts when the exercise is discordantly executed. Specifically, research that is data driven (as opposed to protocol driven) perturbs estimates of effect size and standard error. Therefore, any function of these estimators must also be affected. While it is generally accepted that p-values are problematic in this process, the confidence interval, also derived from the same skewed estimates, are also disturbed. Thus, the practice of setting aside p-values in this type of research is valid and well accepted; however, substitution of this flawed estimate for an equally flawed confidence interval must be avoided.

5.8.2 War Too Important to be Left to the Generals?

As we have seen, some workers have argued that significance testing is not an essential part of statistics, and that epidemiologists and statisticians should not be involved in decision-making. Their job is to report and tabulate the data and turn it over to others to make the difficult choices. These others would use their own metrics developed over the years, based on their experience in the field. This tack removes statisticians from the decision process altogether, leaving the interpretation of the research results to others, as in the following example.

Late last century, a new Florida law required that children in every preschool day-care facility listen to the music of Beethoven each day.[*] The genesis of this law was a powerful, influential Florida state legislator who came across a study suggesting that exposure to this music caused a child's brainpower to be increased. Never mind that the finding demonstrated only a transient increase (approximately 20 minutes) in cognitive ability nor that it was not reproduced in other studies. The legislator believing that exposure to Beethoven's music (eventually expanded to classical music in general) was beneficial, pushed the

---

[*] Florida Senate Bill 0660 was signed into law in 1998.

notion through the legislature to become state law. When asked about the dearth of supporting scientific data, the legislator responded, "What harm can it do?"*

The French politician Georges Clemenceau when asked to comment upon the evolution of armed conflict between nations in the twentieth century, said, "war is too important to be left to the generals"; we cannot afford to let this paradigm characterize the role of statisticians and epidemiologists in research interpretation. Things may not be so great when statisticians and epidemiologists are involved, but unwarranted decisions commonly occur when they are not.

Those who entertained the naïve hope that they can find an easy way out of critical discussion in science by reflexively accepting *p*-values have earned their fare share of criticism. However, it would be wrong to conclude that thoughtless decisions must inescapably accompany significance testing.

5.9 Proper Research Interpretation

Significance testing continues to have vigorous detractors, and opposition to its use still runs deep in the epidemiology community. Nevertheless, the use of *p*-values in general, and the 0.05 threshold of significance in particular, continues to have staunch defenders in the research community. Most recently it has been argued by Efron [23] that the

> ...0.05 significance cutoff has been used literally millions of times since Fisher proposed it in the early 1900's. It has become a standard of objective comparison in all areas of science. I don't think that the .05 could stand up to such intense use it wasn't producing basically correct scientific inferences most of the time.

If statisticians and epidemiologists are to have a shared role in research interpretation the appropriate role of significance testing in research efforts has to be identified. Perhaps it can be found in the following line of reasoning.

It is undeniable that sampling error must be addressed in sample-based research. The compromise investigators make in selecting a sample (mandating that they give up the ability to answer the research question with certainty) injects sample-to-sample variability in their work.† The tendency of a population with one effect size to produce different samples each with a different effect size presents an important obstacle to generalizing sample findings back to the population.

Both the confidence interval and *p*-value quantify the component of sampling error in a research effort's results. The confidence interval, by providing a range of values for the population parameter, gives an overt expression of this variability. Alternatively, by providing only one number, the *p*-value lends itself to dichotomous decisions regarding the strength of evidence that an analysis provides for a particular scientific hypothesis. This estimate is more succinct than that of the confidence interval.

---

* No one has demonstrated any direct, adverse effect on the children. However, purchasing the music required resources, and time spend listening to classical music was time that could not be applied to other activities that had demonstrated their educational value.
† This is discussed at length in Chapter One.

It is this final distillation that is one of the roots of difficulty with significance testing. The concentration of a research result down to a single number is the foundation of the p-value. The p-value is itself constructed from several components: (1) sample size, (2) effect size, (3) the precision of the estimate, and (4) a sampling error assessment.[*] Each of these ingredients is important in the assessment of research interpretation.

However, by integrating them all into the p-value, the investigator commonly succumbs to the temptation of not interpreting each component for itself. Instead he withholds assessment of the research effort until these important components are mathematically integrated into the p-value and judges only the magnitude of the p-value. He has permitted a multidimensional problem (made up of sample size, effect size, effect size precision, and sampling error) to be reduced down to a one-dimensional problem (simply assessing the magnitude of the p-value). Like trying to understand a company by simply examining its yearly income tax bill, much useful information is lost in this incomplete assessment (Figure 5.1).

Much is lost in this dimensionality reduction. The mathematical combination of these four components into the p-value has led to the commonly held belief that the p-value is greater than the sum of its parts. Actually, it is less than this sum. Sample size, effect size, effect size variability, and sampling error go into the p-value. What emerges is not a balanced assessment of each, but instead only a measure of the role of sampling error. Four ingredients go in, and one very different product emerges. This is the basis for much of the criticism of the p-value [24].

Therefore, p-values can be fine descriptors of the role of sampling error. However, they are quite deficient in summarizing an analysis and must be supplemented by additional information, specifically research methodology, sample size, effect size, and effect size precision. The joint consideration of each of these is necessary in order for the study to have a fair and balanced interpretation.

The methodology of the research effort is an important, perhaps, the most important consideration in drawing conclusions from a research effort. If the research is poorly designed or is executed discordantly,[†] then statistical estimators are flawed. In this circumstance, effect size estimators, estimates of its variability, p-values, and confidence intervals are distorted. In this unfortunate set of circumstances, the research effort cannot be interpreted.

---

[*] This last measure is incorporated by applying a probability assessment to the test statistic, i.e., by computing the probabilty of a value at least as large as the test statistic.

[†] Discordant execution is the process by which the study is not executed in accordance with its protocol, but meanders, changing its endpoints and analyses based on the observed data.

Information Needed for Research Result Interpretation

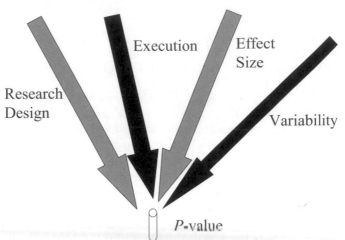

Fig. 5.1. The *p*-value is too small a repository to contain all of the necessary information about the research result.

In concordant research execution, these four statistical estimators have the desirable properties that justify their use. However, they must be interpreted jointly. *P*-value should contribute to, not subsume this integrative process.

This point requires reemphasis. *P*-values receive important attention in applied statistics and epidemiology. However, they provide only an estimate of the role of sampling error in the research effort, nothing more. *P*-values are not the repository of judgment for the study. *P*-values do not measure effect size, nor do they convey the extent of study discordance. These other factors must be determined by a careful critical review of the research effort. Reflexively responding to *p*-values as though it is the sum of all of its ingredients, when in fact it is less than its sum, often leads to inappropriate conclusions from research efforts.

However, the joint consideration of research methodology, sample size, effect size, effect size variability, confidence intervals, and *p*-values, though clearly requiring more effort, are more likely to lead to the proper research interpretation while protecting the *p*-values function as an appropriate reflection of the community and regulatory standard for type I error rate consideration.

References

1. Fiore AE, Nuorti JP, Levine OS et al. (1998) Epidemic Legionnaires' disease two decades later: old sources, new diagnostic methods. *Clinical Infectectious Disease* **26**:426–33.
2. Fisher RA (1925) *Statistical methods for research workers.* Edinburg; Oliver and Boyd.

3. Fisher RA (1926) The arrangement of field experiments. *Journal of the Ministry of Agriculture.* September 503–513.
4. Owen DB (1976) *On the History of Probability and Statistics.* New York; Marcel-Dekker.
5. Edwards A (1972) *Likelihood.* Cambridge; Cambridge University Press.
6. Neyman J, Peason ES (1933) On the problem of the most efficienyt tests of statistical hypotheses. *Philosophical Transactions of the Royal Society (London) Se A.* **231**: 289–337.
7. Pytkowsi W (1932) The dependence of the income in small farms upon their area, the outlay and the capital invested in cows, (Polish, English summaries), Monograph no. 31 of series Bioblioteka Pulawska, publ. Agri. Res. Inst. Pulasy, Poland Wald A (1950) *Statistical Decision Functions* New York; Wiley.
8. Neyman J (1937) Outline of a theoray of statsitical estimation based on the classical theory of probabilitiy. *Philosophical Transactions of the Royal Society (London) Ser A.* **236**:333–380.
9. Neyman J (1938) L'estimation statistique traitée comme un problème classique de probabilité. *Actual. Sceint. Instust* **739**:25–57.
10. Berkson J (1942) Experiences with tests of significance. A reply to R.A. Fisher. *Journal of the American Statistical Association* **37**:242–246.
11. Berkson J (1942) Tests of significance considered as evidence. *Journal of the American Statistical Association* **37**:335–345.
12. Fisher RA (1942) Response to Berkson. *Journal of the American Statistical Association* **37**:103–104.
13. Goodman SN (1999) Toward evidence–based medical statistics. 1: The *p*-value fallacy. *Annals of Internal Medicine* **130**:995–1004.
14. Hill B (1953) Observation and experiment. *New England Journal of Medicine* **248**:995–1001.
15. Kleinbaum DG, Kupper LL, Morgenstern H (1982) *Epidemiologic Research: Principles and Quantitative Methods.* New York; Van Nostrand Reinhold Company.
16. Anonymous (1988) Evidence of casue and efect relationship in major epidemiologic study disputed by judge. *Epidemiology Monitor* **9**:1.
17. Walker AM (1986) Significance tests represent consensus a and standard practice (Letter) *American Journal of Public Health.***76**:1033 (See also journal erratum**76**:1087.
18. Fleiss JL (1986) Significance tests have a role in epidemiologic research; reactions to A.M. Walker (Different Views) *American Journal of Public Health* **76**:559–560.
19. Fleiss JL (1986) Confidence intervals versus significance tests: quantitative interpretation (Letter) *American Journal of Public Health* **76**:587.
20. Fleiss JL Dr. Fleiss response(Letter)(1986) *American Journal of Public Health* **76**:1033–1034.
21. Walker AM (1986) Reporting the results of epidemiologic studies. *American Journal of Public Health* **76**:556–558.
22. Poole C (1987) Beyond the confidence interval. *American Journal of Public Health* **77**. 195–199.
23. Efron B (2005) Bayesians, frequentists, and scientists. *Journal of the American Statistical Association.* **100**:1–5.

24. Lang JM, Rothman KJ, Cann DI (1998) That confounded *p*-value. *Epidemiology* **9**:7–8.

6

P-values, Power, and Efficacy

6.1 Introduction

It is a truism that the purpose of healthcare research is to demonstrate the existence (or nonexistence) of a relationship in the population based on the sample's results. However, this examination presumes that the magnitude of that relationship is worth detecting. If, for example, there is a relationship between genotype and the ability of HMG-CoA reductase inhibitors to reduce low-density lipid (LDL cholesterol levels), then it is a natural assumption that this is an effect that is large enough to bring to the attention of the medical and regulatory community. Demonstrating a 30% improvement in the ability of a statin to reduce LDL cholesterol level in one genotype has important clinical implications. Demonstrating a 3% reduction galvanizes no one. According to the saying, "A difference, to be a difference, must make a difference."

This chapter will demonstrate that the p-value alone does not provide useful information about an effect that is seen in a clinical research effort. It also discusses how one combines event rates, type I error rates, and the anticipated effectiveness of a clinical trial to demonstrate power.

6.2 P-values and Strength of Evidence

As we saw earlier, Fisher's early work in significance testing produced a rigid structure for scientific hypothesis testing. Many statisticians argued for an inflexible null and alternative hypothesis. In this scenario, the data would be used to make a dichotomous decision—rejection or non-rejection of the null hypothesis. Here, one only needed to know whether the p-value was less than the prospectively declared alpha level. Whether it fell in the critical region was more relevant that its actual value.[*]

Fisher argued that the magnitude of the p-value itself, and not just whether it was less than the *a priori* type I error level was useful. To Fisher, the p-value was not about simply rejecting the null hypothesis. It was about strength of evidence.

---

[*] Critical regions are defined in Chapter Three.

The lower the *p*-value was, the less likely it was that a population with no effect between exposure and disease would produce a sample that had the observed effect magnitude. Thus, the smaller the *p*-value the greater the statistical significance of the effect, and the greater the effect size itself.

In response to his vehement arguments, the convention of reporting the findings of significance testing changed. Initially, the results of significance testing were reported by simply stating whether the *p*-value was less than or greater than 0.05. Eventually, this was altered to actually reporting the magnitude of the *p*-value In this circumstance, a *p*-value < 0.001 demonstrated a greater effect size than a *p*-value = 0.01 that in turn represented a greater effect size than a *p*-value of 0.04.

6.2.1 Example

Linking *p*-values and effect size magnitude is often attractive, but is built on the false assumption that the only mutable component of the *p*-value is the effect size.

As an illustration, a randomized controlled clinical trial recruits 500 patients. Half of these patients are recruited to the control group. The remaining 250 are randomized to receive active therapy. In this clinical study, there are two endpoints. One endpoint is the effect of the therapy on the fatal/nonfatal myocardial infarction (MI) rate, and the second endpoint is the effect of therapy on total mortality. The study is well-designed and concordantly executed. The investigator carries out an analysis on each of these two endpoints, reporting the *p*-values for each of these (Table 6.1).

Table 6.1. Effect of therapy on each of total mortality and fatal/nonfatal MI: Sample size and *p*- values from a clinical trial with two endpoints.

Endpoint	N=500	*P*-value
Fatal/Nonfatal MI	250	0.091
Total Mortality	250	0.013

If we use the threshold of 0.05 as statistically significant, then we can observe that the effect of therapy on the total mortality rate is significant, while the effect of therapy on the fatal/nonfatal MI rate is not. Furthermore, if we accept that the magnitude of the *p*-value provides useful information about strength of association, we would also conclude that the therapy had greater effect on the total mortality rate than on the fatal/nonfatal MI endpoint. One could easily construct an argument from the results of Table 3.1 that there was a more important effect of the therapy on reducing total mortality then on the fatal/nonfatal MI rate. This would in turn lead to predictable discussions about the effect of the therapy on causes of death not related to MI, an effect that would be driving the low *p*-value.

These conclusions are wrong, however, and would have to be modulated based on a more complete demonstration of the results of the data (Table 6.2).

Table 6.2. Effect of therapy on each of total mortality and fatal/nonfatal MI. Sample size, p- values and percent reduction in events from a clinical trial with two endpoints.

Endpoint	N=500	Percent Reduction in Events	P-value
Fatal/Nonfatal MI	250	33	0.091
Total Mortality	250	33	0.013

Table 6.2 reveals an unexpected aspect of the results. Even though the p-values for the effect of therapy on each of the two endpoints are dramatically different, and the sample sizes are the same., the percent reduction in events is actually the same for each of the two evaluations.

The active therapy is associated with a 33% reduction in events for total mortality. A large reduction in these events might have been anticipated from the relatively small p-value associated with this effect. However, if we accept the notion that the p-value magnitude is related to the effect size, then the 33% reduction in events associated with the effect of therapy on the fatal/nonfatal MI rate in unanticipated. In fact, the equivalence of sample size and effect size begs the question of why the p-values are not the same. The answer is provided in an evaluation of the event rates for the two endpoints (Table 6.3).

Table 6.3. Effect of therapy on each of total mortality and fatal/nonfatal MI: Sample size, control group event rate, p- values and percent reduction in events from a clinical trial with two endpoints.

Endpoint	N=500	Control Group Event Rate	Percent Reduction in Events	P-value
Fatal/Nonfatal MI		0.15	33	0.091
Total Mortality		0.30	33	0.013

We see that what is difference between the two analyses is the percentage of events. In this trial, there were $(0.15)(250) + (0.15(0.66)(250) = 63$ patients who had either a fatal or nonfatal MI. However, an examination of the total number of deaths in the study reveals that $(0.30)(250) + (0.30)(0.66)(250) = 125$ patients died. The percent reduction was the same for the two therapies, but, because there were more events for the total mortality endpoint, the p-value was substantially smaller. Therefore, in this circumstance, the driving force behind the p-value is not the effect size, but the difference in the underlying number of events.

The point of this example is to show, that, although the effect size is related to the *p*-value, other data-derived measures are also involved. The joint involvement is multidimensional (Figure 6.1).

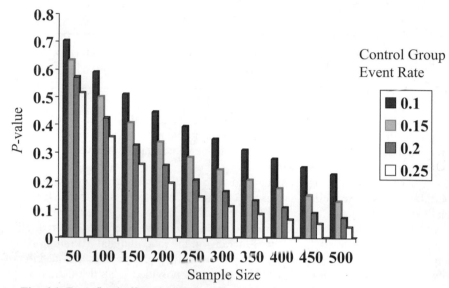

Fig. 6.1. For a fixed effect size (30% reduction in events), the *p*-value is a function of the number of subjects and the control group event rate.

Figure 6.1 reveals the relationship among the *p*-value, the sample size (total number of subjects in the study), and the control group event rate. The effect size (in this case the percent reduction in events produced by the intervention) is 30%. for every computation reflected in this figure. We can see that for the same effect size, the *p*-value will decrease with either (1) an increase in the control group event rate, or (2) an increase in the sample size.

While an examination of the mathematics would quickly reveal why this is so, it may be more helpful to consider the underlying process. If a therapy is being evaluated to decrease a clinical event of interest (such as total mortality), then there must be deaths to evaluate. The greater the number of deaths in the study, the easier it is not only to measure precisely the mortality rate in the control group and the treatment group, but also to be assured that the percent change in deaths produced by the intervention is likely not due to the random aggregation of events. The occurrence of five deaths in a study, three occurring in the active group and two in the control group, reflects a 1/3 reduction in deaths. However, it is also likely that the random aggregation of patients in a sample might have generated this differential when there was no effect of therapy in the population.

Alternatively, if there are 500 deaths in the study, with 300 control group deaths and 200 deaths in the active group, it is much less likely that the difference of 100 deaths is due to chance alone. In general there are three ways to increase the number of events in a study of this kind: the first is to choose an event and a sample such that that the control group event rate is large, and the second is to increase the sample size of the study. A third method is to choose a combined endpoint. These procedures each add endpoints to the data. They therefore improve the interpretability of the experiment by channeling a strong enough signal through the effect size to drown out the background sampling error noise.

6.3 Power

The evaluation of the previous example is a little unnerving. The effect size is the same. Yet as presented above, some circumstances would be treated as a positive result, while other results would be seen as null. Nevertheless, each of them reflect a 30% reduction in the death rate. Are the settings where the *p*-value is greater than 0.05 to be dismissed?

They must not, for the single reason of power. The circumstances where a 30% reduction was identified with a *p*-value of greater than 0.05 does not necessary imply that there is no effect in the population at large. The best interpretation of this finding is based on power.

Recall that there are two type of errors that one can make in the population. One is the likelihood that the treatment effect, obviously apparent in the sample, is not present in the population. At this point, we have come to recognize this as an issue involving type I sampling error and is addressed by an *a priori* allocation of alpha and by the *p*-value at the trial's conclusion. If the experiment is concordantly executed, the *p*-value is interpretable.

However, there is another sampling error issue. What is the correct conclusion of the experiment if the investigator's test statistic did not fall into the critical region, as was the case for many of the settings in Figure 5.1? Does this finding imply that the treatment is not successful and will not produce the required level of efficacy in the population?

This is also a conclusion with important implications, and again the critics home in, armed with a different question. How likely is it that the treatment is effective in the population, but the population has misled the investigator by producing a sample that shows no efficacy? This is type II error.

Let's consider the thought process of this error in more detail. The investigator's significance test falls in the critical region and critics wonder about the spectrum of samples produced from a population in which there is no efficacy. The population produces many samples, some of which will mirror efficacy and some of which will not. In this circumstance, the issue is one of minimizing the probability that the population will produce a sample that appears to suggest efficacy.

However, for the type II error, we shift the paradigm. Before we assumed that there was no efficacy in the population, Now, we assume that population efficacy exists. If this treatment effect is present in the population, we want the sample to reflect it. The probability that the sample does not reflect this positive population finding is termed the probability of type II error, or the beta error.

We saw in Chapter Three that power is simply $1 - \beta$ It has become common for investigators to refer to the beta error subtracted from one. The power of an experiment is the probability that the population in which the treatment is effective produces a sample that mirrors this effect, i.e., that a population with embedded efficacy produces a sample with embedded efficacy. Unlike alpha, power is to be maximized. The greater the power, the more confidence we have that the population has not misled us.

Power is crucial in experimental interpretation. Experiments in which the null hypothesis is rejected are called positive. However, what is the correct conclusion if the null hypothesis is not rejected? This is the circumstance in Figure 5.1 Are the results negative?

The correct answer is — only when there is adequate power. Power is critical in experimental interpretation when the *p*-value is large. In this circumstance, there is sometimes irresistible temptation to call the experiment negative, and the treatments equivalent. However, the lower power level tells us that it is quite possible that the population contains important treatment differences, but produced a sample suggesting no benefit of therapy. Therefore, since the probability of being misled by a nonrepresentative sample is high, treatment equivalence in the sample (i.e., non-rejection of the null hypothesis) does not translate to treatment equivalence in the population. With adequate power, the likelihood of a misleading sample is small, and can be confident in translating sample treatment equivalence to population treatment equivalence (Figure 6.2).

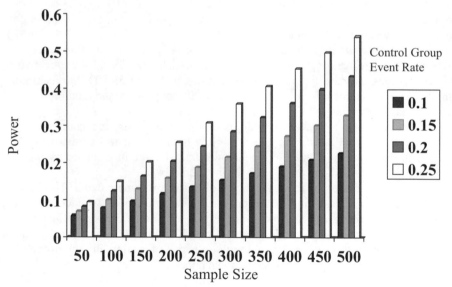

Fig. 6.2. For a fixed effect size (30% reduction in events), the the power is low for combinations of small event rates and sample sizes.

Suppose I tell a friend of mine, "I know that in the basement of this house there is a precious jewel. Go down, find it, and make us both rich." My friend immediately begins the search, but after many minutes, returns, tired and soiled, replying quietly, "My friend, the jewel is not there – but I never turned the light on". Can I believe the jewel is missing? How can I believe the conclusion of the search if the search was flawed? Even if the jewel was there, he would not have found it; so how can I believe there is no jewel just because he says there is none? An underpowered research effort is a search with the lights turned off. We will very likely never find the jewel. For our (re)search to be persuasive, we must have our searchlights on.

6.4 No Way Out?

It is easy to see how a researcher, at the conclusion of his research effort, can feel hemmed in by new and persistent critics. They left him alone during both the design and the execution of the experiment. However, as soon as he attempts to draw con-clusions from his sample, hesitant and circumspect as these conclusions may be, the specter of sampling error rises up. Positive results might be the result of a type I error.

Alternatively, negative results do not open an escape route from these crit-ics. If the test statistic does not fall in the critical region, demonstrating no relation-ship between the treatment and the disease, the critics close in again, now directing their queries to the possibility of a type II error. Isn't it possible that there was an effect in the population, but again through the play of chance, the population pro-duced a sample that demonstrated no relationship. Critics relentlessly remind him that his findings may be nothing at all, merely the freak of chance in the population. Like a weed, sampling error rises up to strangle the early blossom of his result.

We know that the smaller the alpha error, the better. Now we know that the greater the power, the better. However, we saw in Chapter Three that we cannot adjust one without affecting the other. Decreasing the type I error must lead to an increase in the type II error, and trying to reduce the type II error leads to alpha error inflation.[*] We cannot (touching no other part of the experiment), decrease alpha without decreasing power; nor can we increase power without increasing the type I error.

The thought process is very revealing here. Suppose, during the design phase of the study, we wish to adjust the experiment by decreasing the alpha error. By reducing the alpha error, we reduce the probability that the population that has no response to therapy produces a sample that appears to demonstrate a positive response. How do we specifically decrease this probability? We do this by making the criteria for efficacy in the sample very strong, even extreme. However, if we make the criteria too extreme, it is possible that moderate efficacy will be embed-ded in the sample but because it does not meet the extreme criteria, will not be ac-cepted as representative of the population; it will be interpreted as no effect. Thus, the presence of efficacy in the population would not be accepted because the effi-cacy signal from the sample is not extreme enough. This is a beta error. Our attempt to reduce the likelihood of an alpha error has made it easier to miss efficacy in our sample, if there is in fact efficacy in the population. We have overtly diminished alpha but unwittingly have diminished power as well.

However, there is a way out. The only way simultaneously to minimize al-pha and maximize power is to increase the number of observations. By increasing the size of the sample, the investigator improves the precision of the efficacy esti-

---

[*] A review of Figure 3.8 demonstrates that moving the critical region in a way to decrease the type I error must, of necessity, increase the type II error.

mate, making it easier to distinguish between the distribution of the efficacy measurement under the null hypothesis from its distribution under the alternative hypothesis. Thus, sample size computations are critical in insuring that the investigator has the correct balance of alpha and power.

6.5 Sample Size Computations

Sample size computations are a requirement in modern healthcare research. Every
grant, every thesis, every design manuscript purporting to discuss healthcare issues
must contain a detailed set of these computations. They represent more than just
evidence of concern for the optimum utility of scared healthcare resources; in addition, their presence reflects a level of careful forethought about the research effort.

Many textbooks and manuscripts discuss sample size computations[*] Those
most commonly used in clinical research are provided in Appendix B of this text.
This discussion concerns the issues about sample size computations that are not
addressed by the arithmetic.

6.5.1 The Anvil

One of the most important lessons to learn about sample size computation is that
they are often not about sample size at all. The computations may have been initially motivated by stark concerns about type I and type II error. However, they
reflect other pressing considerations as well. Like a political gravity well, the sample size computation attracts important clinical research forces each of which has a
different goal, aligning them so that the research's execution lines up with its goal.

Sample size computations are the table over which important research
agendas meet and collide, ultimately deciding the purpose and direction of the effort. This is not sinister; in fact, it is very appropriate and, when the conversations
are frank and meaningful, give the research effort a much better chance for success.
The discussions must be clear, exposing these agenda's for all to see.

During this period of the design of the experiment, there are several teams
of workers, each dedicated to the success of the research effort, e.g., a clinical trial.
First, there are the investigators; they understand the clinical setting, are familiar
with the types of patients who would be recruited, are knowledgeable about their
availability, and are experienced with the treatment that is to be tested.

Secondly, there is a team of epidemiologists and biostatisticians; they have
the capability of assessing strengths and weaknesses of experimental designs and
can identify the frequency with which the endpoint of the trial will occur. Finally,
there are the administrators, who will be involved in planning the logistics of the
experiment; they must also pay for it.

Early in the trial's design phase, discussions proceed largely within each
of these groups, investigators speaking with other investigators about the potential
risk–benefit balance of the intervention, epidemiologists and biostatisticians discussing event rates, and administrators discussing costs and funding. It is the sample size computation that brings these teams into direct contact. Each group con-

---

[*] References 18 through 23 in Chapter Two are among the most useful in sample size computation.

tributes a critical assumption or data to this discussion revealing its own thought processes to the other teams. It is frank, refreshing and, when collegially handled, results in a strong trial design. The resulting sample size is mathematically consistent and logical but also integrates the necessary logistical and financial considerations.

The sample size computation is the anvil on which the trial design is finally hammered. However, while it is based on mathematics, it also includes a healthy, necessary dose of "political arithmetic."

6.6. Non-statistical Considerations

Sample size formulas explicitly include important statistical concepts. However, their starkness requires them to exclude important influences that must nevertheless be factored into the final sample size consideration. Chief among these non-statistical concerns are material and personnel costs.

The calculations described in Appendix B serve no good purpose if followed blindly. For example, suppose a clinical trial is designed to assess the effect of a therapy to prevent the occurrence of stroke. The investigators believe that the three year incidence of stroke in the age range of interest is 0.10 and that intervention will reduce the incidence by 15%. They prospectively declare a two-sided type I error rate of 0.05 and 90% power. Then the sample size (active and control patients) is

$$N = \frac{2\left[p_c\left(1-p_c\right) + p_t\left(1-p_t\right)\right]\left[Z_{1-\alpha/2} - Z_\beta\right]^2}{\Delta^2}.$$

In this case, the cumulative control group stroke rate is $p_c = 0.10$. Since the medication will reduce this rate by 15%, the treatment group rate is $p_t = (1-0.15)(0.10) = 0.085$. From this we can easily compute

$$\Delta^2 = \left(p_c - p_t\right)^2 = (0.10 - 0.085)^2 = .00023.$$

A two-sided type I error of 0.05 allows us to write $Z_{1-\alpha/2} = 1.96$. Similarly, power of 90% produces $Z_\beta = -1.28$. Thus, the sample size computation becomes

$$N = \frac{2\left[(0.10)(1-0.10) + 0.085(1-0.085)\right]\left[1.96 - (-1.28)\right]^2}{0.00023}$$

$$= \frac{2(0.16778)(10.50)}{0.00023} = 15,320.$$

Thus, 15,320 patients are required for the study, 7,660 in each group. However this calculation is useless when only 5,000 patients total (i.e., control group + active group) are available. Similarly, if only $3,000,000 has been raised to fund the study, defending a sample size that suggests that $8,000,000 is required to execute and analyze it is an exercise in futility. These considerations of resource availability are important, if not paramount; yet, they are not explicitly considered in the sample size design.

The most effective way to inject these concepts into the sample size consideration is to incorporate them indirectly into the discussions about event rates. This is not to say that the event rates are rendered imprecise because of logistical considerations. Quite the contrary, the event rates estimates are clearly sheathed in epidemiology and biostatistics. However, cost and other factors that show up in the sample size computations must have their influence felt in the design, direction and goal of the trial, as demonstrated by the following example. .

6.6.1 The LRC Sample Size

The Lipid Research Clinics (LRC) trial was an important experiment examining the role of cholesterol management and reductions in morbidity and mortality in atherosclerotic cardiovascular disease. The difficulties and compromises achieved during its sample size computation serves as an exemplary example of meshing logistical concerns with sample size computations.

As originally conceived, LRC would test the ability of a cholesterol reducing agent, cholestyramine, to reduce the number of mortal events. Men between 35 and 60 years of age with total cholesterol levels greater than 265 mg/dl would be randomized to receive either diet alone or diet plus cholestyramine for the management of their lipid levels. Patients would be followed for seven years. The end point of the study was coronary heart disease death (primarily fatal myocardial infarction (MI). The sample size estimate returned by the statisticians was, depending upon the assumptions for type I /type II error rates, between 12,000 and 15,000 patients.

This estimate came as shock to the investigators who believed that they could only randomize and follow between 3,000 and 5,000 patients. The sample size required was three to four times greater than their ability to recruit patients. The trial designers appeared to be at an impasse.

It is important in this example to first note what the investigators correctly avoided doing. They did not move forward with the study as originally designed. Specifically, they avoided the temptation to sanction the sample size and then blithely execute the experiment, vowing to "do the best they could" to randomize 15,000 patients when they knew their best evidence suggested they could randomize only a third of that number. Taking this tack would have guaranteed a trial that would not meet its sample size goal and constitute an underpowered examination of the important research question.

Instead, they reconsidered the underlying assumptions of the sample size, focusing on the event rate of the study. They knew that not many patients would die of an MI; this was the major reason why the sample size computed by the statisticians was so large. However, they wondered what would happen if they modified the endpoint, adding to the fatal MI component those patients who sustained a nonfatal MI. Since the total number of fatal and nonfatal MI's was greater than the number of fatal MI's alone, fewer patients could be followed to get a more frequent endpoint, and the sample size would be substantially reduced, In addition, the pathogenesis of nonfatal MI was quite similar to that of fatal MI, so that it was expected that reductions in total cholesterol levels would reduce the number of nonfatal MIs as well. Thus, by changing the endpoint of the study, the investigators reduced the sample size to less than 4,000 while remaining true to their study hypothesis. Good communication between the design teams of the study led to a favorable sample size outcome.[*]

6.7 The "Good Enough for Them" Approach

The laudable re-computation of the LRC sample size during the design phase of the study is an increasingly common occurrence in clinical trials. Schisms between sample size computation and resource availability are best resolved by thoughtful scientists carefully reconsidering experimental programs during their design phase. However, in some experiments, one investigator simply duplicates the sample size of a previous positive study, investing no new thought into the sample size requirement of her own work.

Consider an investigator who is working with the MI model in rats. She notices that a previous investigator has, with 30 mice, demonstrated the efficacy of a compound to improve post-MI heart structure. She wishes to repeat the experiment with a different but related medication. Since the first investigator was able to reject the null hypothesis based on 30 mice, this second investigator plans to study thirty mice as well. After all, it worked for investigator #1.

The difficulty with this approach is that it considers only the positive scenario, and will most likely be uninterpretable if the research effort does not reject the null hypothesis. If the test statistic falls into the critical region, the investigator has essentially "gotten away with it." However, if the second investigator's study is negative, then what is the best conclusion?

At this point in our discussions, we know that a *prima facie* null research finding (i.e., the null hypothesis is not rejected) requires an explicit consideration of the power of the research effort. With inadequate power, the likelihood that the population (of mice) receives benefit but produces a small sample that does not demonstrate this benefit is great. Thus, even if the effect of interest were apparent in the population, it is likely that, in this small sample, the effect would not be produced.

Sample sizes that are based only on an identification of a positive finding and do not explicitly consider power in their computation will be un-interpretable when the null hypothesis is rejected. In this circumstance, the experiment will be interpreted not as null, but instead as "uninformative."

6.8 Efficacy Seduction

A review of Appendix C by the discerning investigator will reveal an interesting relationship between the sample size and the effect size. The sample size decreases as the square of the efficacy increases. Thus, a small increase in the expected strength of the relationship between either (1) the exposure and disease or (2) the

---

[*] Much more will be said about the use of a composite endpoint in Chapter Nine.

intervention and disease reduction produces a relatively large decrease in the sample size.

Thus, just as larger objects require less magnification (and less expensive telescopes) to visualize, larger effect sizes in clinical research require smaller (and less expensive) samples to identify. Thus, the uninitiated investigator, taken aback by an initial large sample size estimate, is commonly tempted to reduce the required sample size by increasing the desired size of the effect he wishes the research to identify.

This well-established relationship resonates with physician-scientists. Investigators involved in clinical trial design can have strong convictions about an intervention's ability to have a beneficial impact on patients. The relationship between effect size and sample size is sometimes taken as an encouragement to make an even bolder statement about the effect of the intervention. Increasing the effectiveness of the intervention from, for example, a 20% reduction in event rate to a 30% reduction can be more closely aligned with their hopes while simultaneously permitting a smaller sample size with its associated lower cost and administrative burden.

For example, consider an experiment in which the investigator believes he has a therapy that reduces the occurrence of stroke in patients at risk of thromboembolic events. His sample size computation is based on a two-sided type I error of 0.05, power of 90%, and a cumulative stroke mortality rate of 0.25 in the placebo group. He believes the therapy will reduce the cumulative stroke rate from 0.25 to 0.20, a 20% reduction. This computation reveals a trial size (patients in active group plus patients in the control group) of 2,922. However, he sees from Appendix B that by assuming a 35% reduction in stroke (leading to a cumulative stroke event rate of 0.163 in the intervention group,) he has reduced the sample size from 2,922 to 890, a 70% reduction!

However, this seductive line of reasoning is quite misleading. Increasing the efficacy with the sole purpose of reducing the sample size denies the investigator the ability to identify more moderate levels of clinical efficacy with statistical signficance.

6.8.1 Efficacy and Sample Size

The effect size is the expected difference in the endpoint event rates between the control and active groups in the clinical trial.[*] Clinical trial designers commonly confront the relationship between the effect size and sample size, on the one hand, and the relationship between effect size and community standard, on the other. Each of these relationships must be understood if the investigators are to use this potent efficacy-sample size relationship without sacrificing the research design they seek to strengthen.

Efficacy is the measure of effect that is derived from the clinical trial. If the primary analysis in the clinical trial is the effect of therapy on a dichotomous endpoint, e.g., total mortality, then the efficacy of the therapy is commonly defined

---

[*] It is frequently measured by percent reduction of efficacy in clinical trials. This is known as the relative risk. In observational studies, it can be measured as either a relative risk, or more commonly as an odds ratio.

as the percent reduction in the event rate produced by the therapy. For example, if the cumulative total mortality rate is 20% in the control group and 15% in the active group of the clinical trial, then the efficacy is $(0.20-0.15)/0.20 = 0.25$ or 25%. If the sample was collected with strict adherence to the inclusion and exclusion criteria and the clinical trial was executed concordantly, then the 25% reduction seen in the primary analysis will be an accurate measure of what could be anticipated in the population.[*] The strength of the finding is further enhanced by the observation that the efficacy produced in the sample is very unlikely to be due to chance alone.

Thus, in order to make the most persuasive argument to the medical and regulatory communities, the designated effect size of a clinical trial must be both clinically meaningful and statistically significant.[†] A clinically meaningful but statistically insignificant finding would be, for example, a study that identified a 40% reduction in total mortality attributable to the therapy, but had an associated p-value of 0.25. Even though the effect size is great, the large p-value suggests that it is quite likely that a population in which the intervention had no beneficial effect could produce a sample with a 40 mortality reduction.

6.8.2. Large P-values and Small Effect Sizes

As we pointed out earlier, clinical trial results are often described in terms of the p-value as though the p-value alone conveys the strength of evidence of the findings. The previous section described the disconnect that can occur when a large p-value is associated with an effect size of clinical significance. However, a small p-value linked to a small effect size is also problematic.

Such a mismatch occurred with the LRC study. As discussed earlier in this chapter,[‡] LRC was designed to demonstrate that the sustained reduction of cholesterol would lower the incidence of fatal and nonfatal MI heart attacks. The investigators, having produced a p-value for the primary analysis of less than 0.05, announced that their study was positive.[§]

However, an examination of the clinical findings raised important questions hidden by a cursory assessment of the p-value. The seven-year cumulative incidence of fatal and nonfatal MI's was 8.6% in the placebo group. In the active group, the cumulative event rate was 7.0. These findings represented a 19% reduction in the fatal/nonfatal MI rate associated with cholestyramine. It is useful to ask what this reduction means for the population to be treated. Simply put, in order to prevent one fatal or nonfatal MI, 63 men would have to be treated for seven years. This is a modest treatment effect at best. In addition, the cost of this treatment would be $12,000 per patient. Thus, $756,000 would be spent on 63 patients to pre-

---

[*] Since samples are subject to sample-to-sample variability or sampling effort, different samples from the same population will produce different estimates of the effect size. While this random, sample-to-sample variability can be measured by the standard deviation of the effect size, it is more commonly reflected in the 95% confidence interval for the effect size.

[†] This assumes, as we will assume throughout the chapter, that the clinical trial was concordantly executed.

[‡] Section 5.6.1.

[§] There was considerable controversy concerning this p-value. See Chapter Five.

vent one heart attack. While the *p*-value was small, the clinical benefit was unfortunately modest.

In a well-designed, concordantly executed experiment, the *p*-value can provide useful information concerning the role sampling error may have played in the study's results. However, additional, thoughtful examinations of the data and the effect size are required to provide an assessment of the benefits of the therapy. The *p*-value does not.

6.9 Number Needed To Treat

To measure the effect of therapy in a clinical trial, a commonly used parameter is the *number needed to treat*, or *NNT*. This is the number of patients that must be exposed to the therapy in order to prevent one event.

For example, assume that in a given clinical trial designed to reduce the risk of fatal and nonfatal stroke, patients are randomized to either the control group or the intervention group and followed for three years. The three year rate of fatal/nonfatal stroke is 0.17 in the control group, and 0.11 in the intervention group. This reflects an absolute difference of $0.17 - 0.11 = 0.06$.

One way to consider this effect size is to say that, if there were 100 patients treated with control therapy only for three years then there would be (100)(0.17) or 17 patients who had a fatal/nonfatal stroke. However, if those patients had instead been treated with the active therapy then (100)(0.11) or only 11 patients would have suffered this event. Thus, the use of intervention therapy in 100 patients, would, on average be associated with the prevention of $17 - 11$ or 6 events. Since treating 100 patients would prevent 6 fatal/nonfatal strokes, then treating $100/6 = 16.7$ patients would have prevented one event. In this example $NNT = 16.7$.

In general, if p_c is the control group event rate and p_t is the treatment group event rate, then

$$NNT = \frac{1}{p_c - p_t}.$$

NNT can easily be computed from knowledge of the control group event rate, p_c and either the efficacy *e* or relative risk *R*.[*]

In general the smaller the number needed to treat, the more effective the medication. Large *NNT* estimates are the result of either (1) a therapy is relatively non-effective, or (2) the event affected by the therapy is relatively rare, or (3) both. From its formulation, it is easy to examine the effect of the influences (Figure 6.3).

---

[*] For example, if one has the control group event rate p_c and the efficacy (i.e., the percent reduction in events associated with the therapy) *e* where $e = (p_c - p_t)/p_c$, then $NNT = 1/ep_c$. Alternatively, if one has p_c and the relative risk *R* where $R = p_t/p_c$, then $NNT = 1/p_c(1 - R)$.

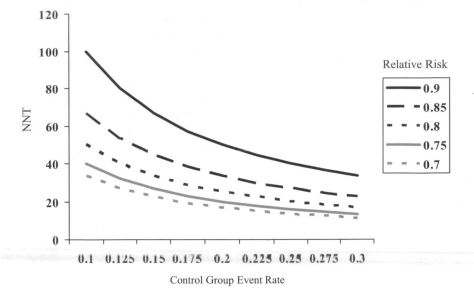

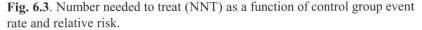

Fig. 6.3. Number needed to treat (NNT) as a function of control group event rate and relative risk.

From Figure 6.3, we see that the number needed to treat decreases as the control group event rate increases. Increasing the control group event rate (everything else being equal) increases the difference between the number of events in the control and active group, decreasing *NNT*. Alternatively a decrease in the relative risk decreases the number of events in the treatment group, again decreasing *NNT*.[*]

6.10 Absolute versus Relative Risk

Figure 6.3 demonstrates that an important ingredient in a low *NNT* is not only a small relative risk but also a large control group event rate. One other way to consider the different ways that effect sizes can be measured in clinical trials with dichotomous endpoints is an examination of the role of relative versus absolute risk. Both relative and absolute risks compare the event rates in the control and intervention group.

Let p_c be the control group event rate in a clinical trial and p_t be the active group event rate. Then the *relative risk reduction* (or *relative risk*) R is computed as $R = p_t / p_c$. The *absolute risk reduction* (or *absolute risk*) A is also easily computed as $A = p_c - p_t$.

---

[*] Similar computations are available in observational studies in which harm is commonly associated with an exposure. In this circumstance, the number needed to harm or NNH is computed.

Each of these computations provides important, complimentary information about the magnitude of the effect of therapy. For example, consider a clinical trial with two primary endpoints: the first is total mortality and the second is the cumulative incidence of fatal stroke. The one-year cumulative total mortality rate in the study is 0.06 in the control group ($p_c = 0.06$); the event rate for the active group is 0.03, reflecting a 50% reduction in the cumulative total mortality event rate that is attributable to therapy (i.e., $R = p_c / p_t = 0.03/0.06 = 0.50$).

The investigators also observe that the fatal ischemic stroke rate for the control group is 0.005. The treatment group rate is 0.0025, producing a relative risk of 0.50 as well. Thus, the therapy produced the same relative risk for each of these two endpoints (Table 6.4)

Table 6.4. Comparison of relative and absolute risks for two endpoints in a clinical trial

Endpoint	Control Group Rate	Treatment Group Rate	Relative Risk Reduction	Absolute Risk Reduction
Total Mortality	0.0600	0.0300	0.5000	0.0300
Fatal Ischemic Stroke	0.0050	0.0025	0.5000	0.0025

Table 6.4 reveals that the relative risk of therapy for each of these two endpoints is identical. However, the absolute risk afforded by the therapies are quite different, with the absolute risk reduction being substantially greater for the total mortality endpoint. This difference in absolute risk reduction is a reflection of the frequency of the two events in the control group. The control group event rate for the total mortality endpoint is 0.06, over ten times greater than the control group event rate for fatal ischemic stroke. The absolute risk reduction is less for fatal ischemic strokes because of the rarity of this event. Thus, from a population point of view, even though the therapy has the same beneficial effect from a relative risk perspective, the impact of this effect will be substantially reduced in the population since the underlying rate of fatal ischemic stroke is so small.

Of course this differential effect can be measured by computing the *NNT*. For total mortality, we compute

$$NNT(mortality) = \frac{1}{p_c - p_t} = \frac{1}{0.06 - 0.03} = 33.$$

Thus, 33 people would have to be treated to prevent one death. The same computation for the second endpoint reveals

$$NNT(fatal\ ischemic\ stroke) = \frac{1}{p_c - p_t} = \frac{1}{0.005 - 0.0025} = 400,$$

demonstrating that 400 people would require treatment to prevent a fatal ischemic stroke.

These numbers will change based on the population in which the therapy is to be used. For example, based on the current analysis, it would be most effective to use the therapy to reduce mortal events. However, this does not preclude the use of therapy in patients who are at greater risk of fatal ischemic stroke. The one caveat is that the therapy may not have been shown to be as effective in these patients, producing different relative risks.

6.11 Matching Statistical with Clinical Significance
The best advice for investigators is that the efficacy around which the sample size is built should be the minimum effect of the intervention that would justify its use in the population. This smallest efficacy of clinical significance will be defined as the *minimum clinical efficacy.* Since larger efficacy levels will produce smaller sample sizes, these smaller sample sizes will not detect the minimum clincial efficacy with statistical signficance.*

Just as it is best first to determine the correct level of magnification before one chooses the microscope lens to use, the investigator must first determine the size of the treatment effect in the population before he chooses the sample size for the trial. This should be carried out carefully. Choosing a sample size that is too big is not only wasteful,† it expends needless resources to identify insignificantly small clinical effects with acceptable but ultimately unhelpful precision. Choosing a sample size for the clinical trial that is too small, on the other hand, denies the investigators the required precision to identify efficacy levels of clinical interest [1] (Figure 6.4).

Figure 6.4 demonstrates the relationship between the p-value and the number needed for treatment as a function of the sample size (the control group event rate is assumed to be 20%). If the investigators are interested in detecting an effect size equivalent to $NNT = 22$, then a sample size of $n = 1,000$ will produce a p-value that is too large if that effect size is achieved in the sample. Thus, a clinically important effect will be rendered statistically insignificant. Alternatively, a sample size of 4000 will not only reach significance for $NNT = 22$; it will also identify as statistically significant a finding corresponding to $NNT = 40$. Since this larger NNT is clinically irrelevant to the investigations, resources should not be expended to identify this smaller level of effect with great precision. A sample size of 1,500 links the range of NNT that is clinically signicant with a range of p-values signfying statistical significance.

---

* We add a caveat to this statement in section 5.12.
† Wasteful not just in time and money, but in the inconvenience and inadvertent harm that is done to patients who volunteer their time to contribute to the scientific process.

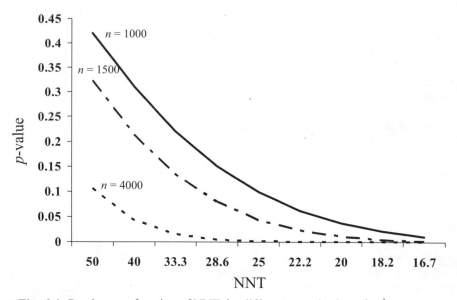

Fig. 6.4. *P*-value as a function of NNT for different sample sizes. As the sample size increases, smaller *p*-values are associated with the same number needed to treat.

The selection of the right level of NNT requires considerable thought from the investigators before the study is designed. In a profession whose professional creed is "First, do no harm," the clinical trial investigators are obligated first to assess the possible problems the therapy can cause in patients who choose to volunteer for their study. These problems include financial hardship as well as the occurrence of undesirable side-effects reasonably believed to be associated with the new intervention. In addition, the current standard of care of the disease for which the medication may be indicated must also be considered. The minimum clinical efficacy is identified after a joint assessment of this standard of care, medication cost, and adverse event profile has been completed. Once these have been carefully evaluated, the minimum clinical efficacy is chosen as the efficacy level that balances these three factors. From this and the anticiapted control group event rate, the number needed to treat can be computed.

Consider, for example, that the intervention is a medication that is proposed to treat a disease for which there are already a panoply of medications. The combination of the available therapies that are already in use are beneficial, well understood, relatively safe, and inexpensive. In this situation where the standard of care is "acceptable," the new medication must demonstrate substantial efficacy in order to justify its use in a clinical environment in which practitioners are comfortable with the risk–benefit balance of the standard treatments. If, in addition, the medication that is being proposed is costly and/or has a new and serious adverse event profile, the efficacy threshold for the medication must be even higher in order to preserve the risk–benefit balance.

On the other hand, consider a clinical trial that is evaluating a medication for the treatment of a condition that has a poorly tolerated standard of care (an example would be acquired immune-deficiency syndrome). Assume that the new medication that the investigators wish to evaluate in a controlled clinical trial has a low frequency of adverse events, and these adverse events are easily recognized and treated. Let us also assume that the financial cost of this medication is small. In this case, the demonstration of overwhelming efficacy by this medication would not be required by the medical community to justify the use of this compound in patients. A risk–benefit assessment would suggest that the demonstration of moderate efficacy by this therapy would be all that was required to offset the low risk and cost associated with its use. This does not imply that a larger effect size is undesirable; clearly the greater the effect size, the greater the attractiveness of the intervention. However, smaller effect sizes would lead to the use of this medication as well.

Thus, the minimum clinical efficacy is the resultant decision of the medical and regulatory communities about the effectiveness of the medication that is required to offset both the adverse events and the cost of the medication while simultaneously considering the current standard of care for the disease. The more dangerous and more costly the medication, the greater the minimum clinical efficacy must be.[*]

6.12 Power for Smaller Efficacy Levels

Consider an experiment designed to establish the efficacy of a medication in patients with severe ischemic heart disease. Patients will be randomized to either placebo therapy or the intervention, and followed for five years. The investigator computes a sample size based on the development in Appendix B using a two-sided alpha of 0.05 and a power of 90%, to detect a 30% reduction in total mortality from the placebo group cumulative mortality rate of 35%. The trial size is 788 patients, 394 each for the placebo and treatment group.

The implications of this design are somewhat subtle but important to examine. A 35% event rate in the placebo group translates to 138 placebo deaths during the course of the trial. If the investigator is correct and there is a 30% reduction from this cumulative mortality rate in the active group, then he can expect a $(0.70)(0.35) = 0.245$ cumulative mortality rate or 97 deaths in the treatment group. What would the test statistic be if these predictions proved to be correct? A quick computation reveals that the test statistic is 3.19 and the two sided p-value is 0.001.

How did this happen? If the study was designed to have a type I error rate of 0.05 and 90% power for the event rates that were observed, why is the test statistic so large and the p-value so much lower than the 0.05 level? The answer is power. The study is designed not just to confirm a positive result, but also to have adequate protection against a type II error. More subjects are required to ensure that type I and type II error rates are low. When the study is positive, concern for the type II error dissolves and the increased number of subjects decrease the p-value.

---

[*] This assumes that the scientists have some reliable information about the safety profile of the intervention to be tested in the study.

The implications are immediate. If the designed efficacy produces not just a *p*-value of 0.05 but of 0.001, then, adequately powering an experiment for a given efficacy allows for slightly smaller efficacies to be considered statistically significant as well. It is the job of the investigator to match this range with the efficacies for which there is critical interest. The best advice is don't overestimate efficacy. Design the research effort to detect modest clinical effectiveness.

6.13 Conclusions

P-values, power, and the effect size of the research effort are all intertwined, and this complicated interrelationship can lead to danger for the unwary research designer. Forcing type I error to extremely low levels, *ceteris paribus* will suck the power from the experiment. Sample size computations in Appendix B demonstrate how to incorporate type I and type II error concerns into an experiment. The investigations should first identify the efficacy level of clinical interest and then choose the sample size that allows this efficacy level to be identified with statistical significance.

However, sample size computations that are only composed of mathematics are subject to the strong persistent undertow exerted by the resource centers of a clinical research effort. This is appropriate, and dialogue between all involved parties should be frank and open, for the good of the research. Once the experiment is underway, discordant concerns preclude major changes in sample size goals. Therefore, honest discussion of logistical and financial issues should be encouraged during the research program's design phase.

References

1. Moyé LA (2003) *Multiple Analyses in Clinical Trials: Fundamentals for Investigators*. New York; Springer.

7

Scientific Reasoning, *P*-values, and the Court

7.1 Introduction

Among the most sensational civil suits in current events are those involving the pharmaceutical industry. Diet drugs, antidepressants, blood pressure medication, anti-diabetic agents, and analgesics are just a few of the many agents that have been implicated in the last ten years with an unacceptably large number of adverse events. Repeated claims that agents developed and disseminated by these drug companies are unsafe rise to prominence as the public becomes increasingly skeptical of the manner in which its public health in overseen.

The resulting litigation is complex; however, at its heart lies a familiar question: Does the exposure cause harm? While this is a scientific question, the science of causality, particularly epidemiology and biostatistics, now finds itself thrust center stage in these civil suits. Commonly, there are pre-trial hearings that take place outside the earshot of the jury, where lawyers argue vehemently for or against the causal relationship. The available scientific literature can be immense and eclectic, spanning case reports, case series, observational studies, and randomized controlled clinical trials.

The court, in order to provide the best environment for the jury to understand the scientific nature of the argument, must understand the nature of the causal relation. The court is obligated to exclude evidence that does not rise to its standard, using federal and state law to guide its deliberations. However, the biostatistical and epidemiologic methodology used to determine the relationship between the drug and related adverse events can be complex, including such esoteric devices as conditional logistic regression, Cox hazard analysis, or structural equation modeling. These modern devices are commonly not specifically covered by existing law, and it is up to the court to first hear arguments for and against the use of this methodology. It then judges their suitability and admissibility using a combination of its own experience and existing law as a metric.

The purpose of this chapter is to discuss at an elementary level the evolution of judicial thinking about epidemiology and biostatistics as it applies to the legal application of scientific causality arguments in the legal system.

7.2 Blood Pressure and Deception: The Frye Test

The first modern attempt to incorporate the role of science into the law was the Frye case. In the 70 years since its formulation, the resulting "general acceptance" rule has been the dominant standard for determining the admissibility of scientific evidence at trial for many years.

In Frye versus US (1923), James Alphonzo Frye was convicted of murder in the second degree. He appealed his conviction, stating that the expert witness prepared to testify in his behalf was improperly excluded by the previous court that had tried his case.

During Mr. Frye's trial, counsel for the defense offered an expert who asserted that he had developed a "deception" test. This deception test was based on the measurement of systolic blood pressure (SBP). The theory, presaging the modern lie detector, asserted that blood pressure is influenced by the changing emotions of the subject. Specifically, the expert argued that when a subject was either lying, concealing facts, or was guilty of the accused crime and working to avoid detection, his SBP would rise in a predictable manner. The expert further asserted that since Mr. Frye had passed this "deception" test, he was not guilty of the crime. The prosecution argued that the test was inadmissible and the trial court agreed.[*]

Mr. Frye appealed, saying that the court has inappropriately excluding the exonerating expert. During the appeal, defense counsel argued that the excluded expert was necessary because both the deception test and its principles were complicated. Since the relationships between emotions, the autonomic nervous system, and blood pressure control were complex and outside of the experience of the jury, they would need to hear advice of an expert who could inform them from his special knowledge and experience.

However, the appeals court was concerned about the reliability of the expert's deception test. Ultimately, they concluded that the SBP test had not yet crossed from the experimental realm to the world of reliability. Their final, operative statement was

> Somewhere in this twilight zone the evidential force of the principle must be recognized, and while courts will go a long way in admitting expert testimony deduced from a well-recognized scientific principle or discovery, the thing from which the deduction is made must be sufficiently established to have gained general acceptance in the particular field in which it belongs.[†]

Because the systolic blood pressure deception test had not yet gained standing and recognition among scientific authorities, evidence based on its results was ruled inadmissible. It was no longer sufficient for admissible scientific evidence merely to be relevant; it must now also be based on generally accepted pro-

---

[*] In an interesting twist, defense counsel offered to have Mr. Frye submit to the test a second time, this time in open court before the jury. The court sustained the prosecution's objection to his action as well.

[†] 54 App. D.C., at 47, 293 F., at 1014

cedures. It is important to note that neither the epidemiologic causality tenets[*] nor statistical inference had been clearly articulated in the scientific literature; thus, it did not pass this "general acceptance" test.

7.3 Rule 402

The Frye test of the 1920s grew in popularity, rising to a judicial de facto standard in many courts. However, the system of rules of evidence in the United States in the early twentieth-century was chaotic. In the absence of an overarching set of procedures, the state courts were relatively free to choose their own rules of evidence, based on a combination of case law (from either their state or others) and common law. Thus, evidence that may have been admissible in one state proved to be inadmissible in another. This incoherence extended to the federal court system where circuit courts operated in a similar state of inconsistency. The resulting uncontrolled heterogeneity of rules of evidence generated a patchwork of law applied in inconsistent and unpredictable ways.

In an early attempt to resolve this problem, the federal bench began a series of corrections. The creation of the Federal Rules of Civil Procedures in 1938 was well received by the legal system, reinforcing interest in the federal court's unification work through the middle of the century. In 1972, the federal court system announced a collection of procedures entitled the Federal Rules of Evidence. After a three-year delay, Congress permitted these rules to become law in 1975.

The stated intent of the Federal Rules of Evidence was to establish a more uniform set of procedures for evidence that in turn would promote a system of fairness, efficiency, clarity, and justice. However, this was not the only motivation. There were many legal opinion leaders who over the years had come to believe that the common law rules of evidence were nonsensical in some cases, and overly judgmental in others. Thus, in the process of establishing a uniform collection of rules of evidence, the more extreme examples of common law were either liberalized or replaced.

The Frye Rule did not escape this transformation, emerging from the Federal Rules of Evidence as Rule 402, that states,

> All relevant evidence is admissible, except as otherwise provided by the Constitution of the United States, by Act of Congress, by these rules, or by other rules prescribed by the Supreme Court pursuant to statutory authority. Evidence which is not relevant is not admissible.

The requirement of general acceptability was removed. Relevant evidence was defined in Rule 401 as evidence that would change the likelihood of a fact that contributes to the court (or jury's) decision. That is, if evidence adds to or subtracts from the plausibility of a useful fact in a case, the evidence is relevant.

---

[*] However, Courts may continue to be guided by the experience of common law. In *United States* v. *Abel*, 469 US 45 (1984), the Supreme Court considered the pertinence of background common law in interpreting the Rules of Evidence.

Thus, after Frye, the test for evidence became one of relevance. The causality arguments in epidemiology as well as principles of statistical inference were admissible under Rule 702, since each met the "relevance" standard.

7.4 The Daubert Rulings

The Daubert case centered around use of the compound Bendectin. The statistical and epidemiologic contentions debated in trial and on appeal allowed the legal system to examine and elaborate on the use of epidemiology and biostatistics in civil cases that focused on the relationship between an exposure and the occurrence of disease.

Bendectin was manufactured by Merrell Dow[*] to combat morning sickness. Marketed in 1957, it was taken by more than 33 million pregnant women before it was withdrawn from the market due to concern about its propensity to produce birth defects.

Jason Daubert and Eric Schuller, children of mothers who ingested Bendectin during pregnancy, were each born with serious birth defects. These two families sued Merrell Dow in California state court, alleging that Bendectin produced these birth defects. Merrell Dow successfully argued that these cases should be removed to federal court.[†]

After the court's extensive examination of all scientific evidence presented by both sides, Merrell Dow's attorneys moved for summary judgment (i.e., for the case to be dismissed), contending that the plaintif's had failed to prove that the drug caused birth defects in humans.

In support of its motion, the drug company submitted an affidavit from Steven H. Lamm, physician and epidemiologist, who was a well-credentialed expert on the risks from exposure to various chemical substances. Doctor Lamm stated that he had reviewed more than 30 published studies involving over 130,000 patients; according to this expert, not one of them proved that Bendectin was a human teratogen. Dr. Lamm concluded that maternal use of Bendectin during the first trimester of pregnancy had not been shown to be a risk factor for human birth defects. The Dauberts responded with the testimony of eight experts of their own, each of whom possessed impressive credentials. In addition, they provided data from animal studies and epidemiologic analyses.

However, the District Court granted Merrell Dow's motion for summary judgment, and its judgment had profound implications for the use of epidemiology and statistics in the court.

First, the court excluded the body of non-human research that had been submitted by the Dauberts. Thus, the animal cell studies, live animal studies, and chemical structure analyses on which the Dauberts had relied could not by themselves raise a reasonably disputable jury issue regarding causation.

---

[*] Now named Merrell Pharmaceuticals and a subsidiary of Hoechst Marion Roussel Inc.
[†] All of the hundreds of Bendectin injury lawsuits brought by plaintiffs against Merrell-Dow have ended in a favor of the company at either trial or appeal.

Turning to the epidemiologic evidence that the Dauberts provided, the court was particularly critical of the type of evaluations that were submitted. These analyses were not original examinations of data, collected with the purpose of elucidating the true nature (i.e., causal, or associative) between Bendectin and birth defects. Instead they were recalculations of data that was already available and already published. Furthermore, the evaluations were based on data that had been published demonstrating no causal link between the drug and birth defects. Thus, the authors of these calculations, in order to persuade the court, attempted to reverse the published null findings in the peer-review literature The court determined that this body of evidence was inadmissible because it had not been published, and thus had not been subjected to the rigors of the peer-review process.

When the Daubert case went to the United States Supreme Court, the Court let stand the lower court rulings in favor of Merrell Dow. The justices also stated that, faced with the possibility of expert scientific testimony, the trial judge must determine at the outset whether the expert is proposing to provide scientific knowledge that will assist the court in understanding or determining the important issues. The court said that this examination would entail a preliminary assessment of whether the reasoning or methodology underlying the testimony was scientifically valid and of whether that reasoning or methodology could properly be applied to the facts at issue.

The trial judge must make this preliminary assessment in what are now known as the Daubert hearings. This inquiry will include many considerations: whether the theory or technique in question can be (and has been) tested, whether it has been subjected to peer review and publication; its known or potential error rate; the existence and maintenance of standards controlling its operation; and whether it has attracted widespread acceptance within a relevant scientific community. The inquiry is a flexible one, and its focus must be solely on principles and methodology, not on the conclusions that they generate. The Supreme Court ruled that judges were competent to undertake this review, and then proceeded to provide some guidance for them. This guidance, known as the Daubert Factors,[*] coupled with information about applying Rule 702, set the stage for the consideration of statistics and *p*-values in courtrooms during pretrial hearings, outside the presence of the jury. If the court ruled that the information was admissible, the statistical and epidemiologic evidence could be presented to the jury.

7.5 The Havner Ruling

After her mother was placed on a course of Bendectin in 1981, Kelly Havner was born with several missing fingers on her right hand. The Havners sued Merrell Dow for negligence, defective design, and defective marketing. The suit took place in Texas, and was never remanded to the federal court system. Thus, both the trial and the appeals occurred within the Texas courts.

As in the Daubert case, the central issue was the scientific reliability of the expert testimony offered to establish causation between the use of Bendectin and

---

[*]Provided in Appendix C.

the occurrence of birth defects. As in the Daubert case, Merrell Dow challenged the evidence brought to trial by the Havner's that alleged causality. The defendant contended that there was no scientifically reliable evidence that Bendectin caused either limb reduction birth defects in general or that it caused Kelly Havner's birth defect.

The basis of the arguments in the trial was the role of epidemiology in biostatistics in establishing the causative link. The Havners' experts were well credentialed, with Dr. Shanna Helen Swan's testimony playing a central role in their case. Dr. Swan, who held a master's degree in biostatistics from Columbia University and a doctorate in statistics from the University of California at Berkeley, was chief of the section of the California Department of Health and Services that determines causes of birth defects; also she served as a consultant to the World Health Organization, the Food and Drug Administration, and the National Institutes of Health. In addition, the Havners called on Dr. Stewart A. Newman, a professor at New York Medical College who had spent over a decade studying the effect of chemicals on limb development.

After exhaustive analyses, these experts had concluded that Bendectin could cause birth defects. Their conclusions were based upon (1) in vitro and in vivo animal studies that found a link between Bendectin and malformations, (2) pharmacological studies of the chemical structure of Bendectin that purported to show similarities between the structure of the drug and that of other substances known to cause birth defects, and (3) the "reanalysis" of previously published epidemiological studies. The question of scientific reliability was raised repeatedly during the liability phase, at the center of which was the role of epidemiology and animal studies.

Both the judgment and the judgment reversals were staggering. At the conclusion of the liability phase, the jury found in favor of the Havners and awarded them $3.75 million. In the punitive damages stage, the jury awarded another $30 million, but that amount was reduced by the trial court to $15 million. However, the manufacturer appealed, and the Texas state appeals court threw out the punitive-damages award and ruled that the Havners were entitled to only the $3.75 million in compensatory damages. Later, the Texas Supreme Court ruled that the Havners were not entitled to any award at all because there had been insufficient evidence linking Bendectin to birth defects.

The issue before the Supreme Court, as in most of the Bendectin cases, was whether the Havners' evidence was scientifically reliable. The Havners did not contend that all limb reduction birth defects were caused by Bendectin or that Bendectin always caused limb reduction birth defects even when taken at the critical time of limb development. Experts for the Havners and Merrell Dow agreed that some limb reduction defects are genetic. These experts also agreed that the cause of a large percentage of limb reduction birth defects is unknown. Given these undisputed facts, the court wrestled with just what a plaintiff must establish to raise the issue of whether Bendectin caused an individual's birth defect (i.e., specific causation).

The Havners relied to a considerable extent on epidemiological studies for proof of general causation. Accordingly, the Supreme Court considered and accepted the use of epidemiological studies and the "more likely than not" burden of proof. The Supreme Court recognized, as does the federal *Reference Manual on Scientific Evidence,* that unfocused data such as the incidence of adverse effects in the exposed population cannot indicate the actual cause of a given individual's disease or condition. The court noted that sound methodology requires that the design and execution of epidemiological studies be examined, especially to control the factor of bias. However, the court stated that epidemiological studies "are subject to many biases and therefore present formidable problems in design and execution and even greater problems in interpretation."

    The Supreme Court identified several reasons why the plaintiffs' expert opinions were scientifically unreliable. First, Dr. Swan provided an odds ratio of 2.8 with no confidence interval. The court stated that, without knowing the significance level or the confidence interval, there was no scientifically reliable basis for saying that the 2.8 result is an indication of anything. Furthermore, the court noted that the expert's choice of the control group could have skewed the results.

    In addition to the statistical shortcomings of the Havners' epidemiological evidence, the court criticized the evidence's reliability because it had never been published or otherwise subjected to peer review, with the exception of Dr. Swan's abstract, which she acknowledged was not the equivalent of a published paper. None of the findings offered by the Havners' five experts in this case have been published, studied, or replicated by the relevant scientific community. As Judge Kozinski said, "The only review the plaintiffs' experts' work has received has been by judges and juries, and the only place their theories and studies have been published is in the pages of federal and state reporters."[*]

    In its review of the Havners' case, the Texas State Supreme Court identified several factors to consider in reviewing the scientific evidence of causation from a legal perspective. These included (1) the rationale for the study (i.e., was the study was prepared only for litigation or used or relied upon outside the courtroom?), (2) whether the methodology was recognized in the scientific community, and (3) has the litigation spawned its own "community" that is not part of the purely scientific community? The court observed that the opinions to which the Havners' witnesses testified had never been offered outside the confines of a courthouse. In doing so, the Court recognized that publication and peer review allow an opportunity for the relevant scientific community to comment on findings and conclusions and to replicate the reported results using different populations and different study designs.

7.6 Relative Risk and the Supreme Court

Although they discounted the specific evidence offered in the Havner case, the Texas State Supreme Court stated that properly designed and executed epidemiological studies may be part of the evidence supporting causation in such a case.

    The court went even further, setting a legal standard for strength of evidence by stating that there was a rational basis for the requirement that there be more than a "doubling of the risk." Thus, the court required a relative risk, or odds ratio, of two.

---

[*] *Daubert,* 43 F.3d at 1318 (commenting on the same five witnesses called by the Havners).

An odds ratio of two corresponds to an effect size of legal interest. In civil court, all that is required for the plaintiff to make their case is that they demonstrate that a preponderance of the evidence supports their contention. This commonly translates to at least 50% of the findings buttressing their arguments. An odds ratio of 2.0 corresponds to an *attributable risk exposed*, or *ARE*, of 0.50. The attributable risk exposed is a well-established concept in epidemiology [1]. The attributable risk exposed is the excess risk that is attributed to the exposure. If one can safely draw the conclusion that the exposure caused the disease, then an odds ratio of greater than 2.0 generates an *ARE* of greater than 50%, signifying that the exposure is more likely than not to have caused the disease, *ceteris paribus*. However, the Court cautioned that the threshold of 2.0 is not a litmus test and that other factors must be considered.

The use of scientifically reliable epidemiological studies and the requirement of more than a doubling of the risk strikes a balance between the needs of our legal system and the limits of science. The court recognized that few courts have embraced the more-than-double-the-risk standard and indicated that in some instances, epidemiological studies with relative risks of less than 2.0 might suffice if there was other evidence of causation. However, it was unwilling to decide in this case whether epidemiological evidence with a relative risk less than 2.0, coupled with other credible and reliable evidence, may be legally sufficient to support causation.* The court did emphasize that evidence of causation from any source must have its scientific reliability considered, and that it would not admit *post hoc* speculative testimony. For example, the court noted that a treating physician or other expert who has seen a skewed data sample, such as one of a few infants who have a birth defect, is not in a position to infer causation.† The scientific community should not accept as methodologically sound a "study" by such an expert, the court concluded. Similarly, an expert's assertion that a physical examination confirmed causation should not be accepted at face value. Further, the court cautioned that an expert cannot dissect a study, picking and choosing data, or "reanalyze" the data to derive a higher relative risk if this process does not comport with sound scientific methodology.

7.7 *P*-values, Confidence Intervals, and the Courts

The court stated that it is unwise to depart from the methodology that is at present generally accepted among epidemiologists. Almost all thoughtful scientists would agree that a significance level of five% is a reasonable general standard. ‡

The court resisted attempts to widen the boundaries at which courts will acknowledge a statistically significant association beyond the 95% level, accepting the notion of significance testing and the Fisher 0.05 standard. In addition, the Court recognized that the establishment of an association does not indicate causality. As the original panel of the court of appeals observed in this case, there is a

---

* For example, see *Daubert*, 43 F.3d at 1321 n.16; *Hall*, 947 F.Supp. at 1398, 1404.
† The reasons for this are discussed in Chapter One.
‡ A fine discussion of this concept appears in the amicus curiae Brief of Professor Alvan R. Feinstein in Support of Respondent at 16, *Daubert v. Merrell Dow Pharms., Inc.*, 509 US 579, 113 S.Ct. 2786, 125 L.Ed.2d 469 (1993) (No. 92-102)))

demonstrable association between summertime and death by drowning, but summertime does not cause drowning.

In the final analysis, the court held there was no scientifically reliable evidence to support the judgment in the Havners' case. Accordingly, it reversed part of the judgment of the lower court and rendered judgment for Merrell Dow. However, the Havner case firmly established the importance of epidemiology, peer-reviewed published results, and, through a statement about confidence intervals, the role of statistical inference in making legal arguments for causation.

7.8 Conclusions

The courts admit that they lag behind science in determining the scientific merit of a legal argument. However, in the past twenty years they have come to rely on the findings of epidemiology and biostatistics, and the court has allowed judges to see for themselves the merits of the scientific argument before a jury hears it. Many of the rules established by the Supreme Court to guide judges in these preliminary hearings are based on reproducibility, timing, and significance of the association.

References

1. Cole P, MacMahon B (1971) Attributable risk percent in case control studies. *British Journal of Prevention Society of Medicine* **25**: 242–244.

8
One-Sided Versus Two-Sided Testing

8.1 Introduction

The charge of unethical conduct stikes at the heart of every physician who takes his or her oath seriously. Ethical conduct does not play an important role in our work in healthcare— in fact it is preeminent. It is present in every conversation we have with patients, in every treatment plan we formulate, and in each of our research efforts. Decisions concerning test sidedness clearly define the battlelines where a researcher's deep-seated belief in therapy effectiveness collides with his obligatory prime concern for patient welfare and protection.

The issue of test sidedness in a clinical experiment may be a technical matter for mathematical statisticians, but for healthcare workers it is an ethical issue. Test sidedness goes to the heart of the patient and community protection responsibilities of physicians.

8.2 Attraction of One-Sided Testing

Students instantly gravitate to one-sided (benefit only) testing, and many, after concluding an introductory section in significance testing, come away with the idea that the one-sided (benefit only) testing is efficient, and that two-sided tests are wasteful.

Consider the example of a test statistic that falls on the benefit side of a two sided critical region. Many investigators argue that the evidence seems clear. The test statistic is positive — why continue to insist on placing alpha in the negative, (opposite) side of the distribution? Be adaptive and flexible, they would say. Respond to the persuasive nature of the data before you. Clearly the test statistic falls in the upper tail — the benefit tail — of the probability distribution. That is where the efficacy measure is. That is where the magnitude of the effect will be measured. Place all of your alpha, like a banner in a newly claimed land, with confidence.

8.3 Belief Versus Knowledge in Healthcare

Physicians may have many reasons for conducting research, but a central motivation is the desire to relieve the suffering of patients. We do not like to harbor the notion that the interventions we have developed for the benefit of our patients can do harm. Nevertheless, harm is often done. Well-meaning physicians, through ignorance, injure their patients commonly. The administration of cutting and bleeding in earlier centuries, and the use of strong purgatives in this century are only two of the most notorious examples. The administration of potent hormone replacement therapy for menstrual symptoms, and the use of surgical lavage and debridement as palliative therapy for osteroarthritic knees are only two of the most recent examples of the well-meaning community of physicians treating patients under mistaken and untested assumptions. What will they say 200 years from now about our current oncologic treatments?

While we must continue to treat our patients with the best combination of intellect, rigor, knowledge, imagination, and discipline, we must also continue to recognize what for us is so difficult to see and accept — the possibility that we may have harmed others.

Physicians often develop strongly held beliefs because of the forces of persuasion we must bring to bear when we discuss options with patients. We find ourselves in the position of advocating therapy choices for patients who rely heavily on our recommendations and opinions. We often must appeal to the better nature of patients who are uncertain in their decisions. We must be persuasive. We educate patients about their options, and then use a combination of tact, firmness, and presige to influence them to act in what we understand to be their best interest.

Of course, patients may select a second opinion but they are the opinions of other physicians, again vehemently expressed. Perhaps the day will come when physicians will be dispassionate dispensers of information about therapy choices, but today is not that day.

However, history teaches us repeatedly that a physician's belief in a therapy does not make that therapy right. Making our belief vehement only makes us vehemently wrong. Physicians must therefore remain ever vigilant about patient harm: the more strongly we believe in the benefit of a therapy, the more we must protect our patients, their families, and our communities from the harm our actions may inadvertently cause. Strong vigilance must accompany strong belief. This is the research role of the two-sided test: to shine bright, directed light on our darkest unspoken fears — that we as physicians and healthcare workers, despite our best efforts, might do harm in research efforts.

8.4 Belief Systems and Research Design

The force behind vehement physician opinion can be magnified by the additional energy required to initiate and nurture an innovative and controversial research program. Relentless enthusiasm sometimes appears necessary to sustain a joint effort. The proponents of the intervention must persuade their colleagues that the experiment is worthy of their time and labor. The investigators must convince sponsors (private or public) that the experiment is worth doing, and their argument often incorportates a forcefully delivered thesis on the prospects for the trial's success. This is necessary, since sponsors, who often must choose among a collection of proposed experiments, are understandably more willing to underwrite trials with a greater chance of demonstrating benefit. It is difficult to lobby for commitments of hundreds of thousands, if not millions of dollars, to gain merely an objective appraisal of the intervention's effect. People invest dollars for success. In this high-stakes environment, the principal investigator must fight the persistent undertow to become the therapy's adamant advocate. The argument for one-sided testing is cogently made by Knotterus [1]

The one-sided (benefit only) test is all available for these strong advocates. The investigators believe the therapy will work, and sometimes they unconciously allow themselves to imperceptibly drift away from the real possibility of harm befalling their patients. The one-sided (benefit only) significance test has the allure of being consistent with their belief and providing some statistical efficiency. This is the great trap.

8.5 Statistical Versus Ethical Optimization

We have pointed out earlier that there is no mathematical preference for one level of type I error over another; the common selection of 0.05 is based merely on tradition. The level of alpha is arbitrary and the mathematical foundation for significance testing is not strengthened or vitiated with the choice of a particular type I error rate. However, the case is different for choosing the sidedness of a significance test. In a strictly mathematical sense, the justification for the one-sided (benefit only) test is slightly stronger than that for two-sided testing. This argument is based solely on the criteria statisticians use to choose from amongst a host of competing statistical tests.

For a given testing circumstance, there are many imaginable ways to construct a significance test for a null and an alternative hypothesis. How does one decide which is best? Statisticians address this important question by comparing the properties of different tests [2].* A uniformly most powerful (UMP) test is a hypothesis test that has superior power (for the same alpha level) than any other competitor test.

When does a UMP test exist? When working with commonly used distributions (e.g., the normal Poisson, binomial distribution), one-sided significance tests concerning the parameters of these distributions are UMP tests. The two-sided tests are not UMP precisely because the type I error has to be apportioned across the two tails. Allocating type I error in each tail when the test statistic from any one experiment can fall in only one tail engenders an inefficiency in the significance test. Thus, strictly from an optimality perspective, the one-sided test is superior.

However, are statistically optimal tests the best criterion in healthcare? Are they of necessity clinically ethical? This is an issue where the tension between the mathematics and the ethics of clinical research.

One-sided (benefit only) testing speaks to our intuition as researchers. We believe we know the tail in which the test statistic will fall. Why not put all of the type I error there? The one-sided test resonates with our own belief in the effective-

---

* This examination is actually very straightforward. Competing tests are compared by keeping alpha constant, and then computing the probability that each test will reject the null hypothesis when the alternative hypothesis is true. The test that has the greatest power is preferred. The theory is easy to understand, although sometimes the mathematics can be complicated. Lehman's text is one of the best elaborations of this work.

ness of the therapy. We have experience with the therapy, and can recognize its effectiveness in patients. We may even come to rely on the therapy in our practices. Why place alpha in the tail of the distribution in which the test statistic will not fall? We are convinced of the importance of managing type I error. Why choose to waste it now? Why should we allocate type I error for an event that we do not believe will occur?

The operative word here is "believe." The best experimental designs have their basis in knowledge — not faith. Research design requires that we separate our beliefs from our knowledge about the therapy. We are convinced of the intervention's efficacy, but we do not know the efficacy. We accept the therapy because of what we have seen in practice. However, our view is not objective, but skewed. We may have seen only those patients who would have improved regardless of the therapy. Those patients who did not respond to therapy may have involved themselves in additional therapy without our knowledge. As convincing as our platform is, it provides only a distorted view of the true effect of the intervention in the community.

We may believe strongly, but our vantage point as practicing physicians assures us that we have not seen clearly. Admitting the necessity of the trial is an important acknowledgment that the investigator does not know what the outcome will be. Therefore, an important requirement in the design of an experiment is that the investigators separate their beliefs from their information. The experiment should be designed based on knowledge of rather than faith in the therapy.

There are many remarkable examples of the surprises that await physician scientists who are not careful with the tails of the distribution. Two singularly notorious illustrations follow.

8.6 "Blinded by the Light": CAST

The "arrhythmia suppression" theory is an example of the difficulties that occur when decisions for patient therapy at the community level are based on untested physician belief rather than on tried and tested fact [3].[*]

In the middle of this century, cardiologists began to understand that heart arrhythmias were not uniform, but instead, occurred in a spectrum with well-differentiated mortality prognoses. Some of these unusual heart rhythms, such as premature atrial contractions and premature ventricular contractions, are in and of themselves benign. Others, such as ventricular tachycardia, are dangerous. Ventricular fibrillation, in which vigorous, coordinated ventricular contractions are reduced to non-contractile, uncoordinated ventricular muscle movement lead to immediate death. The appearance of these dangerous rhythms was often unpredictable; however, they were common in the presence of atherosclerotic cardiovascular disease and, more specifically, were often present after a myocardial infarction.

Drugs had been available to treat heart arrhythmias, but many of these (e.g., quinidine and procainamide) produced severe side effects and were difficult for patients to tolerate. However, scientists were developing a newer generation of drugs (e.g., ecanide, flecanide, and moritzacine) that produced fewer side effects.

---

[*] Much of the discussion is taken from Thomas Moore's book *Deadly Medicine* [3].

The effectiveness and safety of these newer drugs were examined in a collection of case series studies. As the number of patients placed on these drugs increased, the perception was that patients with dangerous arrhythmias taking the new medications were showing some reversal of these deadly heart rhythms and perhaps some clinical improvement.

Unfortunately, the absence of a control group makes case series studies notoriously difficult to assess. When patients survived, their survival was often attributed to drug therapy. However, patient deaths are often not counted against the therapy being tested. When the patient died, investigators suggested that the patient was just too sick to survive i.e., no drug could have helped the patient. Thus the drugs were credited for saving lives, but commonly were not blamed for patient deaths. Despite some debate, a consensus arose that patient survival was also improved.

The consensus that these newer drugs were having a beneficial impact on arrhythmia suppression, and perhaps on mortality gained momentum as prestigious physicians lent their imprimatur to the arrhythmia suppression hypothesis. The sponsors of these drugs, along with established experts in cardiology and cardiac rhythm disturbances, continued to present data to the federal Food and Drug Administration (FDA), pressuring the regulatory body to approve the drugs for use by practicing physicians. This body of evidence presented did not contain a randomized controlled clinical trial to test the efficacy of these compounds – only case series. However, after persistent lobbying, intense advisory committee deliberations, and extensive public and private discussions, the FDA relented and approved the new antiarrhythmic agents. As a consequence of this approval, physicians began to prescribe the drugs not just to patients with severe rhythm disturbances, but also to patients with very mild arrhythmias. This expanded use was consistent with the growing consensus that these drugs were also beneficial in blocking the progression from mild heart arrhythmias to more serious rhythm disturbances. The FDA was extremely uncomfortable with this untested expansion, but was powerless to limit the use of the drugs. Soon, many of the nation's physicians were using the drug to treat the relatively mild ventricular arrhythmia of premature beats.

However, there were researchers who were interested in putting the arrhythmia suppression hypothesis to the test. Working with the National Institute of Health (NIH), they designed an experiment called CAST (Cardiac Arrhythmia Suppression Trial) that would randomize almost 4,400 patients to one of these new antiarrhythmic agents or placebo and follow them over time. Clinical trial specialists with established, prolific experience in clinical trial methodology designed this study. This experiment would be double blind, so that neither the physicians administering the drug nor patients taking the drug would know whether the agent they consumed was active. These workers computed that 450 deaths would be required for them to establish the effect of the therapy. However, they implemented a one-sided trial design, anticipating that only therapy benefit would result from this research effort. As designed, the trial would not be stopped because the therapy was harmful, only for efficacy or the lack of promise of the trial to show efficacy. They had no interest in demonstrating that the therapy might be harmful. Thomas Moore in *Deadly Medicine* states (pps 203–204),

The CAST investigators…wanted a structure that eliminated the possibility of ever proving that the drugs were harmful, even by accident. If the drugs were in fact harmful, convincing proof would not occur because the trial would be halted when the chances of proving benefit had become too remote.

The fact that the investigators implemented a one-sided trial design reveals the degree to which they believed the therapy would reduce mortality. However, the Data and Safety Monitoring Board[*] insisted on reviewing the data using a significance test at the $\alpha = 0.025$ level. This was tantamount to a two-sided hypothesis test for the interim data review. However, the board did not overtly contravene the investigators' desire that this should be a test for benefit.

The CAST investigators' attempts to recruit patients were commonly met by contempt from the medical community. Clinicians were already using these drugs to suppress premature ventricular contractions. Why was a clinical trial needed? Hadn't the FDA already approved these new antiarrhythmic agents? Had not numerous editorials published by distinguished scientists in well-respected journals clarified the benefits of this therapeutic approach? Why do an expensive study at this point? Furthermore, why would a physician who believed in this therapy agree to enter her patients into a clinical trial where there was a fifty-fifty chance that the patient would receive placebo therapy? Vibrant discussions and contentious exchanges occurred during meetings of physicians in which CAST representatives exhorted practicing physicians to recruit their patients into the study. At the conclusion of a presentation by a CAST recruiter, a physician, clearly angry, rose and said of the trial recruiter, "You are immoral," contending that it was improper to deny this drug to half of the randomized participants [1].

However, well before recruitment was scheduled to end, CAST scientists who were mandated to collect and study the data noted an unanticipated effect emerging. After one-third of the required number of patients were recruited for the study, the data analysis provided shocking results. Out of the 730 patients randomized to the active therapy, 56 died. However, of the 725 patients randomized to placebo there were only 22 deaths. In a trial designed to demonstrate only the benefit of antiarrhythmic therapy, active therapy was almost four times as likely to kill patients as placebo. In this one-sided experiment the p-value was 0.0003, in the "other tail" [4].

The investigators reacted to these devastating findings with shock and disbelief. Embracing the arrhythmia suppression hypothesis they had excluded all possibility of identifying a harmful effect. It was difficult to recruit patients to this study because so many practicing physicians believed in suppressing premature ventricular contractions. Yet the findings of the experiment proved them wrong.

There has been much debate on the implications of CAST for the development of antiarrhythmic therapy. However, an important lesson is that physicians

---

[*] The Data and Safety Monitoring Board is a group of external, scientists, separate and apart from the trial's investigators, who periodically review the data in an unblinded fashion. This board's responsibility is to determine if there is early evidence of safety or harm.

cannot form conclusions about population effects by extrapolating their own beliefs.

8.7 LRC Results

CAST exemplified the reaction of investgigators who were forced to confront the findings of harm when they held the full expectation of therapy benefit. The issue in the Lipid Research Clinic (LRC) study was one of efficacy. For these investigators, not even a one-sided test was sufficient to insure success.

As we have seen earlier, LCR studied the role of cholesterol reduction therapies in reducing the risk of clinical events. Designed in the 1970s by lipidologists working in concert with experienced clinical trial methodologists, the LRC trial set out to establish with some finality the importance of cholesterol level reduction in reducing the clinical sequelae of atherosclerotic cardiovascular disease. It was designed to randomize patients either to cholesterol reduction therapy or to no therapy, and then to follow these patients over time, counting the number of fatal and nonfatal myocardial infarctions that occurred. LRC required over 3,500 patients to be followed for seven years to reach its conclusion, incorporated into a prespecified hypothesis test. The final trial test statistic would be assessed using a prospectively declared one-sided hypothesis test at the 0.01 level. If the resulting z-score at the trial's conclusion was greater than 2.33, the investigators would conclude that the therapy was beneficial.

The investigators did not underestimate the importance of their work. They knew the field was contentious and that their study would be criticized regardless of its findings. These researchers therefore designed the effort with great care. Upon its completion, they converted their lucid protocol into a design manuscript, publishing it in the prestigious *Journal of Chronic Diseases* [5]. This was a praiseworthy effort. The investigators prospectively and publicly announced the goals of the research effort and, more importantly, disseminated the rules by which they would decide the success or failure of the experiment for all to review before the data were collected and tabulated. This is one of the best approaches to reducing experimental discordance.

In 1984, the study's conclusion was anticipated with great excitement. When published in the *Journal of the American Medical Association* [6], the researchers revealed that active therapy produced an 8.5% reduction in cholesterol. Furthermore, there were 19% fewer nonfatal myocardial infarctions and 24% fewer deaths from cardiovascular disease in the active group. The final z-score was 1.92. The p-value was less than 0.05. The investigators determined the trial to be positive.

However, the preannounced threshold was $z > 2.33$. Since the achieved z-score of 1.92 did not fall in this critical region, the study should have been judged as null, and therapy unsuccessful by the LRC investigators' own criteria. Yet the investigators concluded that the experiment was positive. Their rationale was that the significance test should now be interpreted not as a one-sided test with a significance level of 0.01 as was planned and announced, but as a one-sided test at the 0.05 level. This adjustment changed the critical region to be $z > 1.645$.

They changed the significance level of the test based on the findings of the trial! The fact that the investigators published a design manuscript prospectively, highlighting the rules by which the trial would be judged and the standards to which the trial should be held, makes the change in the required test significance level singularly ignoble. It is hard to find a clearer example of alpha corruption than this.

As we might expect, there are many plausible explanations for the diluted finding of efficacy for LRC. The cholesterol reduction therapy chosen for the trial, cholestyramine, was difficult for patients to tolerate. This difficulty led to fewer patients taking the medication, vitiating the measured effectiveness of the compound. It must be said that even with this weak cholesterol reduction effect, the investigators were able to identify a trend for a reduction in morbidity and mortality associated with cholestyramine. The study produced new information that would serve as a firm, scientifically based foundation for the next clinical experiment.

However, the investigators chose instead to fly in the face of their own prospective rules for assessing the strength of evidence in their study, resulting not in illumination, but in withering criticism from the scientific community. The LRC investigators had too little objective evidence to believe in the cholesterol reduction hypothesis as strongly as they did at the trial's inception. They believed in it only to the point of excluding a formal examination for the presence of a harmful effect of cholestyramine, choosing instead a one sided (benefit only) evaluation. This belief also led them to take the astounding step of corrupting their study when the type I error appeared larger than they anticipated. Rather than bolster the cholesterol reduction hypothesis, perhaps refining it for the next study, their alpha corrupting maneuver besmirched it. The one-sided test was a symptom of "strong belief disease."

In healthcare, time and again, well-meaning researchers identify an intervention they believe will be effective in alleviating suffering and perhaps prolonging life. This noble motivation is the raison d'être of medical research. Unfortunately, all too often the fervor of this belief spills over, tainting the design and execution of an experiment in order to demonstrate efficacy. These experiments are often encumbrances to medical progress rather than bold steps forward [7] .

The one-sided test is not the disease, only the disease's most prominent sign. The disease is untested investigator belief masquerading as truth.

8.8 Sample Size Issues

Another argument raised in defense of one-sided testing is sample size efficiency. With concern for only one of the two tails of the probability distribution, one might naturally expect there to be a substantial reduction in the size of the sample since the one-sided test focuses on only one tail of the probability distribution of effect.

However, although the savings are apparent, they do not occur at the level one might expect. Figure 8.1 depicts the relationship between the fraction of observations needed in a two-sided test that are required in a one-sided test, from the design of a randomized clinical experiment where the goal is to demonstrate a 20% reduction in clinical event rates from a cumulative control group event rate of 25% with 80% power.

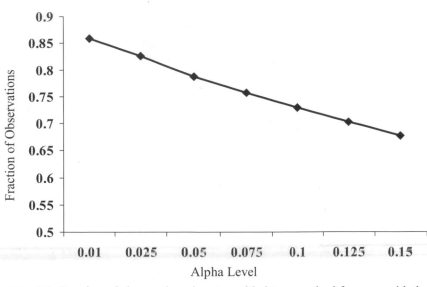

Fig. 8.1. Fraction of observations in a two-sided test required for a one-sided test.

From Figure 8.1, we would expect that if 50% of the observations required for a two-sided test were needed for a one-sided significance test in this example, then the curve would reveal a flat line at $y = 0.50$ for the different levels of alpha. The curve demonstrates something quite different. For example, for an alpha level of 0.075, 76% of the observations required in the two-sided test are needed for the one-sided test. At any level of alpha examined, the 50% value is not achieved. Thus, while some savings are evident, the number of required observations for a one-sided test are more than 50% of that necessary for the two-sided test. The sample size savings for the one tailed test are much smaller than one might naively expect.

8.9 Hoping for the Best, Preparing for the Worst

There are important limitations in carrying out a one-sided test in a clinical research effort. In my view, the major difficulty is that the one-sided testing philosophy reveals a potentially dangerous level of investigator consensus that there will be no possibility of patient harm.

As we have seen in CAST, this sense of invulnerability to harm can ambush well-meaning investigators, delivering them over to stupefaction and confusion as they struggle to assimilate the unexpected, devastating results of their efforts. We physicians don't like to accept the possibility that, well meaning as we are, we may be hurting the patients we work so hard to help; however, a thoughtful consideration of our history persuades us that this is all too often the case. The intelligent application of the two-sided test requires deliberate efforts to consider the possibility of patient harm during the design phase of the experiment. This concern, expressed early and formally in the trial's design, can be very naturally translated into effective steps taken during the course of the experiment. In circumstances where the predesign clinical intuition is overwhelmingly in favor of a finding of benefit, the investigators should go out of their way to assert a level of alpha that will provide community level protection from harm in the research program. It is fine to hope for the best as long as we prepare for the worst.

However, the use of a two-sided test does not in and of itself guarantee adequate community-level protection. In these circumstances, the investigators' mandate for alpha allocation extends beyond the simple stipulation that significance testing be two-sided.

8.10. Symmetrics versus Ethics

Once we have made the decision in the design phase of an experiment for a two-sided significance test, we very naturally and easily divide alpha into two equal components placing half in the tail signifying harm and half in the benefit tail of the probability distribution. This assumption of the symmetric allocation of alpha is perhaps the easiest to justify, but locks us into a reflexive choice involving a community protection issue. It would be useful to examine other options.

Consider, for example, an investigation of the treatment of diabetes mellitus. Diabetes, in addition to its serious renal, microvasculature, lens and retinal complications, is a well-known risk factor for atherosclerotic heart disease. Patients with diabetes mellitus have a greater risk for atherosclerotic disease than the general population. However, the debate over the control of adult onset (type II) diabetes mellitus has persisted for several decades. Should blood glucose be strictly monitored and confined to a narrow range (tight control), or should it be allowed to vary in accordance with a more liberal standard? Suppose an investigator is interested in determining if the tight control of adult onset diabetes mellitus can reduce the risk of death due to cardiovascular disease.

The investigator believes that the risk of cardiovascular disease in a community of type II diabetics can be reduced by 20% with the tight control of diabetes. He plans the following experiment. Select a random sample of patients suffering from adult-onset diabetes from the population at large, allocate them randomly to either standard control or tight control, and follow these patients for five years, counting the number of cardiovascular deaths in each group.

The investigator believes that the tight control group will experience fewer cardiovascular events, but he is also interested in protecting his community. He acknowledges that, despite his belief, the result might not be what he expects. Appropriately separating his belief from his information, he designs a two-sided test. A test statistic that appears in the extreme higher tail of the normal distribution would suggest benefit; one in the lower tail would suggest harm. He does not expect harm to occur as a result of the tight control, but he prepares for it.

This strategy is consistent with the points we have made earlier in this chapter, but is it sufficient? In order to decide in favor of benefit, the investigator needs a cardiovascular event rate to be 20% less in the tight control group than in the standard control group. However, must the tight control intervention be associated with 20% greater cardiovascular mortality before the investigator will conclude that tight control is harmful? Is this symmetric approach of strength of evidence in line with the oath to "first do no harm"? The symmetry argument ensures that the strength of evidence of harm is the same as that required to conclude benefit, but if the ethical concern is harm, perhaps less evidence of harm should be required.

The "first do no harm" principle identifies protection as the primary issue. If we are to protect the patients, we must be especially vigilant for the possibility of harm. We must stop the trial if harm occurs, at the acceptable risk of placing new therapy development on hold. Unfortunately, therapy used for the treatment of type II diabetes mellitus has been associated with harm in the past. Knowing this, the investigator must assure himself and his patients that he will remain vigilant so that the new method of diabetes control he is using will not harm his patients.

Consider the following alternative strategy for alpha allocation. Recognizing that his primary responsibility is to protect the community from a harmful effect of the tight control intervention, the investigator decides that a test statistic suggesting harm should not be as extreme as the test statistic he would accept as suggesting benefit. As a first approximation for the overall alpha for the experiment, the investigator chooses an alpha at 0.05. He apportions 0.03 of this alpha in the harm tail of the distribution and the remaining 0.02 in the benefit arm (Table 8.1).

Table 8.1. Alpha Table: Trial Conclusions

Primary Endpoint	Alpha Allocation	P-value
Harm	0.030	0.030
Benefit	0.020	0.015
Total	0.050	0.045

This leads to the following decision rule (TS is the test statistic).

Reject the null hypothesis in favor of harm if $TS \leq -1.88$.
Reject the null hypothesis in favor of benefit if $TS \geq 2.05$.

The investigator's greater concern for the possibility that he is harming his patients is explicitly expressed in this significance testing. The sample size is chosen to be adequate for the tail of the distribution with the smallest alpha allocation.

Now, at the conclusion of the concordantly executed trial, the test statistic is computed and is seen to be 2.18. What is the p-value for the study? It is the probability that a normal random variable is less than or equal to -1.88 plus the probability that a normal deviate is greater than 2.18 or $P[Z < -1.88] + P[Z > 2.18] = 0.03 + 0.015 = 0.045$. One would correctly conclude that this concordantly executed study is positive. Note that this p-value construction is different from the traditional p-value computation.

as

Traditionally with a test statistic of 2.18, the *p*-value would be computed

$$P[|Z| > 2.18] = P[|Z| < -2.18] + P[|Z| > 2.18] = 2P[|Z| > 2.18]$$
$$= (2)(0.015) = 0.030.$$

In this computation, the probability of a type I error is reduced from the pre-specified level of 0.05, not just on the benefit side of the distribution, but on the harm side as well. How is this justified? Why should we transmute the reduction of the possibility of type I error for benefit into a reduction in the possibility of the type I error for harm? The only justification for this reduction in the harm arm of alpha is the *a priori* notion of symmetry. If the investigator at the trial's inception constructs the two-sided test as symmetrical, he is arguing that the alpha error be channeled symmetrically at the end of the experiment. His best guess at the inception of the study was at the 0.05 level, so he apportions alpha symmetrically as 0.025. At the conclusion of the experiment, although the type I error in the benefit arm decreased from 0.025 to 0.015, the *a priori* assumption of symmetry remains in force. The finding of 0.015 in the benefit side of the distribution results in a total alpha expenditure of 0.030.

However, with the removal of the symmetry constraint *a priori*, there is no longer justification for the symmetric construction of the *p*-value. The possibility of a type I error for harm has not been updated by the experiment and remains unchanged at 0.035. The estimate of the magnitude of type I error in the benefit portion of the efficacy distribution is decreased from 0.035 to 0.015, and the *p*-value for the experiment is 0.030 + 0.015 = 0.045. It would be a mistake to view the results of this experiment as barely significant, as is often done in the reflexive 0.05

Let's return to the design phase of this argument to explore one other consideration. One could make a case that, given the strength of evidence so far suggesting the possibility of long-term harm of the treatment of diabetes, even more alpha should be evidence for harm (Table 8.2)

Table 8.2. Alternative Allocation and Trial Conclusion
(Test Statistic = 2.18)

Primary Endpoint	Alpha Allocation	*P*-value
Harm	0.1000	0.1000
Benefit	0.0250	0.0125
Total	0.1250	0.1125

In this scheme, the overwhelming ethical concern is to identify the possibility of harm. The total alpha for the experiment is 0.125, but only 0.025 is identified for benefit. In this circumstance, the test statistic must be larger than 1.96 to demonstrate evidence of benefit, but only −1.28 to demonstrate evidence of harm.

Suppose now that the test statistic is observed as 2.18 (Table 8.2.). Then the experiment is positive and the total alpha expended

$$P[Z < -1.28] + P[Z > 2.18] = 0.10 + 0.015 = 0.115.$$

The study should be viewed as positive for benefit since the total alpha allocated is less than the alpha allocated at the trial's beginning. Also, adequate population protection was provided for harm. Critics of the study who would minimize the findings of this trial should be reminded that the alpha for significance for benefit = P[Z > 2.18] = 0.015, suggesting that sampling error is an unlikely explanation of the research findings. However, the overriding concern for population protection was the prospectively specified, asymmetric critical region.

In this case, the investigators have allocated alpha prospectively and intelligently, requiring sufficient strength of evidence for benefit while vigorously exercising their mandate for community protection. Nevertheless, many will feel uncomfortable about this nonstandard scheme for alpha allocation. We must keep in mind that the allocation the investigators have chosen stands on good ground, adhering to the following requirements, necessary and sufficient for its clear interpretation. First, alpha is allocated prospectively, in great detail. Secondly, the protocol involved the random selection of subjects from the population and the random allocation of therapy. Finally, the experiment was executed concordantly with no consequent alpha corruption. The investigators have wielded their mandate handsomely, providing adequate community protection while insisting on the same standard of efficacy required by the more traditional scientific community. The experimental findings would be reduced only in the eyes of those with a reflexive requirement of 0.05 with symmetric tails.

8.11 Conclusions

I believe one-sided (benefit only) testing reflects a mindset of physicians and healthcare researchers who believe their intervention can produce no harm, a philosophy that has been shown repeatedly to be faulty, and dangerous to patients and their families. Investigators who agree to the one-sided (benefit only) approach to significance testing in a clinical experiment have closed parts of their minds to the possibility of harm entering into an avoidable flirtation with danger. In this sense, the one-sided test is not the disease, it is only a symptom.

We as physicians and healthcare workers feel strongly about the treatment programs we advocate. This is required in our profession. However, these strong feelings often betray us since our day-to-day experience does not provide an objective view of the treatments. We need every tool we can find to help us gain that objective vantage point. The use of a two-sided significance test is of utmost importance. A forceful, intelligent argument for ethics will argue not only for a two-sided test, but asymmetrical allocation of alpha. Prospective identification of alpha is again critical here, and community protection predominates all other concerns. A sensitive, perceptive, ethical approach to alpha allocation for sidedness can complicate experimental design, but complexity in the name of ethics is no vice.

References

1. Knottnerus JA, Bouter LM (2001) Commentary: The ethics of sample size: two-sided testing and one-sided thinking. *Journal of Clinical Epidemiology* **54**:109–110.
2. Leyman EL (1986) *Testing Statistical Hypotheses.* New York. John Wiley and Sons.
3. Moore T (1995) *Deadly Medicine.* New York Simon and Schuster.
4. The CAST Investigators (1989) Preliminary Report: effect of encainide and flecainide on mortality in a randomized trial of arrhythmia suppression after myocardial infarction. *New England Journal of Medicine.* **3212**:406–412.
5. The Lipid Research Clinic Investigators (1979) The Lipid Research Clinics Program: The Coronary Primary Prevention Trial; Design and implementation. *Journal of Chronic Diseases* **32**:609–631.
6. The Lipid Research Clinic Investigators.(1984)The Lipid Research Clinics Coronary Primary Prevention trial results. *Journal of the Amerian Medical Association* **251**: 351–74.
7. Moyé LA, Tita, A (2002) Defending the Rationale for the Two-Tailed Test in Clinical Research. *Circulation* **105**: 3062–3065.

9

Multiple Testing and Combined Endpoints

9.1 Introduction

In a large research effort, thousands and sometimes tens of thousands of patients can be followed for years. This effort generates hundreds of thousands of data points, carefully collected, verified, entered, and analyzed by many workers, themselves committing thousands of hours to this task. Is all of this effort for just one effect size and a single p-value?

The view that this colossal effort generates one and only one p value for a hypothesis test has long since been discarded. Rising up to replace the original philosophy of research analysis is the multiple-arm, multiple-endpoint research enterprise. Rather than focus on two arms (exposed versus unexposed in an observational study or clinical trial), and one endpoint, these modern, complicated experiments may have several treatment arms (e.g., one arm for each of three doses of therapy and a control arm), and, in addition, several endpoints (e.g., total mortality, total hospitalizations, and quality of life). However, every step out of one problem is a step right into another. The creation of these complicated clinical experiments with their complex endpoints has created a new host of problems in significance testing.

Combined endpoints have surged to popularity as useful research implements. When used appropriately they can provide the identification of an important, clinically relevant effect with great precision and resolving power. The correct use of the combined endpoint improves the clinical trial, by strengthening its capacity to pick out weaker signals of effect from the background noise of sampling error. If larger effect sizes are of interest, then a trial using a combined endpoint can gauge the effect of therapy using a smaller sample size, *ceteris paribus*. However, increasing complexity attends the use of these endpoints. The poorly planned, undisciplined use of these sophisticated tools sows confusion into the research effort, producing only amorphous, unintelligible findings.

This chapter will review the foundation of multiple inference testing in clinical research. Beginning with a discussion of the motivations for the use of the multiple outcomes and the natural sampling error concerns that arise, we will reveal the freedom that investigators have in allocating type I error rates in the multiple endpoint setting. In addition, this chapter will develop and discuss three guiding principles in the use of combined endpoints in clinical research.

Finally, this chapter's focus is on managing type I error rates, particularly *p*-values. This focus does not negate the argument that the joint consideration of research design/execution, effect size, the precision of that effect size, and the *p*-value must be interpreted jointly.

9.2 Definition of Multiple Analyses

Multiple analyses are simply the collection of statistical hypothesis tests that are executed at the conclusion of a research effort. These include, but are not limited to dose response analyses, the examination of multiple endpoints, the use of subgroup analyses, and exploratory evaluations. In reality, these evaluations occur in complicated mixtures. For example, a clinical trial may compare the effect of a single dose intervention to a control group on several different endpoints, and in addition, examine the same effect in subgroups of interest. As another example, a clinical trial may assess the effect of the active intervention on total mortality, while dose response information may be collected on a separate but related combined endpoint. In some circumstances, multiple analyses include not just multiple endpoints, i.e., analyses of different endpoints, but also, multiple analyses, using different procedures of the same endpoint [1].

9.3 Efficiency Versus Parsimony

Significance testing focuses on decision-making; its original motivation was to draw a single conclusion concerning a single effect. In order to accomplish this, one experiment would be executed concordantly,[*] producing one conclusion (such as therapy A yields a better clinical result than placebo). This text thus far has focused on the interpretation of type I error rates derived from these experiments.

However, investigative circumstances have arisen in which the final results of the program involve not just one endpoint, but a collection of endpoints. For example, Chapter Three provided examples in which a concordantly executed experiment tested the ability of a compound to reduce the duration of hospitalization. However, in reality, more than just one variable reflecting the outcome of a patient would be measured. Multiple analyses are a natural byproduct of the complexity of these clinical research efforts. There are three motivations for conducting multiple analyses: they are (1) to provide logistical efficiency, (2) to strengthen the causal argument, and (3) to explore new ideas and establish new relationships between risk (or beneficial) factors and disease. We will briefly discuss each of these in turn.

---

[*] Concordant execution is the execution of an experiment according to its protocol, without a data-based change in the analysis plan (Chapter Two).

9.3.1 Efficiency

One of the motivations that generates multiple analyses is the drive of both the investigator and the sponsor[*] for efficiency. They quite naturally expect the greatest return for resources invested. This translates into ensuring that the clinical trial be as productive as possible, generating a full panoply of results in order to justify the commitment of the logistical and financial resources required for the experiment's execution.

Consider a controlled clinical trial that involves randomizing patients to either the intervention group or the control group, following these patients until they have a fatal or nonfatal stroke, or the predefined follow-up period ends. The investigators focus on this one measure of effectiveness. However, other competing measures are available. For example, the researchers might also measure the number of transient ischemic attacks, duration of hospitalization, or cerebral blood flow studies. The incremental costs of these additional studies are relatively small given that the study is to be carried out to measure the impact of therapy on the fatal/nonfatal stroke rate. Thus, one can triple the number of endpoints and increase the number of statistical analyses (and perhaps increase the likelihood of a positive result on at least one),[†] without tripling the cost of the experiment.

9.3.2 Epidemiologic Strength

The sedulously considered collection of endpoints could be used to elicit further evidence from the data about the true nature of the relationship between exposure and disease (i.e., is it associative or causal?). Imbedding an examination of the evidence that sheds light on Bradford Hill's causality tenets[‡] (particularly those of dose–response, biologic plausibility, consistency, and coherency) could lead to their inclusion within the research enterprise; however, their incorporation would likely include additional endpoints in the study.

For example, an observational study that examines the relationship between the use of an anti-diabetic drug and liver failure may also focus on the relationship between exposure duration and the incidence of acute liver failure. This would require a relative risk (with corresponding confidence interval and p-value) for each dose-duration category. In addition, one could measure the proportion of patients, who have elevated liver enzymes. This collection of evaluations improves the quality of the assessment of the true nature of the exposure–disease relationship. However, each requires an additional analysis.

---

[*] The sponsor of the trial is the organization which funds the study. It could be a government funded study, underwritten by institutes, e.g., the National Eye Institute, or the National Institute of Environmental Health Services. Alternatively, the clinical trial could be funded by a private pharmaceutical company.

[†] We will have much more to say about this concept later.

[‡] These nine tenets are listed in Appendix A.

9.3.3 The Need To Explore

In Chapter Two we discussed the crucial differences between exploratory and confirmatory research. Confirmatory research executes a protocol that was designed to answer a prospectively asked scientific question. Exploratory research is the evaluation of a dataset for new and interesting relationships that were not anticipated.

Clearly, investigators want to cover new ground, and commonly enjoy the exploration process. Exploratory analyses can evaluate the unanticipated, surprising effects of an exposure in an observational study, or a randomly allocated treatment in a controlled clinical trial. These evaluations are powerful motivation for multiple analyses, and make valuable contributions if appropriately relegated to hypothesis-generating arena.

9.4 Hypothesis Testing in Multiple Analyses

The aforementioned concerns of logistical efficiency, in concert with the need to build strong epidemiologic arguments, serve as solid motivation for conducting multiple analyses in a modern healthcare research effort. However, since each of these analyses involves a statistical hypothesis test, and each hypothesis test produces a *p*-value, a relevant question is, How should these *p*-values be interpreted?

This issue has been debated as statistical inference has matured. Some workers contend that many of these *p*-values should be ignored, [2–3] and the reader should focus on the effect size, ignoring sampling error's complicated, serpentine effects. This we must reject, based on the arguments we made in Chapter Two. Others have argued that *p*-values should be interpreted as though the value of 0.05 is the cutoff point for statistical significance, regardless of how many *p*-values have been produced by the study. This is called using "nominal significance testing" or "marginal significance." Others have debated whether investigators should be able to analyze all of the data, and then choose the results they want to disseminate [4 – 6]. This we must also set aside, as again, Chapter Two points out the estimation difficulty when the random data are allowed to determine the analysis plan.

9.4.1 Don't Ask, Don't Tell…

Usually investigators do not prospectively state the analysis rule they will carry out during a research effort. The study results may suggest a multitude of ambiguous conclusions. The investigators believe they have the authority to choose the interpretation of the multiple findings in a way of their choosing. However the resulting interpretation is problematic.

Consider, for example, four analyses from a randomized clinical trial designed to measure the effect of therapy of an intervention in patients with atherosclerotic cardiovascular disease. Let us assume in this hypothetical example the four endpoints are —

P_1 – the effect of therapy on the cumulative total mortality rate,
P_2 – the effect of therapy on the cumulative incidence of fatal/nonfatal strokes.

P_3 – the effect of therapy on the cumulative incidence of fatal/nonfatal MI,
P_4 – the effect of therapy on hospitalizations for cardiovascular disease.

The investigators make no prospective statement about which of these is the most important, but plan to use a nominal 0.05 level to determine significance. At the conclusion of the study, they report the results (Table 9.1).

Table 9.1. Analysis of Four Endpoints and their P-values

Endpoint	Rel Risk	P-value
P_1	0.80	0.015
P_2	0.85	0.049
P_3	0.82	0.025
P_4	0.92	0.076

Table 9.1 provides the relative risk and p-value for each of these evaluations. The relative risks reveals that the therapy has produced an effect that is beneficial in the sample. The investigators want to know which of these is positive.

One tempting approach would be to say that P_1, P_2, and P_3 are positive, accepting that any analysis that produces a p-value ≤ 0.05 is a positive one. This is the nominal approach to p-values. The tack of interpreting each of several p-values from a single experiment, one at a time, based on whether they are greater or less than the traditional threshold of 0.05 may seem like a natural alternative to the *post hoc* decision structure that we rejected in Chapter Two. In fact, the nominal p-value approach is very alluring at first glance. The rule to use nominal p-values is easily stated prospectively at the beginning of the trial and is easy to apply at that trial's end.

However, there are unfortunate consequences of this approach. Should each of these be accepted nominally? That would require us to believe that the population has not produced a misleading sample result for any of the total mortality, fatal/nonfatal stroke, and fatal/nonfatal MI rates. How likely is this "triple positive result" to be true? The probability that no type I error occurs for any of these three evaluations, is easily computed[*] as

no type I error $= (1 - 0.015)(1 - 0.049)(1 - 0.025) = 0.913$.

The probability of at least one type I error is $1 - 0.913 = 0.087$. Thus the probability that the population has mislead us just through by a sampling error is 0.087, larger

---

[*] This computation assumes that the hypothesis tests are independent of each other. Relaxing this assumption leads to computations that are beyond the scope of this text. For an introductory discussion, see [1], chapters 5 and 6.

than the 0.05 level. We cannot accept the triple-veracity in this case because the likelihood of a type I error is too large.

However, the circumstances are even more perilous than that. Why did the investigators choose to focus only on analyses P_1, P_2, and P_3 as positive? Most likely because the *p*-values were all less than 0.05. If, for example, they had chosen P_4 as the most important analysis, the expended type I error would be too large. Thus, looking at the data, they excluded analysis P_4 from further consideration because its *p*-value was too large. Thus, they made their decision to focus on P_1, P_2, and P_3, based on the observed results, and not on a prospective statement declared before the data were collected.

The point is that with no prospective plan, the investigators are drawn to interpret the research endeavor in the most positive, attractive way they can. However, other investigators or readers would interpret the results differently. Why not? With no prospective plan to guide the community, every one falls into the temptation of using analysis rules for the study's interpretation that are based on the data. This is the hallmark of random research.

9.5 Familywise Error [*]

The calculation on the preceding section demonstrates how multiple statistical hypothesis tests propagate type I error rates. With two or more endpoints, the nominal interpretation of *p*-values is unsatisfactory.

If there are two statistical analyses, one on the effect of the intervention on the total mortality rate and the second on the intervention's impact of the fatal and nonfatal stroke rate, then a type I error means that the population has produced (by chance alone) a sample that gives a false and misleading signal that the intervention reduced the cumulative total mortality incidence rate, the fatal/nonfatal stroke rate, or both. The key observation is that there are three errors of which we must now keep track when there are two endpoint analyses, and the misleading events of interest can occur in combination. A comprehensive method to track the magnitude of this combination of sampling errors is the familywise error rate (FWER) [7–8] and will be designated as ξ. This is simply the probability that at least one type I error has occurred across all of the analyses.

There is a critical difference between the standard type I error level for a single endpoint and ξ. The type I error probability for a single, individual endpoint focuses on the occurrence of a misleading positive result for a single analysis. This is the single test error level, or test-specific error level. The familywise error level focuses on the occurrence of at least one type I error in the entire collection of analyses.

9.7 The Bonferroni Inequality

The previous section's discussion provides important motivation to control the type I error level in clinical trial hypothesis testing. One of the most important, easily used methods to accomplish this prospective control over type I error rate is through the use of the Bonferroni procedure [9]. This procedure is very easy to use.

---

[*] The terms *error probability*, *error rate*, and *error levels* will be used interchangeably.

Assume a research effort has K analyses, each analysis consisting of a hypothesis test. Assume also that each hypothesis test is to be carried out with a prospectively defined type I error probability of α; this is the test-specific type I error level or the test-specific α level. We will also make the simplifying assumption that the result of each of the hypothesis tests is independent of the others. This last assumption allows us to multiply type I error rates for the statistical hypothesis tests when we consider their possible joint results.

Our goal in this evaluation is to compute easily the familywise type I error level, ξ. This is simply the probability that there is a least one type I error among the K statistical hypothesis tests. Then ξ, the probability of the occurrence of at least one type I error, is one minus the probability of no type I error among any of the K tests, or

$$\xi = 1 - \prod_{j=1}^{K}(1-\alpha) = 1 - (1-\alpha)^{K}. \tag{9.1}$$

Finding the exact value of ξ requires some computation. However, a simplification provided by Bonferroni demonstrates that

$$\xi \le \sum_{i=1}^{K}\alpha_{i}. \tag{9.2}$$

If each of the test-specific type I error levels is the same value, α, (9.2) reduces to

$$\xi \le K\alpha. \tag{9.3}$$

The correspondence between the Bonferroni approximation and the exact FWER is closest when the type I error for each individual test is very small.[*] Equation (9.3) of course can be rewritten as

$$\alpha \le \frac{\xi}{K}, \tag{9.4}$$

expressing the fact that a reasonable approximation for the α level for each of K hypothesis tests can be computed by dividing the familywise error level by the number of statistical hypothesis tests to be carried out. This is the most common method of applying the Bonferroni procedure.

Note that if a researcher wishes to keep ξ at less than 0.05, the number of analyses whose results can be controlled (i.e., the number of analyses that can be carried out and still keep the familywise error level ≤ 0.05) depends on the significance level at which the individual analyses are to be evaluated. For example, if

---

[*] This is because the higher powers of α (α^{2}, α^{3},...,α^{K}) become very small when α itself is small. When these powers of α are negligible, (9.1) more closely resembles (9.3).

each of the individual analyses is to be judged at the 0.05 level (i.e., the *p*-value resulting from the analyses must be less than 0.05 in order to claim the result is statistically significant), then only one analysis can be controlled, since the family-wise error level for two analyses exceeds the 0.05 threshold. The researcher can control the familywise error level for three analyses if each is judged at the 0.0167 level. If each test is evaluated at the 0.005 level, then ten independent hypothesis tests can be carried out.

9.8 Is Tight Control of the FWER Necessary?

Important criticism of tight control of ξ is commonly based on the fact that the type I error rate for any particular test must be too small in order to control the FWER. For example, if one were to conduct 20 hypothesis tests, the type I error threshold for each test must be $0.05/20 = 0.0025$, a uselessly small type I error rate threshold for many. A difficulty with this line of reasoning is the assumption that all statistical hypothesis tests are essential. In healthcare, pivotal research efforts result from well considered literature reviews. This review and early discussion will commonly produce not twenty, but two or three clinically relevant analyses among which type I error may be dispersed. Casting a wide net for a positive finding is the hallmark of exploratory, not confirmatory research work.

In addition, the main reason for controlling type I error rates in clinical trials is that it represents the probability of a mistaken research conclusion for the treatment of a disease just due to sampling error. This sampling based error has important implications for the population of patients and the medical community. While sample-based research cannot remove the possibility of this mistake, the magnitude of this error rate must be accurately measured and discussed, so that the effectiveness of a therapy can be appropriately balanced against that therapy's risks.[*] This approach is very helpful for interpreting clinical trials designed to assess the risk-benefit ratio of a new therapy.

It is easy for the lay community to focus on the potential efficacy of new interventions for serious diseases [10]. However, it is a truism in medicine that all medications have risks ranging from mild to severe. Sometimes these risks can be identified in relatively small studies carried out before the invention is approved for use in larger populations. However, in addition to the occurrence of specific, anticipated adverse events, there are circumstances in which serious adverse events are generated in large populations without warning. This occurs when the clinical studies (completed before regulatory approval of the compound was granted) are not able to discern the occurrence of these adverse events because the studies contained too few patients.

It is important to acknowledge that regardless of whether the drug is effective, the population will have to bear adverse events. Consider the following illustration: The background rate of primary pulmonary hypertension (PPH) is on the order of 1 case per 1,000,000 patients per year in the United States. Assume that a

---

[*] We are setting aside the kinds of errors in clinical trial design that would produce a reproducible, systematic influence on the results. An example of such a bias would be a study in which compliance is so poor with the active therapy that patients do not receive the required exposure to see its anticipated beneficial effect.

new drug being evaluated in a pre-FDA-approved clinical trial increases this incidence by 20 fold, to 1 case per 50,000 patients exposed per year, representing a 20 fold increase in risk. However, in order to identify this effect, 50,000 patients would have to be exposed to the compound for one year to see one case of PPH. This is a cohort whose size dwarfs the size of studies that are conducted prior to the therapy's approval. The increased risk of PPH remains hidden, revealed only in the marketplace. If this drug were approved and released for general dispersal through the population for which the drug is indicated, patients would unknowingly be exposed to a devastating, unpredicted adverse event.

The fact that a clinical trial, not designed to detect an adverse effect, does not find the adverse effect is characterized by the saying "absence of evidence is not evidence of absence" [11]. This summarizes the point that the absence of evidence within the clinical trial is not evidence that the compound has no serious side effects.[*]

Thus, we expect adverse events to appear in the population regardless of whether the intervention demonstrates benefit or not. Some (perhaps the majority) of these adverse events are predictable; others may not be. In addition, the financial costs of these interventions are commonly considerable and must be weighed in the global risk–benefit assessment. Therefore, regardless of whether the medication is effective, the compound is assured to impose an adverse event and a financial/administrative burden on the patients who receive it. The occurrences of these events represent the risk side of the risk–benefit equation.

The use of the intervention is justified only by the expectation that its benefits outweigh these health and financial costs. The consequence of a type I error for efficacy in a clinical trial that is designed to measure the true risk–benefit balance of a randomly allocated intervention is the reverse of the Hippocratic Oath, succinctly summarized as "First do no harm."[†] In clinical trials, type I errors represent ethical issues as much as they do statistical concerns. In these studies, which are commonly the justification for the use of interventions in large populations, the familywise error level must be controlled within acceptable limits.

An analogous line of reasoning is used in evaluating the relationship between an exposure believed to be dangerous and the occurrence of disease. The large number of evaluations carried out in these studies can commonly produce a plethora of p-values, and the occurrence of any positive p-value out of the collection can be used as evidence of harm. However, the possibility that sampling error has produced the small p-value must be overtly considered in concordant research; control of the FWER is a useful tool in this effort. Ethical considerations can require that the criteria for demonstrating harm be less stringent than the criteria for benefit; however ethical considerations do not negate the need for prospectively declared assessment rules for controlling the familywise error rate.

---

[*] The statistical power computation for this example appears in Appendix D.
[†] This problem is exacerbated by the inability to measure type I error accurately, a situation generated by the random research paradigm.

9.9 Alternative Approaches

One of the many criticisms of the Bonferroni approximation is that it is too conservative. This conservatism leads to an unacceptably high possibility of missing a clinically important finding. There are several alternative approaches to the multiple analysis problem. Two of the most recent developments are sequential rejective procedures, and resampling *p*-values.

9.9.1 Sequentially Rejective Procedures

The sequential procedure approach is easy to apply. Assume that there are K statistical null hypotheses in a clinical trial and each statistical hypothesis generates a *p*-value. Let p_1 be the *p*-value for the first hypothesis test $H_{0,1}$, p_2 be the *p*-value for the second hypothesis test $H_{0,2}$, concluding with p_k as the *p*-value for the Kth and last hypothesis test $H_{0,K}$. These *p*-values must first be ranked from the smallest to largest. We will denote $p_{[1]}$ is the smallest of the K *p*-values, $p_{[2]}$ is the next largest *p*-value ... out to $p_{[K]}$ which is the maximum *p*-value of the K *p*-values from the clinical trial.

Once the *p*-values have been ranked, several evaluation procedures are available to draw a conclusion based on their values. One device proposed by Simes [12] compares the jth smallest *p*-value, $p_{[j]}$ to $\xi j/K$. The procedure is as follows:

(1) Rank order the K *p*-values such that $p_{[1]} \le p_{[2]} \le p_{[3]} \le \dots \le p_{[K]}$.

(2) Compare the smallest *p*-value, $p_{[1]}$ to the threshold ξ/K. If $p_{[1]} \le \xi/K$, then reject the null hypothesis for which $p_{[1]}$ is the *p*-value.

(3) Compare $p_{[2]}$ to $2\xi/K$. If $p_{[2]} \le 2\xi/K$, then reject the null hypothesis for which $p_{[2]}$ is the *p*-value.

(4) Compare $p_{[3]}$ to $3\xi/K$. If $p_{[2]} \le 3\xi/K$, then reject the null hypothesis for which $p_{[3]}$ is the *p*-value.

(5) Continue on, finally comparing $p_{[K]}$ to ξ.. If $p_{[K]} \le \xi$, then reject the null hypothesis for which $p_{[K]}$ is the *p*-value.

The procedure ceases at the first step for which the null hypothesis is not rejected. Thus, as j increases, *p*-values that are increasing are compared to significance levels that are themselves increasing. If the tests are independent one each other, then the familywise error level, ξ, is preserved. This procedure is more powerful than the Bonferroni procedure. Holm [13], Hommel [14], and Shaffer [15] have developed similar procedures. It has been suggested that because these methods are easy to apply and less conservative then the classic Bonferroni procedure, they are preferable for hypothesis testing in which familywise error rate control is critical [16].

9.9.2 Resampling P-values

Another modern device to assist in the assessment of multiple analyses is the use of resampling tools. This approach has been developed by Westfall et al. [17–19] and has figured prominently in the methodologic literature evaluating the multiple analysis issue. These workers focus on the smallest p-value obtained from a collection of hypothesis tests, using the resampling concept as their assessment tool.

Resampling is the process by which smaller samples of data are randomly selected from the research dataset. Essentially, this approach treats the research data sample as a "population" from which samples are obtained. Resampling is allowed to take place thousands of times, each time generating a new "subsample" and a new p-value from that subsample. Combining all of these p-values from these subsamples produces, in the end, a distribution of p-values. The adjusted p-value measures how extreme a given p-value is, relative to the probability distribution of the most extreme p-value.

However, the new ingredient in this approach is that the investigator no longer sets the alpha threshold for each evaluation. Since the data determine the magnitude of the p-values, and therefore the rank ordering of the p-values, the data must determine the order of hypotheses to be tested. We must also recognize that, as the significance level threshold varies from endpoint to endpoint, the link between the endpoint and the significance threshold is not set by the investigator but, again, is set by the data.

This latter point is of critical concern to us. The fact that the sequentially rejective procedures lock the investigator into an analysis procedure is not bad; the problem is that the investigator is locked out of choosing the details of this plan by not being able to set type I error level thresholds. Therefore, while sequentially rejective and resampling procedures might be useful in statistics in general, the fact that they take control of hypothesis testing away from the investigator could severely constrain their utility in healthcare research.

9.10 Analysis Triage

Investigators will follow their nature, examining every endpoint with every analysis procedure they think will provide illumination. However, this intellectually rigourous and curiosity satisfying proclivity must be tempered with discipline so that sampling error can be managed and the research effort is interpretable.

One might integrate each of these actions by triaging analyses in accordance with some prospectively declared guidelines. This strategy of endpoint control permits the investigators the freedom to evaluate and analyze all of their endpoints measures completely; however, they must be clear about their plans for interpreting these.

The process is straightforward. The investigators should first identify each of the endpoints they would like to assess at the study's conclusion. Once this exhaustive process of endpoint identification has been concluded, the investigators should then choose the small number of endpoints for which a type I error rate will be allocated. It is over this final subset of endpoints that the familywise error level will be controlled. Other analyses that cannot be recognized prospectively will fall into the class of exploratory analyses.

9.10.1 Primary Versus Secondary Analyses.

The design phase analysis triage process requires that endpoints be partitioned into two classes: primary analyses, or secondary analyses.

Primary analyses are the primary focus of the study. Their prospective declaration protects them from data-driven changes during the course of the study's execution, thereby preserving the accuracy of the statistical estimators. In addition, since type I error is prospectively allocated to these primary endpoints in a way that controls the familywise error rate, the analysis of these endpoints permits type I error conservation in accordance with community standards. The analyses of these primary endpoints are often described as confirmatory analyses, because the analyses confirm the answer to the scientific question that generated the clinical trial.

9.10.2 Secondary Analyses

Secondary analyses are the prospectively declared evaluations that will be assessed at a nominal 0.05 alpha level. They are not included in the calculations to control the familywise error rate. These endpoints, being prospectively selected, produce trustworthy estimators of effect size, standard error, confidence intervals, and *p*-values, all of which measure the effect of the clinical trial's intervention. However, drawing confirmatory conclusions from these secondary endpoints is not permissible since conclusions based on these secondary endpoints will increase the familywise error level above acceptable levels. The role of secondary endpoints is simply to provide support for the study's conclusions drawn from the trial's primary analyses. For example, they can provide information about the mechanism of action by which an intervention works. Alternatively, they can provide useful data about the dose-response relationship between the intervention and the clinical endpoint of interest.

9.10.3 Example of Endpoint Triaging

As an illustration of these principles, consider a clinical trial that is designed to assess the effect of ultrasound therapy on the evolution of a stroke within three hours of symptoms. Patients diagnosed with an evolving acute stroke are randomly allocated to one of two groups. Patients who enter the control group receive t-PA to reduce the stroke size as well as other state-of-the-art therapy. Patients recruited into the active therapy group undergo ultrasound therapy, that is believed to further reduce the stroke size.

During the design phase of the study, the investigators engage in an energetic debate over the selection of the endpoints of the study. There are many candidate endpoints, including, but not limited to, six-week mortality, duration of hospitalization, Rankin score[*], and change in NIH stroke scale (NIHSS).[†] In addition, estimates of recanalization and reocclusion of the blood vessels are available.

---

[*] Rankin score is a score obtained at the patient's discharge, which assigns a number to each of several clinical outcomes.

[†] NIHSS is a score ranging from 0 (best) to 42 (worst) that assesses the signs and symptoms of a stroke. Repeatedly measured during the course of the stroke, its change is a quantitative assessment of the patient's progress or deterioration.

After lengthy discussions, the researchers identify three primary analyses: (1) duration of hospitalization, (2) Rankin score and (3) six week mortality rates (Table 9.2). They settled on this choice because the neurologic community has traditionally accepted these events as important clinical events. The influence of therapy on these measures would therefore translate into persuasive evidence that the therapy provided an important benefit to stroke patients.

Table 9.2. Endpoint Declaration in a Stroke Intervention Trial

Endpoint	Alpha Allocation
Primary Endpoints	
Duration of Hospitalization	0.02
Rankin Score	0.02
Six Week Mortality	0.01
Secondary Endpoints	
Change in NIHSS	0.05
Complete Recanalization	0.05

The test-specific alpha error rates for these primary analyses are assigned using a simple adaptation of the Bonferroni procedure. The sum of the test specific alpha error rates over the three primary analyses is 0.05, controlling the familywise error rate at the 0.05 level. Controlling the type I error rate in this fashion allows the investigators to assess the trial as positive if any of the analyses for the three primary endpoints is positive. The secondary endpoints are each assessed at the nominal 0.05 type I error level. Since the type I error rates for the secondary evaluations are not set to control the familywise error rates, the findings for the secondary endpoints are only supportive of the findings for the primary endpoints.

Note that the type I error expended for the six week mortality endpoint is smaller than that of the other two primary endpoints. This is not a statement about the relative importance of the endpoints; clearly the demonstration of a beneficial effect on total mortality is of great clinical importance. However, the lower test specific type I error rate for the mortality evaluation is an adaptation based on the logistical reality of the research effort. The investigators believe that the mortality rate for the six-year event rate will be small, implying that the number of deaths in the study will be relatively low. It is difficult to persuade the medical community of the importance of the mortality rate findings unless the findings are decisive. Requiring a smaller type I error rate threshold, implies a stronger magnitude of effect, everything else being equal.

9.11 Combined Endpoints

Combined endpoints have been an important component of clinical trial design for over 40 years. The use of combined endpoints improves the resolving ability of the clinical trial, strengthening its capacity to pick out weaker signals of effect from the background noise of sampling error. A well-designed clinical trial that prospectively embeds a combined endpoint into its primary analysis plan can be appropriately powered to measured clinically relevant but small effects.

Combined endpoints, however, are double-edged swords. In some circumstances, the combined endpoint can be exceedingly difficult to analyze in a straightforward, comprehensible manner. In addition, the components of the endpoint, if not carefully chosen, may produce a conglomerate endpoint that measures different but relatively unrelated aspects of the same disease process. The medical community's resultant difficulty in understanding the meaning of this unequilibrated endpoint can cast a shadow over the effect of the clinical trial's intervention.

A combined endpoint in a clinical trial is a clinically relevant endpoint that is constructed from combinations of other clinically relevant endpoints, termed *component endpoints* or *composite endpoints*. Two examples of component endpoints are (1) the cumulative incidence of stroke and (2) the cumulative incidence of transient ischemic attacks (TIA's). A patient experiences a combined endpoint based on these two component endpoints if the patient has a stroke or experiences a TIA. If a patient experiences either or both of these component events during the course of the clinical trial, then that patient is considered to have experienced the combined endpoint, commonly referred to stroke/TIA or stroke + TIA.

9.12 Why Use Combined Endpoints

There are important motivations for the use of combined endpoints in clinical research. It is a truism that disease, and certainly chronic disease, manifests itself in different ways. As an example, consider CHF which produces death, hospitalization, exercise diminution, and quality-of-life impairment. In addition, it affects cardiac function, including LVEF, end systolic volume, end diastolic volume, stroke volume, cardiac output, and blood pressure. An investigator who wishes to assess the effect of an intervention on CHF must choose from a variety of these effects. Thus, the researcher builds the *combined endpoint* from several of these *component measures* of disease.

Each component measure could stand on its own as an endpoint. However, by building a combined endpoint from several of the signs and symptoms of CHF outlined above, the investigators can simultaneously focus on several manifestations of this disease. Thus, the use of the combined endpoint can represent an earnest attempt by the investigators to construct a "whole" of the disease's varied effects from a collection of its "parts" or components. The final combined endpoint will represent important manifestations of the disease anticipated to be influenced by the selected exposure or treatment.

9.12.1 Epidemiologic Considerations

In addition, epidemiologic assessments of component endpoints reveal that the isolated interpretation of a single component endpoint, while clinically relevant, can be misleading.

As an example, consider the correct interpretation of a clinical trial that is prospectively designed to examine the effect of an intervention on the occurrence of stroke. The one prospectively identified primary analysis in this study is the effect of therapy on the cumulative incidence rate of nonfatal stroke. The experiment is concordantly executed, and, at its conclusion, the study demonstrates both a clinically significant and a statistically significant reduction in the nonfatal stroke rate.

In this illustration, the randomly allocated intervention reduced the occurrence of nonfatal strokes. However, the intervention may not be as effective as it first appeared. By focusing solely on a nonfatal endpoint, the investigators might miss the eventuality that the intervention produced a harmful effect on another measure of this same disease, namely fatal stroke. For example, it is possible that the therapy reduced the incidence of nonfatal strokes by increasing the incidence of fatal strokes. Thus, the therapy decreased the total number of nonfatal strokes but increased the total number of strokes in the active group; the majority of these events were fatal strokes. Because the intervention's influence on mortal events may be hidden if the principle analysis involves the measurement of only a morbidity endpoint, the morbidity endpoint can be combined with the mortality endpoint to provide a more complete depiction of the effect of therapy.

9.12.2 Sample Size Concerns

A common motivation for the use of the combined endpoint is to ensure that there is adequate power for the primary analyses of the study. Combining component endpoints permit their endpoint rates to be accumulated, and this increased event rate can be translated into a reduction in the minimum number of patients required for the clinical trial.

For an exposure to be accurately and precisely related to clinical events, there must be a sufficient number of events. Therefore, one of the critical factors included in the sample size formula is the endpoint event. The larger this rate is, the greater the number of endpoint events that will be accumulated in the study. Thus, if all other assumptions remain constant, we find that the greater the probability of an endpoint, the smaller the number of subjects that will be required to produce an adequate number of those endpoint events.

Construction of a combined endpoint takes advantage of this relationship. In the assembly of the combined endpoint, each component endpoint contributes an additional increase in the event frequency of the combined endpoint. Thus with each new component endpoint, the sample size will decrease because the event rate increases.

9.12.3 Improved Resolving Power

Another advantage of the well-considered use of a combined endpoint follows from the increase in the endpoint's event rate. In the previous section we saw how an increase in the event rate in a clinical trial decreases the sample size required for the study. One other perspective on this multifaceted sample size computation is that the larger event rate provides a more sensitive test of the effectiveness of the therapy. By including a larger number of events, smaller measures of efficacy can be assessed.

9.13 Combined Endpoint Construction

To depict the relationship between the exposure and the disease usefully and accurately, a combined endpoint must be carefully constructed. The important properties of a combined endpoint can be described as (1) coherence, (2) endpoint equivalence, and (3) therapy homogeneity.

9.13.1 Property 1: Coherence

Coherence means that the component endpoints from which the combined endpoint is constructed should measure the same underlying pathophysiologic process and be consistent with the best understanding of the causes of the disease. Consideration of coherence requires an examination of the degree to which different component endpoints may measure related pathology.

Each component endpoint must measure not just the same disease process, but the same underlying pathophysiology. When each component endpoint is measuring the progression of the same pathology, the investigator can be assured that the component endpoint is measuring the process that is best understood to excite the production of the disease's manifestations. However, the component endpoints should not be so closely related that a single patient is too likely to experience all of them. These types of component endpoints are termed *coincident endpoints*. If a patient experiences one of two coincident endpoints, they are likely to experience the other. In this situation, there is no real advantage in using the combined endpoint instead of one of its component endpoints. Constructing component endpoints that are too interrelated will make the combined endpoint redundant. An example of coincident endpoints would be the (1) blood sugar reductions (in mg/dl) and (2) reduction in glycosylated hemoglobin (HbA1c). A fasting blood glucose measurement reports the current level of blood sugar, a level that is transient and changes from day to day. The HbA1c level evaluation provides a more stable measure of blood sugar levels over approximately three months. However, each of these assessments measure too much of the same thing, and it would be unhelpful to join these two measures into a combined endpoint.

This might suggest that *mutually exclusive endpoints*, i.e., collections of endpoints with the property that the occurrence of one precludes the occurrence of the others in the same individual, may be preferable. However, if the endpoints are mutually exclusive, then they can measure characteristics of the disease that physicians are unaccustomed to linking together. This can produce serious problems in the interpretation of the results. Thus, even though the choice of mutually exclusive component endpoints minimizes the required sample size for an evaluation of the effect of the intervention on the combined endpoint, care should be taken to ensure that the component endpoints are not too disparate.

Component endpoints in clinical trials are usually not mutually exclusive; patients can experience combinations of the component endpoints. However, the component endpoints of a combined endpoint should be contributory and coherent — they must make sense. Each of the component endpoints should measure the same underlying pathophysiology, but be different enough that they add a dimension to the measurement of the disease process that has not been contributed by any other component endpoint (Figure 9.1).

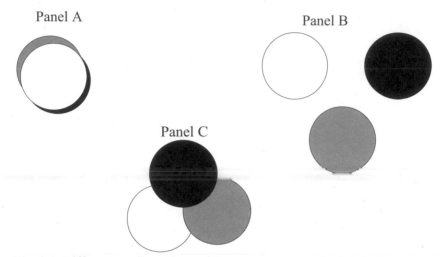

Fig. 9.1. Different configurations of three component endpoints in the construction of a combined endpoint. Panel A (coincident configuration) and Panel B (mutually exclusive) are inferior to the balance of Panel C.

9.13.2 Property 2: Equivalence

The techniques and tools of analysis of these endpoints can be complex. In some circumstances, the complications induced by the analyses of these complicated endpoints can undermine and even negate any advantage the combined endpoint itself offered.

Analysis tools for component endpoints that are either continuous or dichotomous are well described [20–21]. However, analysis tools for combinations of these endpoints can be complex and sometimes may not be generally accepted. Even in the simplest cases, the analysis of the combined endpoint may make some questionable assumptions. As an illustration, consider the circumstance of a clinical trial whose prospectively defined combined endpoint is assembled from two dichotomous component endpoints. The first component endpoint is death and the second component is hospitalization. The patient is considered to have met the criteria for the combined endpoint (said to have "reached" the combined endpoint) if he or she has either died during the course of the trial, or survived the trial but were hospitalized during the study. In the case of a patient who is hospitalized and then dies during the clinical trial, only the first endpoint is counted. As described earlier, this analytic tool avoids the problem of counting patients more than once if they have experienced multiple hospitalizations.

While this analysis is useful, it makes the explicit assumption that each of the two components of this combined endpoint is analytically equivalent to the other. Whether a patient meets the hospitalization part of the endpoint or the mortality part of the endpoint doesn't matter as far as the analysis is concerned. But is a hospitalization the same as a death? Is this assumption of equivalence a true reflection of clinical reality? While one might argue that a patient who is admitted to a hospital in stage IV heart failure is close to death, an investigator would not need to look very far to find someone who disagrees with the assumption that this complicated hospitalization is equivalent to death. In addition, less sick patients can be hospitalized but survive to lead productive lives, a circumstance that is clearly not the clinical equivalent of death.

A similar debate might be sparked in the consideration of the equivalence assumption for patients who reach the prospectively defined combined endpoint of fatal or nonfatal stroke. Since patients who suffer and survive strokes can live for years, be involved in gainful employment, participate in community activities, enjoy their families, and even be enrolled in subsequent clinical trials whose entry criteria require a prior stroke, is it reasonable to assume that stroke and subsequent survival is equivalent to stroke with immediate death?

This equivalence can be a troubling assumption and can complicate acceptability of the combined endpoint. Of course, there are alternative algorithms available that would provide different "weights" for the occurrence of the various component endpoints of a combined endpoint. For example, one might assume that for the combined endpoint of death + hospitalizations, a death is three times as influential as a hospitalization. However, it is very difficult for investigators to reach a consensus on the correct weighting scheme to use, and any selection of weights that the investigators choose that is different from equal weighting of the components is difficult to defend. Unfortunately, at this point there is no commonly accepted way out of this analytic conundrum in clinical research.

The situation only worsens when continuous and dichotomous component endpoints are joined into a combined endpoint. How would one construct an analysis tool for the combined endpoint that has two component endpoints: (1) death or (2) reduction by at least ten units in LVEF? Not only is there the equivalence issue, but there is also the fact that while the exact date of the patient's death is known, the date when the patient first experienced a ten unit reduction in their ejection fraction after they were randomized is not known.* Complicated analysis procedures that address this issue have been developed [22]. However, as revealed at conversations held by the Cardiovascular and Renal Drugs Advisory Committee of the FDA, these endpoints can be difficult to understand and their acceptance by the medical community is guarded at best [23].

9.13.3 Therapy Homogeneity

As pointed out in the previous section, an important trait of a combined endpoint is that each of its component endpoints should reflect an important clinical manifesta-

---

* This could only be known if the patient had an ejection fraction measured each day of the trial.

tion of the disease. However, it would be most useful if the combined endpoint is sensitive to the therapy that will be assessed in the clinical study. This situation is most likely to occur if each of the component endpoints that make up the combined endpoint is itself responsive to the therapy to be tested in the clinical trial. In addition, therapy homogeneity helps to avoid interpretative difficulties when the medical community considers the intervention's effect at the conclusion of the study.

9.14 Measuring Combined Endpoints

The previous sections of this chapter discussed the considerations that the investigators must give to the details of the combined endpoint's construction. However, there are additional requirements that must be satisfied for the successful incorporation of a combined endpoint into a clinical trial. These additional requisites will now be reviewed.

9.14.1 Prospective Identification

As described in the earlier chapters of this book, the incorporation of an endpoint into the primary analysis of a clinical trial must follow certain principles. These principles require the prospective identification of the endpoint and the plan for its analysis. The motivations for this rule have been discussed in detail in Chapter Two. Although that discussion focused on a single endpoint (e.g., total mortality), the guiding concept also applies to the evaluation of the effect of a randomly allocated intervention in a clinical trial on a combined endpoint.

As was the case for the single endpoint, the combined endpoint must be specified in great detail during the design phase of the trial. This description must include how each of the combined endpoint's components will be ascertained. In addition, a committee of investigators is commonly chosen to determine whether a component endpoint has occurred. The procedures put in place to blind or mask these investigators from the identity of the randomly allocated therapy for each patient should be elucidated. In addition, the analysis plan for the combined endpoint must also be detailed. Any weighting scheme that will be used in assessing the contribution each component endpoint makes to the combined endpoint must be determined *a priori*, and should be acceptable to the medical and regulatory communities. If there are plans to submit the results of the clinical trial to a regulatory agency, that agency should be completely and fully informed about the details of both the construction of the combined endpoints and its analysis before the experiment begins.

The requirement of concordant trial execution is critical to the successful implementation of the combined endpoint in a study. Just as it is unacceptable to change the definition of the endpoints used in a study's principle analyses, it is equally crucial to keep the constitution of the clinical trial's combined endpoint fixed. Specifically, the component endpoints of a combined endpoint should be prospectively chosen and locked in. New component endpoints should not be added nor should established component be removed. The same chaotic effects[*] that can

---

[*] These effects are described in Chapter Two.

weaken and destroy the interpretation of a clinical trial whose principle analyses involve a single endpoint can also wreak havoc on the evaluation of a combined endpoint primary analysis.

9.14.2 Ascertaining Endpoints

An accurate assessment of the component endpoint's interpretation in a clinical trial is both critical and complicated. To understand this new complexity introduced by the use of a combined endpoint, first consider a clinical trial that has the effect of the intervention on the cumulative incidence of fatal stroke as its sole primary analysis. At the conclusion of the research, the study's investigators must classify the experience of each of the randomized patients as one of (1) survival, (2) death due to a non-stroke cause, or (3) death due to stroke.

In well-conducted clinical trials, specific documentation is collected to confirm that a patient reported by an investigator to have died is actually dead, and to confirm the cause of that death. These confirmatory steps are taken in order to ensure that living patients are not mistakenly assumed to have died. However, the investigators must also collect data confirming that a patient believed to be alive is in fact alive, a check that avoids the opposite mistake of assuming that a dead patient is actually living. While this last step is a straightforward matter for patients who have attended each visit, there is commonly a subset of patients who have missed several of the most recent visits and from whom no information has been collected. For these patients, intense activity is exerted to determine if they are either alive (as suspected) or dead.

The situation is much more complicated when a combined endpoint is to be part of the primary analysis of a clinical trial. If, in the above illustration, the investigators chose as a primary endpoint not just stroke death, but stroke death + nonfatal stroke, the investigators have an additional inspection to complete. Not only must they assure themselves of the vital status of each patient; they must also determine whether a stroke has occurred in all patients. Of course, specific documentation will be collected from patients who volunteer the information that they have suffered a stroke. However not every patient who experiences a stroke reports the event to the investigators.[*] Mistakenly assuming that patients who had not claimed to have a stroke were stroke-free would lead to an inaccurate count of the number of patients who had this event.

As a final complication, consider the task awaiting investigators who have prospectively chosen the combined endpoint of fatal MI/nonfatal MI/unstable angina pectoris. The evaluation of the unstable angina component, whose occurrence is commonly unrecognized and unreported, can add an overwhelming logistical burden onto the clinical trial apparatus. Nevertheless, the study's investigators must complete this difficult task. Since the occurrence of unstable angina is just as critical as the occurrence of the other two components of the combined endpoint, each must be measured with the same high standard of accuracy and precision. Clearly, the greater the number of component endpoints in the study, the more work the

---

[*] For example, the MI and associated hospitalization might have occurred while the patient was on vacation and the patient was out of contact with the clinical trial's investigator.

investigators must complete in order to assure themselves, the medical community, and the regulatory community that they have an accurate count of the number of endpoints that have taken place during the course of the study.

9.15 Conclusions

The implementation of combined endpoints in clinical trials holds both great promise and great danger. A carefully constructed combined endpoint can helpfully broaden the definition of a clinical endpoint when the disease being studied has different clinical consequences. This expansion commonly increases the incidence rate of the endpoint, reducing the sample size of the trial. Alternatively, if the larger sample size is maintained, the combined endpoint serves to decrease the sensitivity of the experiment to detect moderate levels of therapy effectiveness. However, if the combined endpoint is too broad, it can become uninterpretable and ultimately meaningless to the medical and regulatory communities. Thus, the combined endpoint should be broad and simultaneously retain its interpretability. Additionally, there should be some experiental evidence or at least theoretical motivation justifying the expectation that the therapy to be studied will have the same effect on each of the component endpoints of the combined endpoint. This we have termed the homogeneity of therapy effect. These can be elaborated as a collection of principles, (adapted from [1]:

Principle 1. Both the combined endpoint and each of its component endpoints must be clinically relevant and prospectively specified in detail *(principle of prospective deployment)*.

Principle 2. Each component of the combined endpoint must be carefully chosen to add coherence to the combined endpoint. The component endpoint that is under consideration must not be so similar to other components that it adds nothing new to the mixture of component endpoints make up the combined endpoint; yet, it should not be so dissimilar that it provides a measure that is customarily not clinically linked to the other component endpoints *(principle of coherence)*.

Principle 3. The component endpoints that constitute the combined endpoint are commonly given the same weight in the statistical analysis of the clinical trial. Therefore, each of the component endpoints must be measured with the same scrupulous attention to detail. For each component endpoint, it is important to provide documentation not just that the endpoint occurred, but also to confirm the absence of the component endpoint *(principle of precision)*.

Principle 4. The analysis of the effect of therapy on the combined endpoint should be accompanied by a tabulation of the effect of the therapy for each of the component endpoints. This allows the reader to determine if there has been any domination of the combined endpoint by any one of its components, or if the findings of the effect of therapy for component endpoints are not consistent *(principle of full disclosure)*.

References

1. Moyé LA (2003) *Multiple Analyses in Clinical Trials: Fundamentals for Investigators* New York: Springer.
2. Nester, MR, (1996) An applied statistician's creed *Applied Statistics* **45**: 4401–410.
3. Rothman, RJ (1990) No adjustments are needed for multiple comparisons *Epidemiology* **1**:43–46.
4. Fisher, LD, Moyé LA (1999) Carvedilol and the Food and Drug Administration Approval Process: An Introduction *Controlled Clinical Trials* **20**:1–15.
5. Fisher LD (1999) Carvedilol and the FDA approval process: the FDA paradigm and reflections upon hypothesis testing *Controlled Clinical Trials* **20**:16–39.
6. Moyé LA (1999) P–Value Interpretation in Clinical Trials The Case for Discipline *Controlled Clinical Trials* **20**:40–49.
7. Hochberg Y, Tamhane AC (1987) *Multiple Comparison Procedures*, New York , Wiley.
8. Westfall PH, Young SS (1993) *Resampling Based Multiple Testing: Examples and Methods for P-Value Adjustment* New York: Wiley.
9. Miller RG (1981) *Simultaneous Statistical Inference*, 2nd ed. New York Springer.
10. Adams C (2002) At FDA, approving cancer treatments can be an ordeal *The Wall Street Journal* December 11, p 1.
11. Senn S (1997) *Statistical Issues in Drug Development* Chichester, Wiley, section 15.2.1.
12. Simes, RJ (1986) An improved Bonferroni procedure for multiple tests of significance *Biometrika* **73**:819–827.
13. Holm, S (1979) A simple sequentially rejective multiple test procedures *Scandinavian Journal of Statistics* **6**:65–70.
14. Hommel, G (1988) A stepwise rejective multiple test procedure based on a modified Bonferroni test *Biometrika* **75**:383–386.
15. Shaffer, JP (1986) Modified sequentially rejective multiple test procedures. *Journal of the American Statistical Association* **81**:826–831.
16 . Zhang J, Qwuan H, Ng J, Stapanavage ME (1997) Some statistical methods for multiple endpoints in clinical trials *Controlled Clinical Trials* **18**: 204-221.
17. Westfall PH, Young SS, Wright SP (1993) Adjusting *p*-values for multiplicity *Biometrics* **49**:941–945.
18. Westfall, PH, Young, S *P*-value adjustments for mulitple tests in multivariate binomial models *Journal of the American Statistical Association* **84**:780–786.

19. Westfall PH, Krishnen A, Young, SS (1998) Using prior information to allocate significance levels for multiple endpoints *Statistics in Medicine* **17**:2107–2119.
20. Meinert, CL (1986) *Clinical Trials Design, Conduct, and Analysis*, New York: Oxford University Press.
21. Piantadosi, S (1997), *Clinical Trials: A Methodologic Perspective* New York: John Wiley.
22. Moyé LA, Davis BR, Hawkins CM (1992) Analysis of a clinical trial involving a combined mortality and adherence dependent interval censored endpoint. *Statistics in Medicine* **11**:1705–1717.
23 . Transcript of the Cardiovascular and Renal Drugs Advisory Committee to the FDA Captopril. February 16, 1993.

10

Subgroup Analyses

10.1 Bona Fide Gems or Fool's Gold

Well-trained research investigators diligently work to identify every potentially valuable result. Having invested great time and effort in their studies, these scientists want and need to examine the data systematically and completely. They are well aware that interesting findings await them in non-prospectively declared analyses. Investigators believe that like real gems, these tantalizing surprises lie just below the surface, hidden from view, waiting to be unearthed. If the experiment demonstrated that an intervention reduces the incidence of heart attacks, then ethnicity or gender may affect the relationship between therapy and heart attacks.

Others can also raise these same intriguing questions. In the process of publication, reviewers and editors of the manuscript will sometimes ask that additional analyses be carried out. These analyses may warrant the consideration of the effect of the intervention in subsets of the data. Does the therapy work equally well in the young and old? Does it work equally in different regions of the world? What about in patients with a previous heart attack? These analyses are demanded by others but are also not prospectively stated. Similar inquiries can come from the manuscript's readers.

The research program's cost-effectiveness and the investigator's desire for thoroughness require that all facets of a research effort's data be thoroughly examined. After all, why collect the data if it will not be considered in an analysis? However, as we have seen earlier, the interpretation of non-prospective analyses is fraught with difficulty. The need to protect the community from the dissemination of mistaken results runs head-on into the need to make maximum use of the data that has been so carefully collected. These problems are exemplified in subgroup analyses.

As we will see, there may be no better maxim for guiding the interpretation of subgroup analyses in this setting than "Look, but don't touch."

10.2 What Are Subgroups?

A subgroup analysis is the evaluation of the exposure–disease relationship within a fraction of the recruited subjects. The analysis of subgroups is a popular, necessary, and controversial component of the complete evaluation of a research effort. Indeed, it is difficult to find a manuscript that reports the results of a large observational study or clinical trial that does not report findings within selected subgroups.

Subgroup analysis as currently utilized in clinical research is tantalizing and controversial. As described in the beginning of Chapter Three, the results from subgroup assessments have traditionally been used to augment the persuasive power of a clinical trial's overall results by demonstrating the uniform effect of the therapy in patients with different demographic and risk factor profiles. This uniformity leads to the development of easily understood and implemented rules to guide the use of therapy[*]. Some clinical trials report these results in the manuscript announcing the trial's overall results [1–4]. Others have separate manuscripts dealing exclusively with subgroup analyses [5 – 7]. Such subgroup analyses potentially provide new information about an unanticipated benefit (or hazard) of the clinical trial's randomly allocated intervention.

However useful and provocative these results can be, it is well established that subgroup analyses are often misleading [8 – 11]. Assmann et al. [12] have demonstrated how commonly subgroup analyses are misused, while others point out the dangers of accepting subgroup analyses as confirmatory [13]. Consider the amlodipine controversy.

10.3 The Amlopidine Controversy

In the 1980s, the use of calcium channel blocking agents in patients with CHF was problematic. While initial studies suggested that patients with CHF experienced increased morbidity and mortality associated with these agents [14], additional developmental work on this class of medications proceeded. In the early 1990s, new calcium channel blocking agents appeared, and early events suggested they might be beneficial.

To evaluate this possibility formally, the Prospective Randomized Amlodipine Survival Evaluation (PRAISE) [15] trial was designed. PRAISE's long-term objective was the assessment of the channel blocker amlodipine's effect on morbidity and mortality in patients with advanced heart failure. The primary measurement in PRAISE was the composite endpoint of all-cause mortality and/or hospitalization. The protocol also stipulated that there would be analyses in the following subgroups of patients: sex, ejection fraction, NYHA class, serum sodium concentration, angina pectoris, and hypertension.

PRAISE began recruiting patients in March 1992. Patients with CHF (NYHA functional class IIIb/IV and LVEF < 30%) were randomized to receive either amlodipine or placebo therapy. Suspecting that the effect of amlodipine might depend on the cause of the patient's CHF, the investigators stratified randomization into two groups, patients with ischemic cardiomyopathy and patients

---

[*]The finding that a particular lipid lowering drug works better in women than in men can complicate the already complex decisions that practitioners must make as the number of available compounds increase.

who had non-ischemic cardiomyopathy.[*] PRAISE followed 1153 patients for 33 months. At the conclusion of PRAISE, the investigators determined that amlodipine was not effective in the overall cohort for either the primary or secondary analyses.

The evaluation then turned to the etiology-specific CHF subgroups. PRAISE recruited 732 patients with an ischemic cause for their CHF and 421 patients with a non-ischemic cause. The analysis of the effect of therapy in these strata revealed that treatment with amlodipine reduced the frequency of primary and secondary endpoints in patients with non-ischemic dilated cardiomyopathy (58 fatal or nonfatal events in the amlodipine group and 78 in the placebo group, 31% risk reduction; 95% CI 2 to 51% reduction; $p = 0.04$). Further evaluation of these events revealed that there were only 45 deaths in the amlodipine group while there were 74 deaths in the placebo group, representing a 46% reduction in the mortality risk in the amlodipine group (95% CI $21 - 63\%$ reduction, $p < 0.001$).

The therapy appeared to be effective in the non-ischemic cardiomyopathy stratum. Treatment with amlodipine did not affect the combined risk of morbidity and mortality in the ischemic cardiomyopathy group.

Thus, although amlodipine did not produce an overall beneficial effect, it reduced the combined incidence rate of all cause hospitalization/total mortality, and the total mortality rate in patients with non-ischemic dilated cardiomyopathy.

A second trial, PRAISE-2 [16], was conducted to verify the beneficial effect on mortality seen in the subgroup analysis of patients in PRAISE-1. PRAISE-2 was similar in design in design to PRAISE-1, the exception being its focus on patients with non-ischemic cardiomyopathy. The PRAISE-2 investigators randomized 1,650 patients to either amlodipine or placebo, following them for up to 4 years. However, the results of PRAISE-2 were quite different from PRAISE-1. Unlike the first study, there was no difference in mortality between the two groups (33.7% in the amlodipine arm and 31.7% in the placebo arm; odds ratio 1.09, $p = 0.28$) in PRAISE-2. Thus, the marked mortality benefit seen in the subgroup analysis in PRAISE-1 for amlodipine was not confirmed in PRAISE-2. The positive subgroup analysis could not be confirmed.

Another example of the misleading results that subgroup analyses can provide are from MRFIT, discussed in Chapter Two. In that case, a misleading finding in a subgroup analysis suggested that the use of antihypertensive medications in a subgroup of hypertensive men who had ECG abnormalities at baseline would be harmful.

Nevertheless, the medical community continues to be tantalized by spectacular subgroup findings from clinical trials. A recent example is the subgroup analysis-based suggestion that medication efficacy is a function of race; this has appeared in both peer-reviewed journals [17–18] and the lay press [19].

---

[*] Stratified randomization is an adaptation of the random allocation to therapy process. In general, the random allocation of therapy ensures that each patient has the same chance of receiving active therapy as any other patient. Stratified randomization is randomization confined to a small subgroup of patients. Without it the small size of the subgroup may not permit the overall randomization process to be balanced.

In this chapter, we will review the definitions, concepts, and limitations of subgroup utilization in clinical trials.

10.4 Definitions

While the concept of subgroup analyses is straightforward, the terminology can sometimes be confusing.

A *subgroup* is the description of patient based characteristic, e.g., gender, that can be subdivided into categories. For example, if an investigator is interested in creating a gender subgroup, patients are classified into one of two groups —male or female. These groups are referred to as levels or *strata*. There is one stratum for each category.

The traditional subgroup analysis is an evaluation of the effect of therapy within each of the subgroup strata. In a gender-based subgroup, the subgroup analysis consists of an evaluation of the effect of therapy for males and an evaluation of the effect of therapy for females. Thus. each stratum analysis produces an effect size with standard error, a confidence interval, and p-value.

The definition of a subgroup can be complicated. Consider the categories for a subgroup entitled race. In the 1970s, US-based healthcare research commonly (although somewhat inappropriately) divided their participants into one of two strata: white or black. However, these strata were forced to expand, evolving with the changing US demographics. They now rarely include less than the four categories—white, black (or African-American), Hispanic, and Asian. However, commonly, contemporary research takes a more expansive view of this issue, expanding the consideration to not just race, but ethnicity as well. The nature of the research helps to guide the choice for the number of subgroup strata.

The most useful rules of thumb in developing subgroup strata are to (1) know the demography of the group from whom subjects will be recruited, and (2) understand how the subgroup analysis will be used in interpreting the research result.

10.5 Interpretation Difficulties

The illustrations of the previous sections have demonstrated that there are many possible ways to group patients. Investigators work to identify subgroup classifications that are meaningful. When examination of the therapy effect within a subgroup appears, it is only natural for the investigator to believe the rationale for the choice of the subgroup is justified. Furthermore, the scientist may think that the stratum-specific therapy effect is due to some effect-mediation ability produced by the subgroup trait. However, the very fact that patients are classified and divided can induce a subgroup effect of its own. Subgroup analyses commonly classify and reclassify patients making the attribution of effect unclear.

10.5.1 Re-evaluating the Same Patients

In addition, we must keep in mind that in a collection of subgroup analyses, patients may be stratified, then re-stratified in different ways. This observation can complicate the interpretation of a subgroup evaluations.

For example, consider a randomized, controlled clinical trial that is in its analysis phase. At this time, all of the patients are grouped into either having or not having diabetes mellitus. Once the stratum membership assignment is finished, the effect of the randomly allocated intervention is assessed in each of the two strata. The analyses reveal that the therapy has a greater effect in non-diabetic patients than in those with diabetes.

When completed, these same patients are then re-aggregated based not on diabetes but on age. Subjects are placed into one of the following three age strata: (1) less than 30 years of age, (2) between 30 and 60 years of age, and (3) greater than 60 years of age. When the subgroup analysis is carried out for the age strata, it appears that the effect of therapy is reduced in the older age group.

The investigators report that both age and diabetes modify the effect of therapy. Holding aside the complexities of generalizing from the sample to the population, focus just on the sample, and consider how we know which of these subgroups is responsible for the observed effects? All the investigator has done is to reclassify the same patients in two different ways. Perhaps the older patients are more likely to be diabetic. If this is the case, the diabetes subgroup effect may simply be another manifestation of the age effect. Thus the findings reported out as two different effects may simply be one effect, expressing itself in two different analyses.

It can be misleading to report both, because the investigator has simply reclassified the same patients. The results from these two subgroup analyses essentially demonstrate that the same patients when characterized one way (by diabetes) provide a different result than when characterized another way (by age). Was it really diabetes that modified the effect of therapy or was it the chance collection of patients that made it appear that diabetes gender was an influence? Since we can expect that the effect of treatment within a subgroup stratum depends on the patients within that stratum, then the value of the subgroup analysis must be tightly linked to the ability to demonstrate that the stratum characteristic (and not the random aggregation of patients) is producing the interesting effect.

10.5.2. Random Findings
It is difficult to separate a true stratum-specific "signal" from the random background "noise."

Consider the following simple experiment. A classroom chosen at random has a capacity of seating 80 students. These 80 seats are divided by a central aisle, with 40 seats on each of the left-hand and right-hand side of the courtroom. Eighty students seat themselves as they choose, distributing themselves in an unrestricted manner among the seats on each side of the class. When all are seated, we measure the height of each person, finding that the average height is exactly 69 inches. Does that mean that the average height of those seated on the left-hand side of the classroom will be 69 inches? No, because the 69 inch measurement was produced from all eighty students in the room, not just the forty on the left-hand side. The sample of forty has a different mean simply because they are only part of and not the entire population of 80.

If the average height on the left-hand side of the classroom is greater than 69 inches, then those seated on the right-hand side will have an average height less than 69 inches.[*] Thus, those sitting on the left-hand side have a greater height than those on the right-hand side. While that fact is undeniable in this one classroom during this one seating, would it be fair to generalize this conclusion to the population at large?

No. The random aggregation of observations has induced a subgroup effect that is based only on the play of chance here. Specifically, the "subgroup effect" was induced by selectively excluding individuals from the computation of the mean.

An illustration of this principle is how subgroups are induced by the process of sampling. Consider the result of a hypothetical clinical trial in which the investigators report that the randomly allocated intervention produced a 25% reduction in the prospectively defined endpoint of total mortality. The initial reaction to the demonstration of a beneficial effect of therapy in a well-designed, well executed clinical trial is naturally to assume that the effect of therapy is homogenous. Our first response is therefore to believe that all collections of patients in the active group were beneficiaries of this 25% benefit, and that the beneficial effect of therapy provides protection that is broadly distributed (Figure 10.1, panel 1.) This treatment effect uniformity is the truth about the population at large. However, the examination of the same therapy effect within different subgroups of the clinical trial sample reveals a mosaic of treatment effect magnitudes (Figure 10.1, panel 2).

At first glance, it appears that the uniform mortality benefit has been replaced by a much more heterogeneous response. The uniform 25% reduction in the total mortality effect is still there; the population from which the research sample was derived still experienced a 25% reduction in the proportion of deaths. However, when that uniform effect is viewed through the prism of a small sample, the uniform effect is distorted. The same process that produced a difference in average height on either side of the room, i.e., the exclusion of individuals from the computation of the treatment effect, generates the differences in subgroup effect sizes in Figure 10.1, panel 2. Much as the random aggregation of students in the class from the previous example produced a subgroup effect, the random aggregation of patients in research efforts will induce a heterogeneity of responses.

An investigator, unaware of this effect-distorting phenomenon and having only the data from Figure 10.1, panel 2, believes that the response to treatment is heterogeneous since his data demonstrates variability between, for example, men and women, or African-Americans and Caucasians. However, this variability is not induced by a complex interrelationship among genetics, environment, and therapy response. It is induced solely by the sampling process.

We must also keep in mind that the reverse effect is possible. The sample may suggest that there is no differential effect of therapy between subgroup strata when in fact one is present, again, because of sampling error.

---

[*] If the average height of all in the classroom is 69 inches, and the average height on the left side is greater than 69 inches, then the average height on the right-hand side must be less than 69 inches in order for the average of all to be 69 inches.

The random selection of data from the population produces sampling error. Its presence will produce false findings and "red herrings", just through the random aggregation of subjects in the population. However the data will also accurately reflect relationships that are embedded in the population. This random subgroup effect appears in all subgroup analyses, and we will have to integrate it into our interpretation of any subgroup effect that we see.

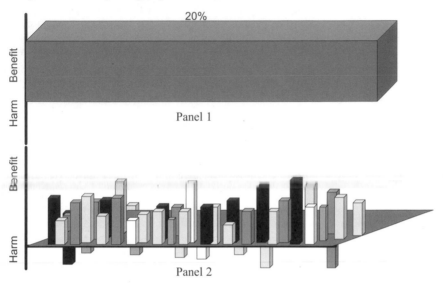

Fig. 10.1. Homogenous population effect (Panel 1)appears as a variable treatment effect in the sample (Panel 2).

It therefore is difficult correctly to classify a relationship that is observed in the data. Unfortunately, exploratory subgroup analysis is an imprecise means of classification. For example, in the MRFIT trial, the identification of a relationship that suggested that the treatment of hypertension may be harmful in men with abnormal hearts confused the medical community for several years.[*] In the end, this finding was attributed to sampling error. These occurrences help to justify the admonition that the best descriptor of the effect in a subgroup is the finding that is observed in the overall cohort.

10.5.3 Clinical Trial-Mediated Subgroup "Effects"

As another example, consider the effect of therapy in a clinical trial designed to assess the role of LDL cholesterol level modification in reducing the incidence of fatal heart attack/nonfatal heart attack/revascularization. The analysis of the effect of therapy on this endpoint in the entire cohort was overwhelmingly positive. The effect of therapy in a variety of *post hoc* subgroups was also examined (Table 10.1).

Table 10.1 reveals the effect of therapy within each of five subgroups (A through E) in the clinical trial. Each subgroup contains two different strata. For

---

[*] See Chapter Two.

each stratum, the number of patients in the subgroup at risk for the disease, the number of patients in the subgroup who have the disease, and the cumulative incidence rate of the endpoint are provided To assess the effect of therapy, both the relative risk of therapy and the p-value are included. For example, subgroup A contains two strata: I and II. In strata I, there are 576 patients; 126 of them experienced the endpoint. The cumulative incidence of the endpoint in the placebo group was 27.59 (i.e., 27.59% of these patients experienced a clinical endpoint), and 16.08 in the active group. The relative risk due to therapy was 0.54, i.e., the risk of an event in the active group was 54% of the risk of that event in the placebo group, suggesting that there was some benefit was associated with therapy. The p-value for this protective effect is 0.001. In this subgroup, the effect of therapy was notable in each of the two strata, (relative risk of 0.54 in stratum I versus 0.80 in strata II) with a further suggestion that patients in strata I received a greater benefit from therapy than patients in stratum II.

Examination of the data suggest that the therapy effect is not uniform across the subgroup strata, providing benefit for some and hazard for others. In subgroup C, for example, the relative risk for the event is 1.02 (p-value = 0.916) for strata I, suggesting no benefit. In stratum II of this subgroup, the relative risk is 0.71 (p-value < 0.001). Does this suggest that patients in subgroup C, strata I should not receive the therapy? If true, this would be an important message to disseminate, especially if the therapy was associated with significant cost or side effects.

There is a similar finding for subgroup D: again, stratum I demonstrates no effect of therapy while strata II demonstrates a possibly important effect. The analyses in subgroups C and D suggest that there may be a stratum dependent therapy, while subgroup E demonstrates that the effect of therapy was the same in each of its strata.

However, we have only the relative risk and the p-value to convey the significance of the therapy effect within subgroups, and our assessment of their joint message tempts us to draw conclusions about which of the subgroup strata demonstrated a therapy effect and which did not. In fact, it's not hard to envision the explanations of imaginative investigators that would be offered to explain the different subgroup effects.

Table 10.2 reveals a more useful explanation. This table contains the same data as Table 10.1 and also the identities of the subgroups. We see that subgroups A, B, and C are clinical subgroups of direct relevance to the clinical investigation. However, subgroups D and E are completely random subgroups, i.e., a random number was used to generate the strata membership for these two subgroups. Nevertheless, the statistical findings of these random subgroups are equally as persuasive as the findings in the subgroups of clinical relevance. The results in the random subgroups mimic the findings in the "real subgroup." From a comparison of Table 10.1 and 10.2, we see that one cannot differentiate a meaningful effect of therapy from just the random play of chance by examining the results.

Table 10.1. Effect of therapy on endpoint incidence within unknown subgroups: Fatal and nonfatal MI plus revascularizations

	Subgroup	Placebo	Active	Total	P-value	Rel Risk
		Patients				
A	I					
	Endpoint	80	46	126		
	Total	290	286	576		
	Cum. Inc Rate *100	27.59	16.08	21.88	0.001	0.54
	II					
	Endpoint	469	384	853		
	Total	1788	1795	3583		
	Cum. Inc Rate *100	26.23	21.39	23.81	0.001	0.80
B	I					
	Endpoint	258	217	475		
	Total	1003	1027	2030		
	Cum. Inc Rate *100	25.72	21.13	23.40	0.018	0.80
	II					
	Endpoint	291	213	504		
	Total	1075	1054	2129		
	Cum. Inc Rate *100	27.07	20.21	23.67	<0.001	0.73
C	I					
	Endpoint	98	95	193		
	Total	461	439	900		
	Cum. Inc Rate *100	21.26	21.64	21.44	0.916	1.02
	II					
	Endpoint	451	335	786		
	Total	1617	1642	3259		
	Cum. Inc Rate *100	27.89	20.40	24.12	<0.001	0.71
D	I					
	Endpoint	105	91	196		
	Total	397	402	799		
	Cum. Inc Rate *100	26.45	22.64	24.53	0.210	0.84
	II					
	Endpoint	444	339	783		
	Total	1681	1679	3360		
	Cum. Inc Rate *100	26.41	20.19	23.30	<0.001	0.75
E	I					
	Endpoint	186	137	323		
	Total	653	639	1292		
	Cum. Inc Rate *100	28.48	21.44	25.00	0.011	0.75
	II					
	Endpoint	363	293	656		
	Total	1425	1442	2867		
	Cum. Inc Rate *100	25.47	20.32	22.88	0.001	0.77

Table 10.2 Effect of therapy on endpoint incidence within known subgroups:
Fatal and nonfatal MI plus revascularizations

	Subgroup	Placebo	Active	Total	P-value	Rel Risk
		Patients				
Gender	I					
	Endpoint	80	46	126		
	Total	290	286	576		
	Cum. Inc Rate *100	27.59	16.08	21.88	0.001	0.54
	II					
	Endpoint	469	384	853		
	Total	1788	1795	3583		
	Cum. Inc Rate *100	26.23	21.39	23.81	0.001	0.80
Age	I					
	Endpoint	258	217	475		
	Total	1003	1027	2030		
	Cum. Inc Rate *100	25.72	21.13	23.40	0.018	0.80
	II					
	Endpoint	291	213	504		
	Total	1075	1054	2129		
	Cum. Inc Rate *100	27.07	20.21	23.67	<0.001	0.73
LDL Cholesterol	I					
	Endpoint	98	95	193		
	Total	461	439	900		
	Cum. Inc Rate *100	21.26	21.64	21.44	0.916	1.02
	II					
	Endpoint	451	335	786		
	Total	1617	1642	3259		
	Cum. Inc Rate *100	27.89	20.40	24.12	<0.001	0.71
Random D	I					
	Endpoint	105	91	196		
	Total	397	402	799		
	Cum. Inc Rate *100	26.45	22.64	24.53	0.210	0.84
	II					
	Endpoint	444	339	783		
	Total	1681	1679	3360		
	Cum. Inc Rate *100	26.41	20.19	23.30	<0.001	0.75
Random E	I					
	Endpoint	186	137	323		
	Total	653	639	1292		
	Cum. Inc Rate *100	28.48	21.44	25.00	0.011	0.75
	II					
	Endpoint	363	293	656		
	Total	1425	1442	2867		
	Cum. Inc Rate *100	25.47	20.32	22.88	0.001	0.77

Two points are to be made from this evaluation. The first is that neither the *p*-value nor the relative risk discriminated between the clinical versus the random subgroup. Relying on these measures can be quite misleading in subgroup analysis. Secondly, it is not so much that the random subgroup looked like the clinical subgroup. It is more to the point to say that the clinical subgroups are more likely to produce random findings just through the aggregation of events.

Even if we concentrate on the first three subgroups whose subgroup definitions are plausible and have scientific meaning, we still cannot be sure that the effects demonstrated in Table 10.2 truly represent the findings in the population. The gender examination suggests that women derive a greater benefit from cholesterol reduction therapy then do men. There appears to be no real difference in effect of therapy across the different age strata. Also, it appears that patients with baseline LDL cholesterol greater than 125 mg/dl derive a profound effect from therapy while those patients with a baseline LDL cholesterol $\leq$ 125 mg/dl obtain no benefit from therapy.

10.5.4 The Importance of Replication

These findings for women and patients with baseline LDL cholesterol $\leq$ 125 mg/dl were obtained from the CARE clinical trial and published by Sacks et al. [2], producing much discussion among lipidologists. A follow-up manuscript elaborating on the effect of cholesterol reduction therapy in women was published by Lewis et al [6]. A manuscript examining the relationship between LDL cholesterol and clinical endpoints was also published in 1998 [7]. The subgroup findings from CARE and the subsequent published manuscripts based on these findings were surprising and useful, generating much debate. In neither case was the hypothesis stated prospectively (with alpha allocation) in the protocol.* Yet, in each case the subgroup analysis was relevant and insisted upon by the scientific community. How can one interpret the findings of these required but non-prospective evaluations?

One relevant tool for assessing subgroup results is the criterion of confirmation or replication of an experiment's results. In its narrowest form, study replication involves the slavish reproduction of previous numeric results using the original experimental protocol; its goal is to limit investigator error (either inadvertent or intentional). More broadly, replication involves the systematic variation of research conditions to determine whether an earlier result can be observed under new conditions. This is particularly important when a number of different study designs are used. The variety of study designs, each with its own unique strengths and weaknesses, minimizes the chance that all of the studies are making the same mistake. Consistency is demonstrated when several of these studies giving the same results [20].

It is this broader, more useful interpretation that would be most helpful in interpreting the results from CARE. An independent clinical trial carried out in Australia [4], completed after the end of CARE, examined the effect of the same cholesterol reducing therapy. This second study differed in that (1) the Australian

---

* The protocol is the prospectively written plan which outlines the goal, design, execution, and analysis of the experiment.

study (known by the acronym LIPID) was twice as large as CARE, (2) the entry criteria were somewhat different, and (3) the clinical endpoint LIPID was coronary heart disease death, a stronger endpoint than the well-accepted combined endpoint of fatal heart attack/nonfatal heart attack/revascularization used in the CARE subgroup analysis. The LIPID investigators carried out the subgroup analyses in women and in patients with low levels of baseline LDL cholesterol. They found no differential effect of therapy in women, a finding that contradicted the observation of CARE. However, the Australian study did replicate the baseline LDL cholesterol subgroup findings first identified in CARE. Thus, one would give more credence to the replicated finding involving baseline LDL cholesterol than to the finding involving women. The lesson is that subgroup analyses from one study are difficult to interpret on their own; they should be reproduced in an independent study before they are considered reliable.

10.6 Stratified Randomization

Another difficulty in the interpretation of subgroup analyses in clinical trials is that the patient classification process can undo one of the most important features of these research experiments — the ability to attribute differences in observed endpoints to the randomly allocated intervention. The absence of this key feature complicates the interpretation of the subgroup analysis.

Consider a clinical trial that has a control group and a treatment group. The random allocation of therapy can clarify a study's results by requiring each of its patients have their therapy assignment based on factors separate from his/her own traits. Frequently, this means that each patient has the same probability of receiving the active intervention as the next patient.* This feature distributes patients between the control and active group in such a way that the only difference between the two groups is that one group received active therapy and the other received control group therapy. There are not likely to be any important demographic, sociologic, or risk factor differences between the two groups. Therefore, differences between endpoint rates that occur at the end of the trial can be attributed to the only difference between the two groups — the randomly allocated therapy.

These finely balanced circumstances are perturbed when subgroups are analyzed. Unfortunately, membership in the subgroup stratum of interest may be very low, and randomization may not have had a real opportunity to balance patient distribution in this stratum.† Thus, the effect of therapy within that particular subgroup stratum may be confounded, i.e., confused and intertwined with other characteristics that are different between the treatment groups. It can be virtually impossible to persuasively attribute any differences between the treatment groups to the therapy within this one stratum.

---

* Adaptations of this procedure can be executed to ensure that there is an exact balance between the number recruited to each of the control and treatment arms. However, therapy is not assigned based on a patient's characteristic.
† The importance of prospectively declared scientific questions was addressed in Chapter Two.

Knowledgeable investigators anticipate the distribution of patients across the subgroup and the resultant small number of patients within some of the subgroup's strata. These investigators sometimes actually force the random allocation therapy to work. That is, they adjust the randomization algorithm so that there are an equal number of patients allocated to each of the control and active groups of the trial within the subgroup stratum. This randomization within the strata, or *stratified randomization,* ensures that even though there is a small number of patients within the stratum, the allocation of therapy will be more effectively balanced. While not compensating for the different endpoint event rates stemming from the relatively small number of patients in the stratum, this adaptation does substantially improve the balance of baseline characteristics between the treatment groups. By doing this, investigators strengthen their ability to ascribe differences in the mortality rate to the randomly allocated therapy.

10.7 Proper Versus Improper Subgroups

A critical preliminary task in subgroup analysis is the proper classification of patients into each of the subgroup strata. Although membership determination may appear to be a trivial task, there are circumstances in which this classification is problematic. These concerns revolve around the timing of the subgroup membership determination.

There are two important possibilities for determining of the timing of subgroup membership. The first is the classification of patients into the correct subgroup stratum when the patients are randomized. The second choice is to classify patients into subgroup strata at some time during the execution of the trial. While each has advantages, the determination of subgroup membership at the beginning of the study is preferred.

Determining subgroup membership at the beginning of the trial requires not only that the subgroup must be defined at the beginning of the study, but also that the subgroup strata membership should be defined prospectively as well. This is a straightforward procedure to apply to the gender subgroup with its two strata. However, for other subgroups of clinical interest, the process can be complex. For example, while it can be relatively straightforward to evaluate the relationship between cholesterol levels subgroup strata 1) less than 175 mg/dl, and 2) greater than 175 mg/dl and the cumulative incidence of stroke, the evaluation of these strata when they are based in follow-up levels of cholesterol is problematic.

The problems arise for two reasons. The first is that patients can change subgroup strata as the study progresses and the their cholesterol levels fluctuate. This makes it difficult to determine definitively and convincingly subgroup membership, and the analysis can suffer from the observation that changing the subgroup membership of just a few patients can change the results of the subgroup analysis. Such brittle evaluations are unpersuasive.

Secondly, there are many influences that effect lipid measurements over time. If the exposure being evaluated reduces cholesterol levels, then patients with lower cholesterol levels are more likely to have received active therapy, and patients with the higher levels would have a greater chance of being in the control group. Thus the evaluation of lipid levels will be confounded with exposure to the agents after the study was initiated, confounding (i.e., confusing) the attribution of the observed effect on the endpoint.

In our first example in this section, we acknowledged that there were many factors that influence baseline lipid levels. Race, gender, family history, and prior treatment are but a few of them. However, the randomly assigned intervention did not influence baseline LDL-cholesterol levels. It is the absence of any relationship between the randomly allocated therapy and the baseline LDL-cholesterol level that allows a clear examination of the effect of LDL-cholesterol level on the relationship between the intervention and stroke. A subgroup whose strata membership criteria are based on baseline characteristics of the patient is called a *proper subgroup* [21]. Improper subgroups are those whose strata membership can only be determined after the patient has been randomized. Membership based on follow-up data is influenced by randomly allocated therapy and the interpretation is complicated.

There are circumstances in which this type of analysis is nevertheless carried out. If the investigators are interested in an evaluation of the effect of lower blood pressure on the incidence of stroke, regardless of how the blood pressure was lowered, then analysis procedures are available.[*] However these evaluations are exceedingly complicated and the results must be interpreted with great caution. Similar evaluations have examined the relationship between lipid lowering medications and atherosclerotic morbidity and mortality [22–24].

Finally, we will hold aside the issue of the analysis of a proper subgroup defined *post hoc*. In that circumstance, the subgroup criteria using baseline variables is defined at the end of the study. Since the subgroup analysis was planned after the data were examined, the analysis is exploratory.

10.8 "Intention-to-Treat" Versus "As Treated"

Consider a clinical trial in which patients are randomized to receive an intervention to reduce the total mortality rate from end-stage renal disease. At the inception of the study, patients are randomized to receive either control group therapy or the intervention. At the conclusion of the study, the investigators will compare the cumulative mortality rates of patients in each of the two treatment groups. However, how will the investigators decide which patients should be assigned to each group in the final analysis? The commonly used approach is to assign treatment group membership simply as the group to which the patient was randomized. This is the "intention to treat" principle.

The "intention-to-treat" principle of analysis is the standard analysis procedure for the evaluation of clinical trial results. Undoubtedly, this analysis tends to be a conservative one, since not every patient is treated as they were "intended." For example, some patients randomized to the active group may not take their medication. These patients, although randomized to the active group, will have the control group experience and produce endpoints at rates similar to that of the control group. However, they would be included in the active group since they were randomized to and "intended to be treated" like active group patients. The inclusion of these patients in the active group for analysis purposes tends to make the active

---

[*] Cox hazard analysis with time-dependent covariates has been one useful tool in this regard.

group experience look more like the control group experience, increasing the over-all active group event rate.[*]

Similarly, patients who are randomized to the control group may neverthe-less be exposed to active group medication. These patients will experience event rates similar to the rates of the active group, but since they are considered as part of the control group, the inclusion of these patients will produce an event rate for the control group that is closer to that of the active group.

Thus the control group rate will approach that of the active group, while the cumulative event rate in the active group will be closer to that of the control group (described in the previous paragraph). This effect of these combined rate alterations reduces the magnitude of the treatment effect, thereby diminishing the power of the clinical trial.[†]

An alternative analysis to the "intent to treat" principle is one that analyzes the endpoint results using an "as-treated" analysis. In this case, although patients are still randomized to receive either placebo or active therapy, they are classified for analysis purposes based on whether they actually took their medication. Since this is determined after the patient was randomized to the medication, and the effect (both perceived beneficial and adverse effects) of the medication may determine whether the patient takes the medication, the "as-treated" evaluation is a con-founded analysis. A clearly detailed examination of this issue is available [25].

10.9 Effect Domination Principle

The examination of individual subgroup strata effects in healthcare research can be misleading for reasons that have been elaborated. If we cannot believe the event rates that are present in the stratum are the best measures of that stratum's response to the exposure, what then is the best measure of the effect of an exposure on a sub-group stratum?

The classroom illustration provided in section 9.5.1 reveals the answer. In that circumstance where the average height was greater for those sitting on one side of the room than the other, the best estimate of the average height of those who sit on the left side of the room is the overall average height of all in the class.

We are not saying that the average height should replace the actual heights of those on each side of the room. Clearly, the best estimator of the average height of those sitting on the left side of the room is the average height of precisely those people. However, we are saying that if one wished to generalize results to the popu-lation at large, the best generalization of the average height of people who sit on the Allowing the overall measure of effect in the entire cohort to supersede the sub-group stratum effects can be termed the *effect domination principle* and is attribut-able to Yusuf et al. [21]

---

[*] There are occasional complications in an "intention-to-treat" analysis. In some cases, a patient is tested and randomized, but then, subsequent to the randomization the test result reveals that the patient is not eligible for the trial for a prospectively stated reason. In this case, there was no "intent" to randomize this patient when the test result was known, and the patient is removed from the study.
[†] The effect of the magnitude of the treatment effect on the power of a study for fixed sample size is elaborated in Appendix B.

Thus, in the example from the PRAISE I clinical trial discussed in section 10.3, the generalizable effect of therapy in those with non-ischemic cardiomyopathy was the overall effect of therapy in general. This was borne-out in the PRAISE II findings. This principle of effect domination is not very provocative and contains none of the excitement of exploratory analyses. However, it is far more reliable, given the general non-confirmatory analyses that the majority of subgroup analyses constitute in healthcare results.

10.10 Confirmatory Subgroup Analyses

Since subgroup analyses have and will, in all likelihood, continue to engender the interest of the medical community, it is logical to ask why there aren't more confirmatory analyses involving subgroup evaluations. This is an especially interesting question since there are clear circumstances in which subgroup evaluations can produce confirmatory results of a therapy effect within (or across) subgroup strata. When executed, these confirmatory results stand on their own, separate and apart from the result of the effect of therapy in the overall cohort. The criteria for these evaluations are clearly characterized by and are coincident with our development of confirmatory analyses in this text.

The first of these criteria for the development of confirmatory analyses in clinical trials is that the subgroup analysis must be prospectively designed and proper. This structure is required so that (1) the therapy effect size estimators that the subgroup analysis produces are trustworthy; and (2) that the effect of therapy to be evaluated in a subgroup is not confounded by (i.e., bound up with) post-randomization events as discussed in the previous chapter. In general, there has been no difficulty with meeting this requirement of confirmatory subgroup analyses. Many clinical trials make statements in their protocols describing the plans of investigators to evaluate the effect of therapy within their subgroups of interest. These subgroups are, proper subgroups, e.g., demographic traits, or the presence of risk characteristics at baseline.

However, the final requirement for a confirmatory subgroup analysis is the prospective allocation of type I and type II error rates. This last criterion has proved to be especially troublesome because of the severe sample size constraints this places on subgroup analyses. As we have pointed out earlier, the allocation of type I error rates for confirmatory testing must be such that the FWER, ξ, is conserved. This requires that statistical testing at the level of subgroup analyses be governed by test-specific α error rates that are generally less than 0.05.

The difficulty of executing subgroup analyses in the presence of FWER control and adequate statistical power is not difficult to understand. In fact, resources are generally strained to the breaking point for the analysis of the effect of therapy in the overall cohort. This overall analysis is typically carried out with the minimum acceptable power (80%) because of either financial constraints or patient recruitment difficulties. By definition, subgroup analyses (and certainly within-stratum subgroup analyses) will involve a smaller number of patients; it is a daunting task to allocate prospectively type I and type II error rates at acceptable levels in a smaller number of patients, although the methodology for the accurate computation of sample size is available [26]. Thus, the growth of the use of subgroups as

confirmatory tools has, to some extent, been stunted by the difficulty of constructing a prospective clinical trial with an embedded, prospectively defined proper subgroup for which tight statistical control is provided for type I and type II statistical
errors.

10.11 Assessment of Subgroup Effects

The evaluation of subgroup effects in clinical trials focuses on the effect of the randomly allocated therapy on the subgroup of interest. However this assessment can
be carried out in two complementary manners. The first is the determination of a
differential effect of therapy across subgroup strata. The second is the evaluation of
the effect of therapy within a single subgroup stratum. Each approach, when prospectively planned and concordantly executed, can supplement the information
provided by the evaluation of the main effect of a clinical trial.

10.11.1 Effect Modification and Interactions

We commonly think of the effect of the randomly allocated intervention in a clinical trial as an effect across the entire research cohort. The examination of u dataset
for this effect, while complicated, has become a routine part of the evaluation of the
randomly allocated therapy's influence in a clinical trial. The finding of both clinical and statistical significance for this analysis suggests that the effect of therapy is
different for one subgroup stratum than for another.

This type of subgroup effect is commonly referred to as a *treatment by
subgroup* interaction; a notable product of this analysis is the *p*-value for interaction. Typically, the analysis result is described as identifying how the subgroup
strata interacts with the therapy to alter the occurrence of the endpoint, and the
evaluation is called an *interaction analysis*. Alternatively, this approach is described as *effect modification*, i.e., it examines the degree to which the subgroup
stratum modifies the effect of treatment on the endpoint.

We should not be surprised by the observation that statistically significant
effect modification analyses in research are uncommon. The subgroup analyses
involve an evaluation of an effect difference between smaller subsets of patients
within the research cohort. Everything else being equal, the smaller sample sizes
reduce the statistical power of the hypothesis tests. The presence of a test statistic
that does not fall in the critical region in a low-power environment is not a null
finding, but instead is merely uninformative; many of these subgroup analyses are
unhelpful.

Alternatively, the occurrence of a statistically significant effect size can be
particularly noteworthy. An example of such a finding occurred in the Cholesterol
and Recurrent Events (CARE) clinical trial. CARE was designed to demonstrate
that the reduction in LDL cholesterol in patients with moderate lipid levels would
reduce the incidence of cardiovascular disease in patients with a history of MI. In
that study, an examination of the effect of the HMG-CoA reductase inhibitor
pravastatin was assessed in the gender subgroup. The relevant analysis was the effect of pravastatin on the cumulative incidence rate of the *post hoc* composite endpoint of CAD death + nonfatal MI + coronary revascularization [7]. There were
4,159 patients recruited in the CARE study; of these, 576 (13.8%) were women and

3,583 (86.2%) were men. During the course of the trial the effect of the randomly allocated intervention pravastatin on lipids appeared to be the same in women and men, producing equivalent reductions in total cholesterol (20% in women, 19% in men), low density lipid (LDL) cholesterol (28% in women, 28% in men), and triglycerides (13% in women, 14% in men). There were also equivalent elevations in high-density lipoprotein (HDL) cholesterol (4% in women, 5% in men).

However, the subgroup analysis revealed an apparent difference in the effect of pravastatin therapy on the expanded endpoint in men and women (Table 10.3).

Table 10.3. Gender-moderated effect* of therapy in CARE

Gender Strata	Relative Risk	Interaction P-value
Males	0.761	
Females	0.545	
		0.050

*CHD disease death + nonfatal MI + coronary revascularization.

Men in CARE experienced a relative risk of 0.761 on pravastatin therapy, while women who were randomly chosen to receive pravastatin therapy experienced a 0.545 relative risk. The p-value that assesses the difference in the effect for men and women was 0.05. Within CARE, the effect of therapy appeared to be modified by gender, women being the greater beneficiary of this effect than men.

However, care must be exercised in the interpretation of the analysis. This evaluation was but one of a number of secondary analyses executed in the study, and as such, was not subjected to a correction in the type I error rate for multiplicity. Thus its findings serve as merely supportive of the overall finding of cardioprotection from statin-based LDL reduction from CARE.

10.11.2 Within-Stratum Effects

The evaluation of a subgroup mediated effect modification may not directly address the question the investigators have raised about the subgroup. This is because the investigators' interest may not be in the entire subgroup, but only in selected subgroup strata. Specifically, the investigators may not ask whether the effect of therapy is the same across subgroups, but instead ask whether there is an explicit effect of the intervention in the prospectively defined subgroup stratum of interest. This is a different question than that addressed by an interaction analysis.

One such situation would be when the stratum is composed of patients who have a very different prognosis from that of patients in other strata of the subgroup. While investigators may be most interested in the effect of a new intervention on thyroid cancer, they may be particularly interested in the effect of the therapy in patients with an advanced stage of the disease. This interest does not require the investigators to ask whether the effect of therapy in patients with less advanced thyroid cancer is different from that of patients with advanced thyroid cancer; they wish to know only whether the therapy has been shown to have explicit efficacy in patients with advanced thyroid cancer.

Similarly, a new therapy for the treatment of CHF may hold promise for reducing mortality in all patients with CHF, but the investigator is motivated to demonstrate the effect of this therapy in patients with CHF whose etiology is non-ischemic. She is not interested in comparing or contrasting the efficacy of the intervention between ischemic versus non-ischemic etiologies of CHF. She is instead focused on two questions: (1) Is the therapy effective in the entire cohort and (2) Can the effect of this therapy be confirmed in the subcohort with CHF-non-ischemic etiology?

Is it possible that the therapy could be effective in the entire cohort but not the subcohort of interest? Yes. Consider the possibility that the therapy in fact is effective for patients with CHF-ischemic etiology but ineffective for patients with a non-ischemic etiology for their CHF. Let the research sample primarily contain patients with CHF-ischemic etiology with only a small number of patients who have a non-ischemic etiology for their heart failure. Since the research sample contains primarily those patients who will respond to the therapy, the result of the concordantly executed clinical trial will be positive (barring an effect that is driven by sampling error). The investigator will then argue that, since the trial is positive, this positive finding will apply to the CHF-non-ischemic subgroup as well. Essentially, the conclusion about the non-ischemic subcohort is based primarily on the findings of patients who are not in that subcohort at all.

This is the consequence of the effect domination principle, in which the findings in the overall cohort devolve on each of the subgroup strata. In this example, the principle produces the wrong conclusion; nevertheless, it is the best conclusion available in the absence of a confirmatory subgroup analysis. In order to avoid this possibility, the investigator is interested in reaching a confirmatory conclusion.

As another illustration of a circumstance in which prospectively specified, stratum-specific subgroup analyses can make an important contribution, consider the situation in which the adverse event profile of a therapy that is being studied in a controlled clinical trial is known to be different between women and men. As an illustration, consider a cholesterol-reducing drug that produces benign breast disease in women. In this circumstance, the risk–benefit profile of this drug is different for women than it is for men. Since women will be exposed to a greater risk with this therapy, it is reasonable to require investigators to produce a statistically valid demonstration of efficacy in women. The investigators are not disinterested in an effect in men; however, the relatively low risk of the drug in men allows the investigators to be satisfied with deducing the effect of the therapy in men from the effect of therapy in the overall cohort. It is the greater adverse event risk in women that requires an explicit demonstration of efficacy in them.

There are different questions that can be asked of subgroups. Some of these questions can be addressed by a heterogeneity of effect evaluation with its accompanying interaction analysis; however, there are others that are addressed by the direct demonstration of efficacy in a single subgroup stratum. Numerous examples and scenarios of the execution of subgroup stratum-specific analyses are available [27, 28].

10.12 Data Dredging — Caveat Emptor

Data dredging is the methodologic examination of a database for all significant relationships. These database evaluations are thorough, and the analysis procedures are wide ranging, spanning the gamut from simple t-testing to more complex time to event evaluations, repeated measures assessments, and structure equation modeling. Typically, little thought is given to endpoint triage as discussed in Chapter Nine.

The notion that if they look hard enough, work long enough, and dig deep enough they will dig up something "significant" in the database drives the data dredgers. Indeed, the investigators may identify a relationship that will ultimately be of great value to the medical community. However, while it is possible to discover a jewel in this "strip-mining" operation, for every rare jewel identified, there will be many false finds, fakes, and shams. As Miles pointed out, datasets that are tortured long enough will provide the answers that the investigators seek, whether the answers are helpful, truthful, or not [29].

Unfortunately, many of the important principles of good experimental methodology are missing in the direct examination of interesting subgroups. Inadequate sample size, poorly performing estimators,* low power, and the generation of multiple p-values combine to create an environment in which the findings of the data dredging operation are commonly not generalizable. Accepting the "significant" results of these data-dredging activates can misdirect researchers into expending critical research resources in fruitless pursuits, a phenomenon described by Johnson [30]. In his 1849 text *Experimenta Agriculture*, Johnson stated that a badly conceived experiment was not only wasted time and money, but led to both the adoption of incorrect results and the neglect of further research along more productive lines. It can therefore take tremendous effort for the medical and research community to sort out the wheat from the data-dredged chaff, often at great expense.

10.13 Conclusions

Subgroup analyses are most likely here to stay. As long as physicians focus on the treatment of individual patients, factoring in those patients' unique and distinguishing characteristics when fashioning therapy, they will be interested in the results of subgroup analyses. This is an honest attempt to reduce the number of unknowns in the prediction of an individual patient's response to treatment, and will continue to stoke the subgroup analysis fire.

This chapter demonstrates some of the contemporary difficulties that subgroup analyses create. Many subgroups evaluations can be misinterpreted because subgroup membership may merely be a surrogate for another, less obvious factor

---

* The observation that the accuracy and precision of commonly used estimators is distorted in exploratory research is discussed in Chapter Two.

that determines efficacy. The investigator must consider this possible explanation for her subgroup specific effect in her interpretation of the analysis.

Yet another force that exerts traction on both investigators and regulators for subgroup interpretation is the lay press. Consider, as an example, an editorial appearing in the Wall Street Journal that purported to have identified an unnecessary obstruction put in place by the FDA's drug approval process [31]. The editorial, complained openly, asking, "Why not allow companies to cull the relevant data from existing studies when a certain subgroup is clearly of help?"

Unfortunately, these calls for directed action that are based on the misdirected and misleading belief that subgroup analyses are not harmless. The genuine, heartfelt desire to come to the aid of ailing people must be tempered with a disciplined research strategy and execution. In the absence of this control, research efforts produce interventions that harm patients.

It is also more than likely that the majority of subgroup analyses will continue to be carried out as either prospectively declared secondary evaluations or as exploratory analyses. Thus the guidelines put forward by Yusuf will continue to be predominant for these evaluations—the best estimate of the effect of a therapy within a subgroup in such an analysis is the effect of the therapy that was seen in the overall cohort. These subgroup evaluations can suggest but not confirm the answers to questions about the risks and benefits of an exposure in clinical research. Fishing expeditions for significance commonly catch only the junk of sampling error.

References

1. Pfeffer MA, Braunwald E, Moyé LA et al (1992) Effect of captopril on mortality and morbidity in patients with left ventricular dysfunction after myocardial infarction–results of the Survival and Ventricular Enlargement Trial. *New England Journal of Medicine* **327**:669–677.

2. Sacks FM, Pfeffer MA, Moyé, LA (1996) The effect of pravastatin on coronary events after myocardial infarction in patients with average cholesterol levels. *New England Journal of Medicine* **335**:1001–1009.

3. The SHEP Cooperative Research Group (1991) Prevention of stroke by antihypertensive drug therapy in older persons with isolated systolic hypertension: final results of the systolic hypertension in the elderly program (SHEP). *Journal of the American Medical Association* **265**:3255–3264

4. The Long-Term Intervention with Pravastatin in Ischaemic Disease (LIPID) Study Group (1998) Prevention of cardiovascular events and death with pravastatin in patients with CAD and a broad range of initial cholesterol levels. *New England Journal of Medicine* **339**:1349–1357.

5. Moyé, LA, Pfeffer, MA, Wun, CC, et. al (1994) Uniformity of captopril benefit in the post infarction population: Subgroup analysis in SAVE. *European Heart Journal* **15**: Supplement B:2–8.

6. Lewis SJ, Moyé LA, Sacks FM, et. al (1998) Effect of pravastatin on cardiovascular events in older patients with myocardial infarction and cholesterol

levels in the average range Results of the Cholesterol and Recurrent Events (CARE) trial. *Annals of Internal Medicine* **129**:681–689.

7. Lewis SJ, Sacks FM, Mitchell JS, et. al (1998) Effect of pravastatin on cardiovascular events in women after myocardial infarction: the cholesterol and recurrent events (CARE) trial. *Journal of the American College of Cardiology* **32**:140–146.

8. Peto R, Collins R, Gray R (1995) Large-cale randomized evidence: Large, simple trials and overviews of trials. *Journal of Clinical Epidemiology* **48**:23–40.

9. MRFIT Investigators (1982) Multiple risk factor intervention trial *Journal of the American Medical Association* **248**:1465–77.

10. ISIS-1 Collaborative Group (1986) Randomized trial of intravenous atenolol among 16027 cases of suspected actue myocardial infarction–ISIS–1 *Lancet* **ii:**57–66.

11. Lee, KL, McNeer F, Starmer CF, Harris PJ, Rosari RA (1980) Clinical judgment and statistics Lessons from a simulated randomized trial in coronary artery disease *Circulation* **61**:508–515.

12. Assmann S, Pocock S, Enos L, Kasten L (2000) Subgroup analysis and other (mis)uses of baseline data in clinical trials. *Lancet* **355**:1064–69.

13. Bulpitt, C (1988) Subgroup Analysis *Lancet*: 31–34 .

14. Multicenter diltiazem post infarction trial research group (1989) The effect of dilitiazem on mortality and reinfarction after myhocardial infarction. *New England Journal of Medicine* **319**:385–392.

15 Packer, M, O'Connor, CM, Ghali, JK, et al for the Prospective Randomized Amlodipine Survival Evaluation Study Group (1996) Effect of amlodipine on morbidity and mortality in severe chronic heart failure. *New England Journal of Medicine* **335**:1107–14.

16. Packer, M (2000) Presentation of the results of the Prospective Randomized Amlodipine Survival Evaluation-2 Trial (PRAISE-2) at the American College of Cardiology Scientific Sessions, Anaheim, CA, March 15, 2000.

17. Exner DV, Dreis DL, Domanski MJ, Cohn, JN (2001) Lesser response to angiotensin–converting enzyme inhibitor therapy in black as compared to white patients with left ventricular dysfunction. *New England Journal of Medicine* **334**:1351–7

18. Yancy CW, Fowler MB, Colucci WS, Gilber EM, Bristow MR, Cohn JN, Luka MA, Young ST, Packer M for the US Carvedilol Heart Failure Study Group (2001) Race and response to adrenergic blockade with carvedilol in patients with chronic heart failure. *New England Journal of Medicine* 334:1358–65.

19. Stolberg SG (2001) Should a pill be colorblind? *New York Times Week in Review* May 13. p1.

20. Cohen AJ (1997) Replication. *Epidemiology* **8**:341–343.

21. Yusuf S, Wittes J, Probstfield J, Tyroler HA (1991) Analysis and interpretation of treatment effects in subgroups of patients in randomized clinical trials. *Journal of the American Medical Association* **266**:93–8.

22. Pedersen TR, Olsson AG, Faergeman O, Kjekshus J, Wedel H, Berg K, Wilhelmensen L, Haghfelt T, Thorgeirsson G, Pyòrälä K, Miettinen T, Christo-

phersen BG, Tobert JA, Musliner TA, Cook TJ for the Scandinavian Simvastatin Survival Study Group (1998) Lipoprotein changes and reduction in the incidence of major CAD events in the scandinavian simvastatin survival study (4S). *Circulation* **97**:1453–1460.

23. West of Scotland Coronary Prevention Study Group (1996) Infleunce of pravastatin and plasma lipids on clinical events in the West of Scotland Coronary Prevention Study (WOSCOPS). *Circulation* **97**:1440–1445.

24. Sacks, FM, Moyé, LA, Davis, BR, Cole, TB, Rouleau, JL, Nash, D Pfeffer, MA, Braunwald, E (1998) Relationship between plama LDL concentrations during treatment with pravastatin and recurrent coronary events in the Cholesterol and Recurrent Events trial. *Circulation* **97**:1446–1452.

25. Peduzzi, P,Wittes, J, Deter, K, Holford, T (1993) Analysis as-randomized and the problem of non-adherence; an example from the veterans affairs randomized trial of coronary artery bypass surgery. *Statistics in Medicine* **12**:1185–1195.

26. Peterson, B, George, SL (1993) Sample size requirements and length of study for testing interaction in a 1 x k factorial design when time to-failure is the outcome *Controlled Clinical Trials* **14**:511–522.

27. Moye LA, Deswal, A (2001) Trials with trials: confirmatory subgroup analyses in controlled clinical experiments. *Controlled Clinical Trials* **22**:605–619.

28. Moyé LA (2003) *Multiple Analyses in Clinical Trials: Fundamentals for Investigators* New York. Springer.

29. Miles JL (1993) Data torturing. *New England Journal of Medicine* **329**: 1196–1199.

30. Cochran WG. Early development of techniques in comparative experimentation. From Owen DB (1976) *On the Hstory of Probability and Statistics* New York and Basal Marcel Dekker, Inc.

31. Editorial: Now for the real cancer vaccines. *The Wall Street Journal* November 26, 2002.

11

P-values and Regression Analyses

11.1 The New Meaning of Regression

Regression analyses and the *p*-values that they produce are everywhere in medical statistical inference. Their omnipresence is no great surprise. At their respective cores, regression analysis and healthcare research focus on the examination of relationships, e.g., "Does a new therapy for hypertension improve clinical outcomes?" Regression analysis is the statistical tool that proves a quantitative assessment of the relationship between variables.

Much of the statistical analysis in healthcare today falls under the rubric of regression analysis. Its explosive growth has been fueled by the computational devices that have evolved over the last 40 years. Increasingly affordable computing stations and software, once only within the reach of the statistical specialist, are now being wielded by non-statisticians. In addition, regression procedures themselves have subsumed other modes of analysis traditionally viewed as related to but separate from regression analysis.

Initially, regression analysis was designed to look at the relationship between two variables, a dependent variable whose value the investigator was interested in predicting and a single explainer* variable used to "explain" the dependent variable. In classical regression analysis, both of these variables were continuous variables.† However, the development of computing techniques and theory have led to a dramatic expansion from this paradigm. Models that have more than one explainer variable are commonly examined (in what is still known as multiple regression analysis). Also, "regression analysis" now includes the examination of relationships between a continuous dependent variable and polychotamous explainer variables (formally known as the analysis of variance), as well as relationships between a continuous dependent variable and a mixture of polychotamous and continuous explainer variables (known in the past as the analysis of covariance). Repeated measure analysis allows each sub-

---

* This type of variable has historically been termed an independent variable. However the term *independence* is a misnomer since it is neither independent of the dependent variable nor independent of other *independent* variables in the model. In this text the term, "explainer variable" will be used.

† A continuous variable, e.g., age, permits integer and fraction values. A dichotomous variable has only two levels (e.g., male and female). A polychotamous variable has multiple levels but no particular value is placed on the order, e.g., 1 = married, 2 = never married, 3 = divorced, and 4 = spouse has died.

ject to have multiple measurements that have been obtained over the course of time to be analyzed. Complicated models mixing within subjects and between subject effects are all also now contained within the domain of regression analysis.[*] In addition, the dependent variable could be dichotomous (logistic regression analysis) or represent information that reflects survival (Cox regression analysis). In fact, the simple two-sample *t*-test discussed in an introductory course in statistics and most commonly not taught as a regression problem can be completely derived and understood as a result from regression analysis.

Thus, through its expansion, regression analysis is now a common analysis in healthcare frequently carried out by non-statisticians. It is a procedure that produces tremendous reams (or screens) of results. Each explainer variable in each model produces a *p*-value. *P*-values are produced in main effect models, in more complicated models that include effect-modifiers, and for co-variates. *P*-values can be generated for unadjusted as well as adjusted effects. The giant statistical software engines of the early twentyfirst century belch forth these *p*-values by the hundreds, and in the absence of intellectual discipline, these *p*-values commonly misdirect.

11.2 Assumptions in Regression Analysis

The hallmark of regression analysis is relationship examination. One of the most common motivations for examining relationships between variables in healthcare is the examination of the causality argument; i.e., is the relationship between the two variables associative or causal? Recall that the tenets of causality have many non-statistical components; i.e., many criteria other than a single analysis relating the putative risk factor to the disease. In healthcare, this relationship dissection can be exploited to predict the value of the dependent (unknown) variable from the value of the explainer (known) variable. The correct use of regression analysis in a well-designed experiment provides solid support to the arguments that address these tenets, constructing a sound causality argument. However, to be convincing, this regression building block must be precisely engineered. This is the core motivations for clearly understanding the assumptions of regression analysis.

We begin with a straightforward model in regression analysis, the simple straight line model. Assume we have collected *n* pairs of observations (x_i, y_i), $i = 1$ to n. Our goal is to demonstrate that changes in the value of *x* are associated with changes in the value of *y*. We will assume that *x* and *y* are linearly related. From this, write the simple linear regression model

$$E[y_i] = \beta_0 + \beta_1 x_i,\tag{11.5}$$

where $E[y_i]$ may be interpreted as "the average value of y_i."

The relationship expressed in equation (11.5) states that the dependent variable *y* is a linear function of the *x*'s. Everything else being equal, the larger the value of the coefficient β_1, the stronger the linear relationship between *x* and *y*. In regression analysis, we assume that the coefficients β_0 and β_1 are parame-

---

[*] In modern statistical treatments. This falls under the rubric of the general linear model.

ters whose true values will never be known since that would require including everyone in the population in the experiment. We will estimate parameters β_0 and β_1 with parameter estimates b_0 and b_1, respectively. The estimates we will use are called least-square estimates, estimates with very pleasing properties.[*]

In order to predict the expected value of y in this model, we will make some common assumptions. They are that

1. **The model is correct**. It serves no purpose to exert time and energy into collecting data and performing an analysis if the underlying relationship between x and y is wrong. The investigator should examine the literature and speak with experts to understand the relationship between x and y. In this example, if the relationship between x and y is not a straight-line relationship, our modeling results are DOA (dead on arrival).

2. **The error terms are independent, have common variance, and are normally distributed**. Despite the rigor of the experimental design, and the precision of the estimates, it is extremely unlikely that each observation's dependent variable will be precisely predicted by that observation's explainer variable. Thus, for our dataset, the equation of interest is

    $$y_i = b_0 + b_1 x_i + e_i,$$

    where e_i is the error term. Similar to a sample of data in which the sample mean will not be exactly equal to the population mean, in regression analysis, the sample parameter estimates b_0 and b_1 will not exactly equal the beta parameters β_0 and β_1. We assume that the error term e_i is independent, with a common variance σ^2. This is the most common assumption in regression analysis.[†] For the sake of all our hypothesis testing, we will assume the e_i's follow a normal distribution.[‡]

11.3 Model Estimation

Let's begin with the model for simple linear regression:

$$E[y_i] = \beta_0 + \beta_1 x_i .$$

---

[*] Least-square estimates have pleasing properties. They are unbiased, which means that there are neither systematic overestimations or underestimations of the population parameters, β_0 and β_1. Also, the variances of the estimates b_0 and b_1 have the smallest variances of any unbiased estimators that are linear functions of the y's for the same model.

[†] In some advanced models, e.g., weighted least squares, this assumption can be relaxed, opening up a wider range of useful experimental designs for which this can be implemented e.g., repeated measure designs.

[‡] The normality assumption is not necessary for parameter estimation, only hypothesis testing.

Since the β's are parameters that can only be known by an analysis of every subject in the population, we attempt to estimate the parameters by drawing a sample (x_i, y_i), $i = 1$ to n. Our job then is to estimate the β_0 and β_1 by b_0 and b_1 from the n equations, $y_i = b_0 + b_1 x_i + e_i$, $i = 1, \dots, n$ where the e_i are the error terms as described in the previous section. Even for a small dataset, having to compute the regression coefficients on a hand calculator is at best inconvenient. Fortunately, easy-to-use statistical software has evolved, sparing us the computational burden, and is almost always accurate in performing the calculations for us.

Consider the following observational study as an example in regression analysis. Two thousand patients are randomly chosen from a population of patients who have heart failure. The investigator is interested in looking at predictors of left ventricular dysfunction. Therefore, at baseline, the investigator collects a substantial amount of information on these patients, including demographic information, measures of morbidity prevalence, and measures of heart function. The investigator begins with a small model that predicts left ventricular ejection fraction (lvef) from age; i.e., he is "regressing" lvef on age. The model is

$$E\left[lvef_i\right] = \beta_0 + \beta_1 age_i .$$

In this model, the investigator assumes that the average lvef is a straight line function of age. He obtains the following results from his favorite software program (Table 11.1).

Table 11.1. Univariate regression of lvef on age

Variable	Parameter Estimate	Standard Error	T- statistic	P-value
Intercept (b_0)	33.593	0.810	41.48	0.0001
Age (b_1)	-0.043	0.013	-3.22	0.0013

The parameter estimate ($\pm$ its standard error or standard deviation) for b_0 is 33.59 ± 0.81 and for b_1 is -0.043 ± 0.013.

Already, we have p-values. The p-value for each parameter is a test of the null hypothesis that the parameter is equal to zero. We see that for each of these, the p-values are small.

11.3.1 Cross-Sectional Versus Longitudinal

This first analysis is very revealing. However, it would be a mistake to conclude that this analysis proves that age produces a smaller ejection fraction. Any comment that states or implies causality must be buttressed by arguments addressing the causality tenets,[*] i.e., arguments that the investigators have not yet posited.

---

[*] The Bradford Hill causality tenets are discussed in Chapter Four.

Similarly, this analysis does not imply that as patients age, they are more likely to have a smaller ejection fraction. We must keep in mind the subtle but important distinction between a cross-sectional analysis, which this evaluation represents, and a longitudinal analysis, which has not been carried out. The latter evaluation requires that we follow a cohort of patients over time, serially measuring their ages and their ejection fractions. Such an analysis would permit a direct examination of the relationship between changes in age over time and subsequent changes in ejection fraction.

In this particular circumstance, only one age and only one ejection fraction were measured as a "snapshot" of each patient. This cross sectional evaluation permits an examination of differences in ejection fraction between people of different ages. The longitudinal perspective examines the effect of the aging process in single individuals.

Thus, for this group, we can say only that there is a relationship between a patient's age and their ejection fraction; older patients appear to have lower ejection fractions than younger patients. Note the passive tone of this comment. We cannot say that age generates lower ejection fractions or that aging produces smaller lvef's. We can only say that patients who were older were found on average to have smaller ejection fractions than patients who were younger. This careful distinction in the characterization of this relationship is a trait of the disciplined researcher who uses regression analysis.

What does the identified p-value of 0.0013 from Table 11.1 mean? Using our community-protection definition, it means that it is very unlikely that a population in which there is no relationship between ejection fraction and patient age would produce a sample in which this relationship is identified. However, the small p-value contributes very little to a causality argument here. Since age cannot be assigned randomly to an individual, we cannot be sure that it is actually age (as opposed to duration of disease which is related to age) to which the ejection fraction is related.

One other possible explanation for this lvef–age relationship is that older patients may have had a history of heart attack; perhaps it is the number of heart attacks that is really related to ejection fraction. Since we have not ruled out these possible explanations for the identified lvef–age relationship, we can only say that age and lvef are associated[*] a very weak message.

11.4 Variance Partitioning

Before we move onto the examination of another variable in this cross-sectional analysis, it would be useful to explain the mathematics underlying the construction of the lvef–age relationship. Regression analysis is a form of variance examination.

In this example, variability is simply the fact that different patients have different ejection fractions. In statistics, variability is either explained or unexplained. We can follow this variance in lvef's as we go through the process of modeling lvef as a function of age.

---

[*] The issue of attribution of effect to clearly assign a reason for an effect when the risk factor is not assigned randomly is discussed in Chapter Four.

When we begin the evaluation of lvef, measuring only the ejection fraction and no other explanatory variable, we see the anticipated scatter in the lvef's over patients (Figure 11.1, panel 1).

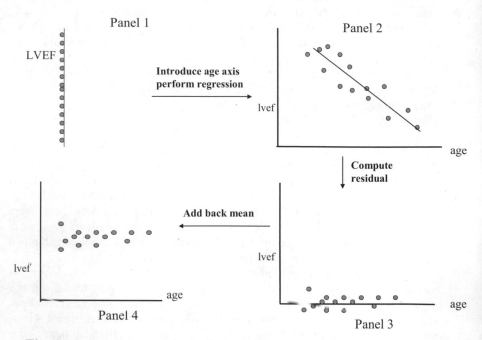

Fig. 11.1. Step-by-step view of regression.

Panel 1 shows only that there is variability in lvef measurements among the patients. At this point, the investigator does not know why these patients have different ejection fractions. The variability in ejection fraction represented in panel one represents the total variability in the system. We may attribute it to random error, but at this point, we don't know that lvef's vary across individuals. We write this total variability as

$$\text{Total variability} = \sum_{i=1}^{n}(y_i - \bar{y})^2.$$

This is the numerator of the familiar expression for the sample variance $s^2 = \sum_{i=1}^{n}(y_i - \bar{y})^2 \Big/ n-1$. With no other explanation for the different ejection fractions in different patients, this quantity is the measure of variability that the investigator uses to generate confidence intervals or create the variance component that goes in to the denominator of a simple test statistic. Similarly, with no other information, the best predicted value of a patient's lvef is the mean lvef of the cohort. We say that that $\hat{y}_i = \bar{y}$.

However, it is possible that another variable would "explain" some of the variability or the spread of the ejection fractions across patients. The investigator's experience suggested that one reason different patients have different measures of ejection fraction is that the patients have different ages. This is depicted in panel 2. With age introduced as an explainer variable, the best predicted value of the individual's ejection fraction depends on their age, which we can now write as $\hat{y}_i = 35.59 - 0.043\, age_i$, denoting the ith patient's age as age_i.

Examining panel 2, we see that there are two sources of variability: 1) the variability between $\hat{y}_i$, the predicted value of a patient's lvef using age, and $\bar{y}$, the predicted value without age, and 2) the difference between $\hat{y}_i$ and y_i. This latter component is the remaining unexplained variability in lvef after removing the role of age. We can write this algebraically as

$$\sum_{i=1}^{n}(y_i - \bar{y})^2 = \sum_{i=1}^{n}(\hat{y}_i - \bar{y})^2 + \sum_{i=1}^{n}(y_i - \hat{y}_i)^2,$$

$$\text{SST} \qquad = \qquad \text{SSR} \quad + \quad \text{SSE}$$

where SST stands for *sum of squares total,* SSR is *sum of squares regression,* and SSE denotes the *sum of squares error.*[*]

This expression is an algebraic depiction of what we saw in Figure 11.1. The total variability of the system is broken into two components. The first is the variation in lvef (y) that is explained by variability in age, i.e., one of the reasons that patients have different lvef's is because they have different ages. This variability is termed the sum of squares regression (SSR) and is the component of the total variability that is explained by the regression line.

The second source of variability is the remaining or residual unexplained variability. It is often called the "sum of squares error" (SSE), reflecting the degree to which the fitted values deviate from the actual values. In regression analysis, using the least-squares approach, we choose the estimates b_0 and b_1 for β_0 and β_1 to minimize the sum of squares error. Since the sum of squares total (SST) is a constant, by minimizing the SSE, the least-squares approach maximizes SSR.

A useful quantity to keep track of in model building is $R^2 = \text{SSR}/\text{SST}$. This may be thought of as the percentage of the total variability explained by the regression model. The range of this measure is from 0 to 1. Models that fit the data well are characterized by small SSE, large SSR, and a large value for R^2. Models that fit the data poorly have large SSEs, small SSRs, and a low R^2. If you hope to draw inferential conclusions from models, you are more persuasive if you draw these conclusions from models with large R^2.

------

[*] The expression appears after some simple algebraic manipulation. Beginning with $\sum_{i=1}^{n}(y_i - \bar{y})^2$, add and subtract $\hat{y}_i$ to produce $\sum_{i=1}^{n}(y_i - \hat{y}_i + \hat{y}_i - \bar{y})^2$. Expand this expression by writing $\sum_{i=1}^{n}(\hat{y}_i - \bar{y})^2 + \sum_{i=1}^{n}(y_i - \hat{y}_i)^2 + 2\sum_{i=1}^{n}(\hat{y}_i - \bar{y})(y_i - \hat{y}_i)$. This last term is zero, providing the desired result.

Panel 3 is an examination of the residue of the regression analysis. Here we subtract from the lvef of each patient the estimated value of lvef predicted by that patient's age. If the best relationship between lvef and age is a straight line, then Panel 3 depicts what the residuals look like. They have a mean value of zero, and variance smaller than the total variance from panel 1 (note that we are focusing on variance of lvef (vertical variance) and not the variance of the ages (horizontal variance)). We would expect this, since much of the variability in lvef was due to age. Adding back the mean lvef gives us the location and scatter of the lvef with the age component removed as depicted in panel 4.

11.5 Enter Dichotomous Explainer Variables

The investigator now wishes to examine the relationship between lvef and the presence of a history of myocardial infarction (MIs, or heart attacks). His suspicion is that patients with a history of MI will have smaller ejection fractions. However, unlike the explainer variable age, which was continuous, the MI history variable takes on only two values, zero and one.[*] The flexibility of regression analysis allows us to incorporate these classes of explainer variables as well. In doing so, we can apply everything we have learned about regression analysis parameter estimates. However, we will need to be very careful about how we interpret the parameter is this model.

For the model we are examining, y_i is the ejection fraction of the ith patient, and x_i reflect the presence of a positive MI history. We let $x_i = 0$ for a patient if they have no prior MI's, and $x_i = 1$ if the patient has a positive MI history. Now write the model

$$E[y_i] = \beta_0 + \beta_1 x_i.$$

Before we go any further, let's consider the implications of this model. We have modeled the lvef as a function of multiple myocardial infarctions. For patients with only one MI, $x_i = 0$, and regardless of the value of β_1, the term that contains x_i will be zero. Thus, for patients with only one MI

$$E[y_i] = \beta_0.$$

For patients with multiple myocardial infarctions, $x_i = 1$, and their expected left ventricular ejection fraction is

$$E[y_i] = \beta_0 + \beta_1.$$

Thus, β_1 is the difference in the expected lvef between patients with only one heart attack and patients with a positive MI history. A statistical hypothesis test conducted for β_1 (by examining parameter estimate b_1) is a test on the impact of positive MI history on lvef in a population of patients with at least one heart attack (Table 11.2).

---

[*] In fact the examination of the relationship between left ventricular ejection fraction and multiple myocardial infarctions is really an unpaired *t*-test. The univariate regression to be executed here will give the exact same result as the *t*-test.

Table 11.2. Univariate regression of lvef on history of MI's

Variable	Parameter Estimate	Standard Error	T-statistic	P-value
Intercept (b_0)	31.846	0.175	182.16	0.0001
Prior MI (b_1)	-2.300	0.293	-7.84	0.0013

This data reveals that patients with multiple myocardial infarctions in general have an ejection fraction that is 2.30 ± 0.29 (parameter estimate ± its standard error) units less than patients with only one heart attack.

However, as in our previous lvef–age assessment, we cannot conclude that the presence of a prior MI causes lower ejection values by simply looking at the regression results. Prior MI is not a randomly assigned value. Thus, the lack of random assignment of the MI history variable to patients (of course this is impossible), precludes the clear attribution of ejection fraction differences to the presence of multiple heart attacks. In addition, the occurrence of a prior MI is associated with many clinical factors such as longstanding atherosclerotic disease, hypertension or genetic influences.[*] We can say only that the presence of a prior MI is associated with lower ejection fraction on average, i.e., patients with a positive MI history have on average lower ejection fractions than patients without.

11.6 The Meaning of "Adjustment"

Each of these univariate models had provided an important piece of information involving the influences on left ventricular ejection fraction. However, the two explainer variables, age and multiple myocardial infarctions, are related. Patients who are older are more likely to have had a prior MI than younger patients. How can the investigator decide which of the two is the driving variable in influencing lvef?

Regression models with more than one explainer variable are commonly considered models that provide adjusted effects for the explainer variables. However, words like "adjustment" have very broad uses in healthcare, so we must be precise when we use them in regression analysis. Consider the previous model focusing on differences in lvef. We know that patients with different values for the MI history variable will on average have different ages (patients with a prior MI tend to be older than those without), and that age is itself related to lvef. How can we get at the actual relationship between age and lvef?

One way to do this would be to "hold the MI variable constant." That would be tantamount to choosing patients in the sample who have the same value for the MI history variable but different ages. While this may be reasonable in some cases, it is, in general, an impractical solution. Consider instead the

---

[*] A *post hoc* examination of the MI–lvef relationship would further weaken any conclusions about the degree to which a prior MI produces lower ejection fraction.

following results the investigator has obtained by regressing lvef on both age
and the MI history variable simultaneously. The model is

$$E[y_i] = \beta_0 + \beta_1 age_i + \beta_2 x_i. \tag{11.6}$$

The results will provide estimates for each of the three parameters (Table 11.3).

Table 11.3. Multivariate regression of lvef on age and MI history.

Variable	Parameter Estimate	Standard Error	T-statistic	P-value
Intercept (b_0)	33.723	0.800	42.15	0.0001
Age (b_1)	-0.032	0.013	-2.41	0.0163
Prior MI's (b_2)	-2.222	0.295	-7.54	0.0013

The data in Table 11.3, reflecting the result of model (11.6), reveals
that each age and prior MI has a notable relationship with left ventricular ejection fraction. However, if we compare coefficients across the Tables 11.1, 11.2,
and 10.3, we find that the relationships have different magnitudes. The coefficient estimate b_1 (reflecting the univariate relationship between lvef and age (-
0.043)) from Table 11.1 is different from the estimate in the multiple variable
regression (– 0.032) from Table 11.3. Similarly, we see that –2.300 from Table
11.2 is the regression estimate for b_1 from the univariate model, but –2.222 is
the analogous estimate from for the multiple regression model from Table 11.3.
What do the new coefficient estimates mean, and which should be reported?

In order to understand the implications of the multiple regression parameter estimates from Table 11.3, we need to examine how these coefficient
estimates were obtained. Consider the relationship between lvef and age. The
underlying theory collapses these computations into three stages to compute the
estimate from Table 11.3:

1. regress lvef on prior MI and compute the residual of lvef,
2. regress age on prior MI and compute the residual of age,
3. regress the lvef residual on the age residual.

If we were to go through each of these three individual steps ourselves,
we would find the result (Table 11.4) that matches perfectly with the results
from Table 11.3, and then interpret the results of the multiple regression model.

Table 11.4: Explicit regression following three-step proecss.

Residual of lvef on residual on age

Variable	Parameter Estimate	Standard Error	T-statistic	P-value
Age (b_1)	−0.0321	0.013	−2.41	0.0162

Fortunately, this three-step calculation is carried out automatically by most regression software. The depicted relationship in the multiple regression model between lvef and age is a relationship with the influence of the prior MI variable "removed." More specifically, we isolated and identified the relationship between lvef and prior MI, and the relationship between age and prior MI, and then removed the influence of prior MI by producing the residuals. Finally, we regressed the residual of lvef (i.e., what was left of lvef after removing the prior MI influence) on the residual of age.

In regression analysis, when we adjust a relationship, we mean we identify, isolate, and remove the influences of the adjusting variable. This is done simultaneously in multiple regression analysis by standard software. In the relationship between prior MI and age in Table 11.3, the influence of age has been isolated, identified, and removed.

So already, we have two sets of p-values — one for unadjusted effects, the other for adjusted effects. Which do we choose? We address this question in the next section.

11.7 Super Fits

Since the multiple regression procedure automatically allows for simultaneously adjusting every explainer variable for every other explainer variable, a great plethora of findings can and are reported. However, the model from which these findings are reported must be persuasive.

One criterion for a model's plausibility is R^2. As we have seen, the greater the sum of squares regression, the better the model's fit to the data. This improved fit has the advantage of increasing the persuasiveness of the model, since the model does a good job of explaining the variability of the dependent variable. A second implication of this criterion is its reduction of the sum of squares error. By reducing this measure of unexplained variability, the power of the test statistic for any of the parameter estimates increases.[*] Thus, a model with a large R^2 has the advantage of greater statistical power. Recognizing this, modern regression software contains tools to build automatically models for a specified dependent variable from a list of candidate explainer variables. These procedures work on the principle of maximizing the variability explained by the regression model.

The investigator could increase R^2 by identifying the variables in the dataset that are most "important" and then adding them to the list of explainer variables included in the model. However, regression procedures will do this for him automatically. They will search among all candidate variables in the model

---

[*] The concept of power is discussed in Chapter Six.

using established criteria to decide if the inclusion of a particular explainer variable will significantly increase R^2.

The algorithms are ruthlessly efficient. Some of these work in a forward direction, considering the additive variable of each candidate variable one at a time, then choosing the one variable that makes the greatest contribution. That variable is accepted as an explainer variable for the model. Once this has occurred, the system cycles through the remaining explainer variables, again finding the variable that makes the best contribution to the model containing the earlier accepted explainer variable chosen on the first round. The cycle repeats, building the model up until all contributory explainer variables are added.

Other procedures work backward, starting with a large model that contains all candidate explainer variables, then searching for the variable that is easiest to drop (i.e., where its loss has the smallest impact on R^2). In this system, the model is "built down" to a smaller collection of variables. Other procedures, termed *stepwise algorithms*, employ a combination of forward and backward examinations. The result is a model that has maximized the variability of the dependent variable that is explained. The more variables, the larger is R^2, the better the fit. The computer "super fits" the model to the data

Thus, modern computing facilities permit the creation of automatically generated models in which each included explainer variable is statistically significant This wholesale automation leads to a sense that the researcher is getting something of great value for a very small price; the press of a button provides the best model. However, these models, so efficiently produced at so little cost, come with the caveat "You get what you pay for."

The difficulty with these fully automated approaches is that they subtlely alter the investigator's purpose. The researchers were initially focused on models that would provide generalizable predictive capacity; they would provide new generalizable information about what helps to determine values of the dependent variable. These automatically determined models produce something quite different, since they are not built on relationships that are known to exist in the population. On the contrary, they are constructed to maximize the sum of square regression and R^2, ignoring the contributions of epidemiology, clinical experience, or powers of observation. The resulting, blind construction of the model often leads to results that make no sense, are uninterpretable, and are often unacceptable. Plausibility, interpretability, and coherence have been sacrificed for computing efficiency.

This point is worthy of amplification. In general, the dataset will have two classes of relationships: those that are truly representative of the relationships in the population, and those are completely spurious. In fact, some relationships that may be present in the population can be absent in the sample. The investigator with a combination of experience in the field and some prospective thought and research will be able to identify these. The automatic variable selection procedures cannot differentiate between an association due to sampling error[*] and an association that mirrors a relation that actually resides in the population.

---

[*] An association due to sampling error is an association between a risk factor and an effect in a sample which does not represent the true relationship between the risk factor and the effect in a population.

Rather then rest on the bedrock of scientific community experience, these heavyweight models are based only on the shifting sands of sampling error. Thus, variables that are found to be significant can suggest relationships that are completely implausible. Guided only by levels of significance, these automatic variable selection algorithms yield weak models that often are not corroborated by findings from other datasets. This is no surprise, since the model is built on sampling error. Another dataset, drawn at random from the same population and teeming with its own sampling error relationships, will provide a different selection of variables. In variable selection, silicon-based algorithms let us down, and we must rely on our own intuition to build the model.

11.8 Pearls of Great Price

The construction of sound regression models begins with the investigators' acknowledgement that their purpose in carrying out regression analysis is not to report on inconsequential, spurious relationships. Their job is take a database, full of relationships and interrelationships, and distill it down to a compact body of knowledge governed by a few master principles. This requires a thoughtful, deliberate approach.

Commonly, the purpose of regression analysis is to evaluate the plausibility of a causal relationship. This purpose often narrows the investigator's focus to a small number of explainer variables (principal explainer variables) and their relationship with the dependent variable. Generally, these principal explainer variables will be related to other variables (called adjusters), that are related to the dependent variable. A full review of the literature will reveal the identity of these adjustors, tempered by discussions with co-investigators.

Because of the likelihood of a type I error, adjustors should not be chosen by an automated mechanism. They should be chosen prospectively by the investigator only after considerable reflection. Furthermore, if the purpose of the effort is to examine the adjusted relationships between the principal explainer variables and the dependent variable, p-values for the adjustors should not be provided in the primary analysis, as they will most likely confuse and mislead. The purpose of the regression is not to evaluate the effect of an adjustor and the dependent variable, but to adjust the relationship between the principal explainer variable and the dependent variable for the adjustor. The adjusted effects of the principal explainer variable are of the greatest important and should be reported.

The more options we have in model building, the more disciplined we must be in using them. Automatic procedures for model building should be avoided in regression analysis in healthcare because they distract and confuse. They are easy to generate, but just because we *can* take an action, does not mean we *must* take it. Investigator-generated models stand to contribute the most to the understanding of the elucidated relationship. Since adjustors were chosen from the literature, they have some basis other than sampling error for inclusion in the model, i.e., they have scientific community support. In addition, other researchers with experience in the field from the literature the potential importance of the adjustors, and will expect them in the analysis. An automatic (silicon-based) approach will use tens and sometimes hundreds of p-values to build a model that rests on only the thin reed of sampling error.

The investigator-based model rests on strength of evidence from the literature and the scientific community, and uses only a small number of p-values to provide an assessment of the statistical significance of the relationships between the principal explainer variables and the dependent variable. Easy to interpret and incorporate into the scientific community's fund of knowledge, such models are pearls of great price.

11.9 Effect Modifiers and Alpha Allocation

We have seen that a disciplined approach to model construction in regression analysis can allow an investigator to report on the effects of principle explainer variables. These effects are reported after adjusting for (i.e., isolating, identifying, and removing) the influences of adjustors. However, regression analysis is not limited to these direct or main effects, but can also assess effect modification. Effect modifiers exerts their influence by modifying the relationship between a principal explainer variable and the dependent variable. They are elegant, but can be complicated. *P*-value interpretation for these effects must be approached with great care.

11.9.1 Effect Modification Models

Thus far, we have used the three Hill criteria of plausibility, consistency, and coherency in the regression model building process. Interpretability of the model is often enhanced with the explicit consideration of effect modification terms.

Consider the model developed in this chapter relating lvef to age and the history of an MI, i.e.,

$$E\left[lvef_i\right] = \beta_0 + \beta_1 age_i + \beta_2 x_i. \tag{11.7}$$

Recall that x_i was equal to 1 if the patient had a prior MI, and 0 if not. As a preamble to studying the role of effect modification, we can examine the direct effect of MI history on lvef by exploring the predicted value of lvef for patients with different MI history. If, for example, a patient has no previous MI's, then the value of x_i is zero, and the model may be written as

$$E\left[lvef_i\right] = \beta_0 + \beta_1 age_i + \beta_2 x_i$$
$$= \beta_0 + \beta_1 age_i + \beta_2(0)$$
$$= \beta_0 + \beta_1 age_i.$$

The last equation simply states that lvef is a function of age. However, if the patient has a positive MI history, the value of x_i becomes one. The model is now

$$E\left[lvef_i\right] = \beta_0 + \beta_1 age_i + \beta_2 x_i$$
$$= \beta_0 + \beta_1 age_i + \beta_2(1)$$
$$= (\beta_0 + \beta_2) + \beta_1 age_i.$$

This is also a model that says that the relationship between lvef and age is a straight line relationship. Thus two relationships are developed depending on the patient's MI history (Figure 11.2).

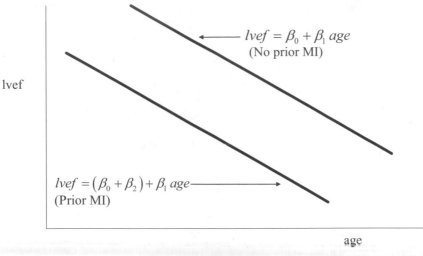

Fig. 11.2. The effect of the presence of prior MI history on the relationship between lvef and age. The parallel lines indicate that age has the same reductive effect on lvef. At all ages, patients with a positive MI history have a lower lvef than those with a negative history.

From Figure 11.2 we see that the relationship between lvef and age, as reflected by equation (11.7), consists of two parallel lines, one for patients with a prior MI history and one for those with no previous heart attacks. The difference between the two parallel lines is captured in the parameter β_2. Thus, if the parameter β_2 is zero, then there is no impact of MI history on lvef (assuming the model depicting the relationship $\left(E[lvef_i] = \beta_0 + \beta_1 age_i + \beta_2 x_i\right)$ is correct. Also, note that the effect of age on lvef is the same, as indicated by the parallel nature of the two lines.

However, equation (11.7) does not depict the only way to relate lvef to age and the presence of a prior MI. Consider the following model:

$$E[lvef_i] = \beta_0 + \beta_1 age_i + \beta_2 x_i + \beta_3 age_i x_i. \tag{11.8}$$

Note that we have added an additional term $\beta_3 age_i x_i$ to the model. For patients with no prior MI, the model expressed by equation (11.8) becomes

No Prior MI : $E[lvef_i] = \beta_0 + \beta_1 age_i$

Prior MI : $\quad E[lvef_i] = (\beta_0 + \beta_2) + (\beta_1 + \beta_3) age_i.$

This reflects an important change from the model relating lvef to age for patients with a prior MI. For all patients, the relationship between age and lvef is a straight line. However, the nature of the straight lines are quite different from each other. Patients with a prior MI not only have a different intercept

$(\beta_0 + \beta_2$ versus $\beta_0)$ but also a different slope $(\beta_1 + \beta_3$ versus $\beta_1)$. The impact of the prior MI history has become more complicated (Figure 11.3).

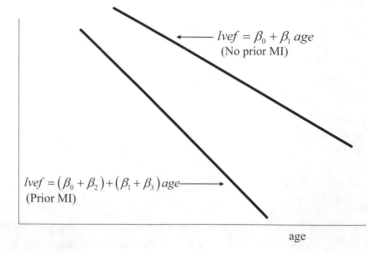

Fig. 11.3. The effect of the presence of prior MI history on the relationship between lvef and age that includes an effect modifier term.The different slopes of the two lines demonstrate how the presence of a prior MI increases the strength of the relationship between age and lvef.

From Figure 11.3, the presence of a prior MI amplifies the effect of age on lvef. We say that prior MI modifies the relationship between age and lvef, and the MI variable is an effect modifier.

Effect modifiers can have multiple effects. They can directly influence lvef (as reflected in the parameter β_2) or they can indirectly effect lvef by modifying the relationship between lvef and age. Historically, these terms have been described as *interaction effects*.

11.9.2 The Difficulty of Effect Modification

Interaction terms in regression models can be very attractive, but the effects they measure can be complicated to explain. In the previous example, the relationship between the explainer variables age and lvef is straightforward in the absence of effect modification. As we have seen earlier in this chapter, older patients tend to have lower ejection fractions than younger patients. However, the inclusion of the product term suggests that this relationship between age and lvef is a function of the prior MI history. This more complicated relationship will require time and effort for the medical community to absorb. Since additional work is required to explain and ultimately to persuade the medical community of the veracity of this complex finding, the investigator should be convinced that this relationship is not likely to be due to chance alone. An important component of this evaluation should therefore assess the strength of *a priori* evidence for including the effect modification term in the model

Unfortunately, this is not often the case. A common approach is that significance levels (i.e., *p*-values) for effect modification terms to be included in the model should be on the order of 0.10 or even larger. This is driven by the sense that the identification of an effect modification is worth the greater risk of a type I error i.e., the investigators don't want to miss anything. Unfortunately, what they commonly catch is sampling error. The effect modification term that appears in one sample disappears in others, that themselves produce novel and irreproducible effect modification terms on their own. Trying to explain a complicated interaction term based on a weak finding at a level of significance of 0.10 or higher is often a futile attempt to explain shifting patterns in the sampling error sands.

As an alternative approach, consider the following cross sectional evaluation. An investigator has obtained demographic and lipid data on 4,159 patients who have sustained a heart attack. He is interested in identifying demographic measures that may be related to LDL cholesterol levels. He will do this using a cross-sectional design.[*]

Before his evaluation begins, the investigator thoroughly reviews the literature and consults with other lipid specialists. His review suggests that each of the main effects of age, gender, race, country, and family history of heart disease are related to LDL cholesterol levels. The investigator also notes that others have suggested that each of smoking history, alcohol consumption, exercise level diabetes, hypertension, and use of beta blockers may exert influence as well, although the evidence for these latter variables is somewhat weaker.

In addition, the investigator's own assimilation of the available information suggests that several effect modifications may be of interest. One is that age may influence the relationship between gender and baseline LDL cholesterol. A second effect modification of interest is exercise and gender (i.e., gender influences the relationship between LDL and exercise). Several other effect modifiers have been suggested by co-investigators; however, there is no literature-based evidence supporting their existence.

The investigator must consider his decision strategy and alpha allocation decisions carefully. He believes *a priori* that the catalog of effect modifiers may be present, but he also understands the difficulty of arguing persuasively for them since a relationship modifying effect is more difficult to explain than a main effect. For example, explaining that the effect of exercise on LDL cholesterol levels is related to gender, and that women may have to exercise more than men to achieve an equivalent reduction in LDL is a complicated message to deliver to a scientific community and patient population that is already overwhelmed by advice (sometimes contradictory) on reducing risk factors for heart disease. Recognizing this, the investigator will argue for an effect modification term only if its "signal" is strong enough. If the type I error is too great, he is unwilling to attempt to make a persuasive argument for an effect size. He chooses to apportion type I error as described in Table 11.5.

---

[*] The strengths and weaknesses of cross-sectional designs were discussed in Chapter Four.

Table 11.5. Prospective alpha allocation for predictors of LDL

Effect	Allocated Alpha
Effect Modifiers	
Age –gender interaction	0.003
Exercise-gender interaction	0.003
All other externally suggested interactions	0.003
Main Effects	
Age	0.024
Gender	0.04
Race	0.04
Family History of CVD	0.04
Country	0.04
Smoking	0.024
Alcohol	0.024
Exercise	0.024
Diabetes	0.024
Hypertension	0.024
Beta blocker use	0.024

The investigator apportions 0.003 alpha to each effect modifier of interest and an additional 0.003 to the group of interactions suggested by others. For the main effects, he allocates 0.04 each to gender, race, country and family history of heart disease, with 0.024 for the other main effects. At the conclusion of the research, the investigator reports his results (Table 11.6).

This table shows the interaction effects first, since main effects cannot be assessed in the presence of effect modification. Since none of the effect-modifiers met the criteria of significance, they may now be removed from the model. The remainder of table displays the unadjusted and adjusted effects of the candidate risk factors on LDL cholesterol levels. Z-scores and p-values are shown only for the adjusted effects, because attribution of effect size will be easily confused or confounded among these correlated main effects. The results may be summarized as follows.

In exploratory evaluations of baseline LDL cholesterol correlates, no model explained more than 1.5% of the total variability of LDL cholesterol. No effect modification term made a significant contribution to the ability of any covariate to explain LDL cholesterol variability. Gender and the presence of diabetes mellitus provides significant reductions in unexplained LDL cholesterol variability. Women had a 0.05 mg/dl lower LDL cholesterol than men after adjusting for age, race, history of atherosclerotic cardiovascular disease, country, smoking, alcohol, exercise, diabetes, hypertension, and beta blockers ($p =$

0.020). Diabetics had a 0.08 mg/dl lower baseline LDL cholesterol than non-diabetics after adjustment ($p < 0.001$).

11.10 Conclusions

Regression analysis provides a powerful tool for exploring the relationships between potentially influential factors and dependent variables. However, the careful investigator must be sensitive to the extent to which he relinquishes control of the analysis to the computer. Software can provide important useful information, such as effect size and variance estimates. However, the investigator should wrest control of variable selection from automatic search procedures that work to build maximum R^2 models. Since population-based relationships as well as sampling error-based relationships are embedded in the analysis sample, the investigator needs a tool to differentiate these influences. The best discriminatory tool is not the computer, but the investigators themselves. By diligently reviewing the literature, the investigator is in the best position to distinguish the real relationships from the spurious ones.

Alpha allocation plays an important role in interpreting regression analyses. Effect modification influences should be carefully considered before the analysis is undertaken. If the purpose of the research is to tease out an effect modifier, the investigator may justifiably increase alpha. However, if the interactions are not expected, then their biologic non-plausibility and tangled explanations argue for a small type I error level. Finally, by understanding the role of adjustment (identification, isolation, and removal of the adjustor's effects) in regression analysis, the investigator can usefully disentangle confounded effects. However, the lack of the use of randomization tightly circumscribes the contribution such regression models can make to causality arguments.

Finally, consider the stethoscope. It is a well–designed, finely tuned tool for physicians and others to interpret body sounds. Yet, despite its high level of craftsmanship, the most important part of this instrument is the part between our ears. That is where the most important part of computer–based regression analysis is located.

Table 11.6. Results of baseline LDL evaluation

Total Alpha	0.30

Alpha for Interaction	0.01

Interactions	Allocated Alpha	P-value	Conclusion
Age group	0.003	> 0.5	Insignificant
Exercise group	0.003	> 0.5	Insignificant
Others	0.003	> 0.5	Insignificant

Alpha for main effects	0.29

| | | | Main Effects | | | | | |
| | | | Unadjusted | | Adjusted | | | |
Variable	Allocated Alpha		Effect Size	Std Error of Effect Size	Effect Size	Std Error of Effect Size	P-value	Conclusions
Age	0.024		-0.068	0.024	-0.002	0.001	0.027	Insignificant
Gender	0.040		-1.254	0.654	-0.050	0.026	0.020	Significant
Race	0.040		1.278	0.863	0.051	0.035	0.543	Insignificant
Family History	0.040		0.168	0.461	0.007	0.018	0.090	Insignificant
Country	0.024		-1.250	0.477	-0.030	0.011	0.090	Insignificant
Smoking	0.024		1.115	0.614	0.027	0.015	0.325	Insignificant
Alcohol	0.024		0.236	0.492	0.006	0.012	0.638	Insignificant
Exercise	0.024		0.795	0.457	0.019	0.011	0.028	Insignificant
Diabetes	0.024		-3.361	0.647	-0.081	0.016	<0.001	Significant
Hypertension	0.024		-0.560	0.457	-0.013	0.011	0.241	Insignificant
Beta Blockers	0.024		-0.631	0.462	-0.015	0.011	0.699	Insignificant

12

Bayesian Analysis: Posterior *P*-values

12.1 An Arbitrary Process

P-values continue to play an important role in data-based decision–making, and their appropriate use requires deliberate thought. Even in the simplest of experiments, investigators are encouraged to provide a prospectively determined, clear statement about the level of type I and type II errors that their research will generate. The circumstances were even more complex in Chapter Nine when there were more than two treatment arms and multiple analyses in the same experiment. These more complicated research endeavors required more intricate decisions involving multiple *p*-values.

Whether the circumstances are simple or complex, the process is certainly arbitrary. The best, most community-oriented physician-scientist possessing firm knowledge of the possible efficacy and side effects of the intervention must eventually settle on alpha levels for each of their experiment's primary analyses. How does one finally decide on 0.024 for one endpoint, 0.015 for another, and 0.011 for a third? What precisely is the reasoning process?

The arbitrary nature of the choice in the absence of firm rules for the selection (apart from the reflexive 0.05 choice) is a singular handicap of this process. In fact, one of the reasons that the 0.05 threshold has maintained its popularity is because a competitor choice would have to be accompanied by compelling motivation; so far, no such generally accepted rationale is available. The choice would be less problematic if there were some specific, broadly accepted guidelines one could follow that responded to the complex interaction of the intervention and the characteristic features of the subject population being studied. However, there are no such conventions. It is therefore no surprise that consumers of the medical literature are commonly flummoxed by the *p*-value and its accompanying selection procedure.[*]

Recently, there has been a good deal of discussion about the Bayesian approach to statistical reasoning in medicine. The Bayes philosophy places less em-

---

[*] Dr. Kassell's reaction in the Introduction is a fine example of the exasperation that the 0.05 dilemma produces.

phasis on pre-experimental selections of alpha levels, focusing instead on the process of updating information. Prior information is updated by the research data, resulting in a posterior assessment.

This concept is relatively new to statistical reasoning in healthcare research and is part of a diverse and growing field. Like grass growth in the spring (although its critics would say that its not grass at all, but weeds), Bayes procedures are making new inroads into many aspects of statistics, providing a fresh perspective on estimation and hypothesis testing in statistics, with important implications for *p*-value interpretation.

In this chapter, we will discuss the difference between classical and Bayesian statistics, explain the new features offered by Bayesian statistics, and provide an example of the use of Bayesian statistics in a hypothesis–testing situation. However, we must note that, just as for the classical approach, the correct use of Bayes procedures requires disciplined, prospective thought.

12.2 The Frequentists

Historically, the Bayesian philosophy has generated a negative, even visceral reaction among traditional biostatisticians (who have come to be known as frequentists). The computational underpinnings of Bayes procedures rely on the straightforward application of well-established, conditional probability theory. However, the philosophical foundation of the Bayes approach, with its frank and explicit use of prior information in concert with the invocation of loss functions, is often the subject of heated controversy. In order to understand the point of view offered by Bayesians, we must first review the perspective of the frequentist school of thought.

12.2.1 The Frequentist and Long-Term Accuracy

Classical statistics is the collection of statistical techniques and devices whose justification is its long-term, repetitive accuracy [1]. The *p*-value is a familiar example of this approach. If, for example, the *p*-value for a well-conducted, well executed research effort is 0.03, then its small value does not guarantee that a type I error was avoided in the research effort. The result simply means that, in the long run, the overwhelming majority of experiments (97% of them) that generated $p = 0.03$ would produce no type I error for the hypothesis test. Thus, the virtue of the *p*-value is its accuracy in a series of repeated experiments, and not its veracity in a single research effort. This leaves the investigator to only hope that his single experiment is one of the efforts that falls within this majority.

12.2.2 Reverse Perspective

One price the frequentist pays for this point of view is in the construction of the significance test. The entire formulation of the hypothesis–testing paradigm to non-statisticians appears backward. In significance testing, statisticians are only allowed to reject conclusions, not accept them. For example, if the test statistic does not fall in the critical region, they do not accept the null hypothesis; they just are unable to reject it. Alternatively, if the test statistic falls in the critical region, they do not accept the alternative hypothesis, they just reject the null hypothesis.

Significance testing is based on rejection. However, the investigators are interested in affirmation. Specifically, they would like to know the probability that their scientific hypothesis is correct, not the reverse probability that the idea they do not believe is incorrect. To many workers in healthcare, the mathematics of statistics is complicated enough without engaging in this awkward and indirect reasoning process.

12.2.3 The Likelihood Principle

Another problem of classical statistics is its concentration on not just what has occurred, but also on what has *not* occurred in a research program. How these non-occurrences are handled can have a dramatic impact on the answer to the hypothesis test, and preoccupation with them can bedevil the result interpreter.

12.2.4.1 Frustration

Consider the following example, adapted from Lindley [2]. A physician who staffs a cardiology clinic believes that more than half of his patients have hypertension. He is interested in carrying out an observational study to test this hypothesis. The cardiologist proceeds by counting the number of patients who come into the clinic, keeping track of how many patients have hypertension.

There are several acceptable ways to do this. One would be to first count patients until a given number of normotensive patients are observed. If hypertension is as prevalent as he suspects, this count will be relatively high. The investigator carries this out one morning, counting the number of patients, n, until there are three patients who are normotensive ($y = 3$). He finds that $n = 12$. These results reveal a hypertension prevalence of $9/12 = 0.75$ or 75%.

Observing that these results are clinically significant, the cardiologist engages a statistician to assess whether these findings are statistically significant. The investigator lays out the rationale and method of his research, providing his findings. After hearing how the study was executed, the statistician computes the probability of the results given the null hypothesis is true. Under the null hypothesis, the prevalence of hypertension in the clinic, represented as θ, is 0.50. Thus, he computes the probability of seeing n patients until there are 3 normotensive patients as

$$P\left[n = 12, y = 3 \mid \theta = 0.50\right] + P\left[n = 13, y = 3 \mid \theta = 0.50\right] + P\left[n = 14, y = 3 \mid \theta = 0.50\right] + \ldots$$

The cardiologist is perplexed.

"Why are all of these terms necessary?" he asks the statistician. "I understand why the first term, $P[n = 12, y = 3]$, has to be included, since it represents my data. But where do these other terms come from: $P[n = 13, y = 3]$, $P[n = 14, y = 3]$, etc.?' Come on! I didn't observe 13 or 14 patients, only 12. I don't want to misrepresent my findings, so why should I include probabilities for events that did not take place?"

"Well," the statistician replies evenly, "the *p*-value construction is based not only on the results as they occurred but also on results that are more extreme."

"What do you mean by that?" replies the doctor, a little agitated.

"Well, I mean that its possible you could have observed more patients, be-fore you saw three who were hypertension-free, right?" the statistician asks.

"But I didn't see more patients," the cardiologist complains.

"But you might have," retorts the statistician. "At the beginning of the study, you didn't know how many patients it would take before you observed three who were hypertension-free. It might have been 15, 20, or even more. That possi-bility must be factored into the answer."

"The results are my results, " the cardiologist responds stiffly. "You're telling me that I have to expand them to include findings that I didn't observe."

"I'm not changing your results. But the *p*-value is based on more than your results," the statistician responds.

"Hmmm," the unconvinced cardiologist mutters.

The statistician then turns back to compute the sum of these probabilities, that is 0.0327. The small *p*-value, generated under the assumption that $\theta = 0.50$ is evidence that this assumption about the hypertension prevalence is incorrect. Thus the null hypothesis is rejected.

The cardiologist, although pleased with the outcome, nevertheless harbors some suspicion about the computations. Still concerned about the practice of in-cluding "results" in the computation that did not occur in his research effort, he does not understand why is wasn't enough to simply compute $P[n = 12, y = 3]$ (which equals 0.013). He simply wants to know whether the data he observed (not the data that he didn't observe) supports the thesis that hypertension has a high prevalence.

Since he is in the clinic the next day, the cardiologist decides to carry out another observational study, consulting another statistician. The next day, he chooses to observe his clinic for a specified period. This time, be decides to count a sequence of 12 patients, then identify the number of patients among these 12 who have hypertension. The cardiologist observes that twelve patients have appeared in clinic, 9 of whom have high blood pressure. This is again a prevalence of 0.75. The consistency of these results with those of the previous day bolsters the cardiologist's confidence that the prevalence of hypertension is indeed high.

Taking his results to a second statistician, he watches as she begins. Letting θ be the prevalence of hypertension in this population, and x the number of patients with hypertension, she computes the probability that the test statistic falls in the criti-cal region when the null hypothesis is true]:

$$P[x = 9 \mid \theta = 0.50] + P[x = 10 \mid \theta = 0.50] + P[x = 11 \mid \theta = 0.50] + P[x = 12 \mid \theta = 0.50].$$

Again, the cardiologist is vexed. This statistician, like the other, starts with the observed result (9 patients with hypertension out of 12 patients seen), but con-tinues by considering more extreme findings. This time however, the cardiologist is shocked to find that the sum of these probabilities is 0.075, much greater than the 0.0327 produced by the first statistician. In fact the first term in this expression, $P[n = 9, x = 3 \mid \theta = 0.50]$, the probability of his observed result, is equal to 0.054, and is already larger than the computation from the first experiment, as well as be-ing greater than 0.050. Thus the findings for the second day's results, although they yielded the same hypertension prevalence as from the first day, produce a different result in the statistical analysis.

The cardiologist is staggered. Not only has the second day generated different results, but the computation is dependent on events that did not occur. In fact, the issue is somewhat worse. Under the null hypothesis, these non-occurring, extreme events were very unlikely anyway. So, the *p*-value is dependent not only on events that did not occur, but it is dependent on events that would not have been expected to occur. Constructing a decision rule based on the nonoccurrence of unlikely events commonly makes no sense to the non-statistician. This cardiologist relates his problem to an internist, who describes the following experience in her own clinic (adapted from Pratt [3]):

> I was just interested in producing a confidence interval for diastolic blood pressures in my clinic. That's all I wanted to do! I had an automated device that would read blood pressure very accurately and produce data that appeared to be normally distributed with a mean of 87 and a standard deviation of 5. I turned the data over to a statistician for a simple analysis.
>
> When the statistician came to my clinic to share his findings, he had a conversation with the staff nurse who told him that the automated blood-pressure-measuring device did not read above 100 mm Hg. When I confirmed this, the statistician said that he now had to do a new analysis, removing the underlying assumption of a normal distribution, since the blood pressure cuff would read any diastolic blood pressures greater than 100 mm Hg as 100 mm Hg, I understood his point, but assured him that in my data, no patient had a diastolic blood pressure greater than 97 mm Hg. Also, if there had been one, I would have called another clinic for a backup automated device equally sensitive to BP readings greater than 100 mm Hg.
>
> The statistician was relieved, thanked me, and returned to his office. However, after he left, I noticed that my backup unit was broken, and e-mailed this circumstance to him. He e-mailed me back, saying that he would have to redo the analysis after all! I was astonished and called him immediately. Why should the analysis be redone? No blood pressure was greater than 100 mm Hg, so the broken backup device would not have had to be used. My measurements were just as precise and accurate as they would have been if all instruments were working fine. The results would have been no different. Soon he would be asking me about my stethoscope!

These two examples illustrate an important underpinning of the frequentist approach. Its analysis relies not just on what has occurred, but what has not occurred. Both more extreme results in the first example, and the inability to measure diastolic blood pressures that were never observed to occur in the other demonstrate the frequentists' focus on the non-occurrence of events.[*]

12.2.4.2 Implications of the Likelihood Principle

The likelihood principle itself states that the only relevant information about an experiment's results is contained in the observed data. The implications of this principle are that it encourages a post-experimental way of thinking as opposed to the more traditional pre-experimental result. It is this latter perspective that is the basis for the two-tailed versus the one-tailed test.

Consider a two-armed, placebo-controlled clinical trial designed to test an intervention for its effect on all-cause mortality. The rationale for the two-sided test is that during the design phase of the research effort, the clinical researcher does not know whether the findings of the study will be favorable or unfavorable. The investigators may have a firm belief in the beneficial impact of the intervention, but at this stage it is only a belief. She is therefore compelled to divide the type I error, distributing it across the two tails of the test statistic's distribution, e.g., in Figure 3.15.

When the study is concluded, and the result is known, the type I error for the research effort is computed using the same two-sided distribution. For example if the test statistic at the conclusion of the study is 1.85, the *p*-value is

$$p - \text{value} = P[Z < 1.80] + P[Z > 1.80] = 2P[Z > 1.80] = 2(0.036) = 0.072.$$

This standard computation is a violation of the likelihood principle. The observed data produces a Z-score of 1.80, clearly demonstrating benefit. The possibility of harm is no longer a real consideration, and is not supported by the results. Nevertheless, the *p*-value computation includes the component $P[Z < -1.80]$ in the final calculation, even though the test statistic is on the other "benefit" side of the distribution. The motivation for this inclusion is simply that at the experiment's inception, the researchers didn't know if the effect would be beneficial or harmful. Thus, the pre-experimental view injects itself into the post-experimental computation when it has become clear that the pre-experimental view has been negated by the data. The likelihood principle states that only $P[Z > 1.80] = 0.036$ need be considered as the *p*-value.

---

[*] In their defense, frequentists would quite correctly argue that the point is not just to measure sample results accurately, but to extend them to the population. In the case of the second example, it was just the freak of chance that restricted patients to DBP's less than 100. Another sample could equally produce DBP's in the range where they could not be measured. In this circumstance, truncation of the normal distribution would have been necessary. The statistician was focused on a methodology that would work for every sample, not just the sample that happened to be on hand.

12.3 The Bayesian Philosophy

These examples reveal an important cornerstone of the classical statistician or frequentist; events that did not occur influence the interpretation of actual results. Alternatively, the Bayesian formulation is based on the likelihood principle, which states a decision should have its foundation in what has occurred, not in what has not occurred.

Like classical statistics, Bayes theory is applicable to problems of parameter estimation and hypothesis testing. Before turning to hypothesis testing, we will spend just a moment discussing Bayesian parameter estimation. Unlike frequentists who believe that the parameter (e.g., the population mean μ) is constant, Bayesians treat the parameter as though it itself has a probability distribution. This is called the *prior distribution,* signified as $\pi(\theta)$.

Once the prior distribution is identified, the Bayesian next identifies the probability distribution of the data given the value of the parameter. This distribution is described as the *conditional distribution* (because it is the distribution of the data conditional on the value of the unknown parameter) and is denoted as $f(x_1, x_2, x_3, ..., x_n | \theta)$. This second step is not unlike that of the frequentist. When attempting to identify the mean change in blood pressure for a collection of individuals, both the frequentist and the Bayesian may assume that the distribution of blood pressures for this sample of individuals follows a normal distribution with an unknown mean, whose estimation is the goal. However, the frequentist treats this unknown mean as a fixed parameter. The Bayesian assumes that the parameter is not constant, but changes over time.

The Bayes process continues by combining the prior distribution with this conditional distribution to create a *posterior distribution*, or the distribution of the parameter θ given the observed sample, denoted as $\pi(\theta | x_1, x_2, x_3, ..., x_n)$. From the Bayes perspective, the prior distribution reflects knowledge about the location and variability of θ before the experiment is carried out. After the experiment is executed, the researcher has new information in the form of the conditional distribution. These two sources of information are combined to obtain a new estimate of θ. To help in interpreting the posterior distribution, some Bayesians will construct a loss function, which identifies the penalty that they pay for underestimating or overestimating the population parameter. Bayesian hypothesis testing on the location of the parameter is based on the posterior distribution.

12.3.1 Bayes and Heart Failure

Consider the following illustration of the use of Bayes analysis in heart failure. A serum assay, useful only in patients with known heart failure offers the clinician a way of differentiating between ischemic and non-ischemic causes of CHF. If the patient has ischemic CHF, the probability of a positive assay is 0.90. If the patient has non-ischemic CHF, the probability of a negative test is 0.60. Each of two clinicians carry out the test on a patient of theirs. The test is positive for each patient.

While the test result is the same, conveying identical information about the likelihood that their patients' CHF is ischemic in nature, the utility of the information can be quite different. For example, suppose that Clinician A believed, based on the history and physical examination of her patient, that there is an overwhelming likelihood that her patient had a non-ischemic etiology for her heart failure. The positive test, indicating an ischemic cause for her patient's CHF does not change her mind. It may require her to re-consider the possibility of an ischemic etiology, but given the totality of the information available about the patient, she remains committed to the belief that her patient has non-ischemic CHF.

Alternatively, Clinician B is uncertain about the cause of his patient's CHF, believing that it is just as likely that the patient's disease has an ischemic versus a non-ischemic cause. In this circumstance we may expect a positive test to be helpful to this clinician, moving him closer to a definitive diagnosis.

It is this style of thinking that is formally encapsulated in the Bayesian perspective. In each of these two cases, the clinicians bring to the test result important prior information about their patient's disease state. This prior information is updated by the test result to produce a posterior (i.e., "posterior to" or "after the test result is available") conclusion. In addition, different prior assumptions lead to different posterior conclusions.

A Bayesian might formalize the argument in the following way. Let θ represent the state of the patient's CHF. Let $\theta = 1$ denote the presence of ischemic CHF, and $\theta = 0$ denote a non-ischemic case. Each clinician wishes to know the value of θ for their patient. In the same vein, let x denote the test result; $x = 1$ supports ischemic CHF and $x = 0$ supports a non-ischemic cause. This information about the test result we will refer to as the conditional distribution of x given θ. We also have been told how well this test works i.e., $P[x = 1 | \theta = 1] = 0.90$, and additionally, $P[x = 0 | \theta = 0] = 0.60$. What we would like to know is the probability of ischemic CHF, or $P[\theta = 1 | x = 1]$. The application of simple conditional probability reveals

$$P[\theta = 1 | x = 1] = \frac{P[\theta = 1 \text{ and } x = 1]}{P[x = 1]} = \frac{P[x = 1 | \theta = 1] P[\theta = 1]}{P[x = 1]}. \quad (12.1)$$

Note that equation (12.1) contains two conditional probabilities. The conditional probability that we desire, $P[\theta = 1 | x = 1]$, is expressed in terms of a conditional probability that we know, $P[x = 1 | \theta = 1]$.

Examining the denominator on the right-hand side of equation (12.1), we now focus on rewriting $P[x = 1]$ (i.e., the probability of a positive test result). This can be written as the probability of a positive test result when the patient has ischemic CHF plus the probability of a positive test result in the presence of non-ischemic CHF, i.e.,

$$P[x = 1] = P[x = 1 | \theta = 1] P[\theta = 1] + P[x = 1 | \theta = 0](1 - P[\theta = 1])$$

Substituting this result into equation (12.1), we find

$$P[\theta = 1 \mid x = 1] = \frac{P[x = 1 \mid \theta = 1] P[\theta = 1]}{P[x = 1 \mid \theta = 1] P[\theta = 1] \; + \; P[x = 1 \mid \theta = 0](1 \; - \; P[\theta = 1])}.$$

Since $P[x = 1 \mid \theta = 1] = 0.90$, and $P[x = 0 \mid \theta = 0] = 0.60$, we may write the conditional probability $P[\theta = 1 \mid x = 1]$ as

$$P[\theta = 1 \mid x = 1] = \frac{0.90 \, P[\theta = 1]}{0.90 \, P[\theta = 1] \; + \; 0.60(1 \; - \; P[\theta = 1])}. \qquad (12.2)$$

We now have the posterior probability of ischemic CHF as a function of the clinician's prior information $P[\theta = 1]$ (Figure 12.1).

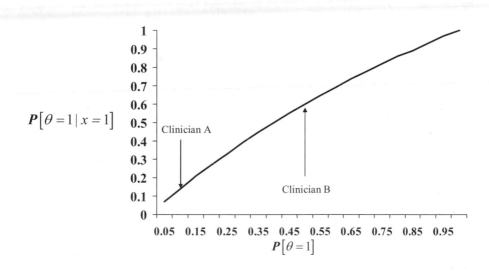

Figure 12.1. The posterior distribution of the probability of ischemic CHF
As a function of the prior belief $P[\theta = 1]$.

Figure 12.1 illustrates the strong relationship between the posterior probability of ischemic CHF and the prior information about the occurrence of ischemic CHF. On that curve, we can locate the posterior probability for Clinician A and B. For Clinician A, whose prior knowledge was determined as $\theta = 0.10$, the posterior probability of an ischemic cause for the patient's CHF is 0.14. As we might have expected, this strong prior knowledge suggesting a non-ischemic etiology was not negated by the positive value of the test result. Alternatively, for Clinician B, whose prior information was $\theta = 0.50$, the update provided by the test result produces a posterior probability of 0.60, providing a useful, although it might be argued a non-substantial, increase in the likelihood of on ischemic cause for their CHF.

It would be illuminating to assess the degree to which the clinician's prior information is updated by the test. If the test does not make a substantial change in the clinician's prior information, then the test may not be worth considering in the evaluation of the patient. We define *absolute update strength* S_A as the absolute value of the difference between the posterior and prior probability of an event (in this case the occurrence of ischemic CHF), i.e.,

$$S_A = \Big| P[\theta = 1 | x = 1] \ - \ P[\theta = 1] \Big|. \tag{12.3}$$

Similarly, we will define S_R as the relative update strength of the test. This is just the percent change in the probability of the test, and is easily written as

$$S_R = \frac{\Big| P[\theta = 1 | x = 1] \ - \ P[\theta = 1] \Big|}{P[\theta = 1]} = \frac{S_A}{P[\theta = 1]}. \tag{12.4}$$

These values are easily determined from the ischemic CHF example (Figure 12.2)

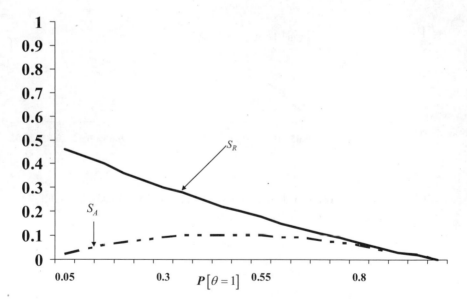

Figure 12.2. The ability of the posterior distribution to update the prior information Using the concept of absolute (S_A) and relative (S_R) update strength.

If the test is valuable, the investigator should be able to see large values of S_A and

S_R over the range of prior information. For this test, we see that absolute update strength is at its largest for intermediate values of the prior information about θ. For patients in whom the prior information suggests that the patient has ischemic CHF, i.e., $P[\theta = 1]$ is high — both S_A and S_R are low, suggesting that the test would not provide useful updated information about the likelihood of an ischemic cause of heart failure when the prior belief about an ischemic cause is high.

However the values of S_A and S_R are functions of the conditional probabilities $P[x=1|\theta=1]$ and $P[x=0|\theta=0]$. The quantity $P[x=1|\theta=1]$ is known as the sensitivity of the test, i.e., how likely is the test to determine an ischemic cause, when an ischemic cause is in fact the case. The quantity $P[x=0|\theta=0]$ is the specificity of the test. Both S_A and S_R are functions of the sensitivity and specificity. For the example of a second insensitive $\left(P[x=1|\theta=1]=0.04\right)$ but very specific $\left(P[x=0|\theta=0]=0.99\right)$ test the characteristics of S_A and S_R are quite different (Figure 12.3).

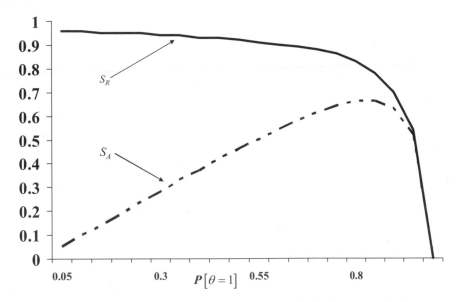

Figure 12.3. Absolute (S_A) and relative (S_R) update strength for a test with low Sensitivity (0.04) and high specificity (0.99).

In this case, the optimum range of prior information for the utility of this test is $P[\theta = 1]$ from 0.50 to 0.95.

The use of Bayes procedures can provide useful insights into the performance of tests. It explicitly considers available prior distribution information and allows construction of a loss function that directly and clearly states the loss (or gain) for each decision. However, the requirement of a specification of the prior

distribution can be a burden if there is not much good information about the parameter to be estimated. In this case, the two clinicians were clear about what they
knew (or did not know) about the likelihood of their patient who had ischemic congestive heart failure. However, there are some type of prior information that reflect another degree of vagueness about the likelihood of ischemic CHF.

     In addition, tests commonly are not negative or positive but instead provide a
range of values. Striking differences between the values for different disease states
provide important discriminating ability for the tests (Figure 12.4).

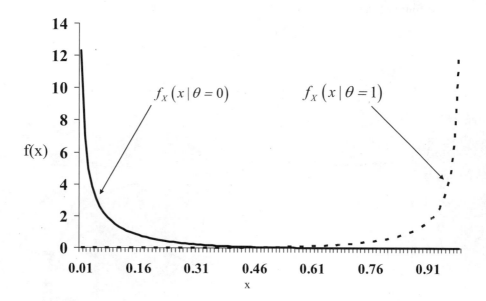

Fig. 12.4. Testing characteristics of CHF test. The probability distribution of the
values of the test depends on whether the patient has ischemic ($\theta = 1$) or non-
ischemic ($\theta = 0$) CHF.

In this circumstance, test results that are small ($x \leq 0.15$) are most common for patients
with non-ischemic CHF, while large test values (e.g., $x \geq 0.85$) are likely when the
patient has ischemic CHF. Computation of the posterior probability follows the previous development, and we may write

$$P[\theta = 1 \mid x \geq 0.85] = \frac{P[x \geq 0.85]P[\theta = 1]}{P[x \geq 0.85]P[\theta = 1] + P[x \geq 0.85][1 - P[\theta = 1]]}, (12.5)$$

where $P[x \geq 0.85]$ is computed from the area under the curves from Figure 12.4.

     Yet another layer of sophistication can be added through a reevaluation of
the assumptions concerning the underlying disease process. Up to this point, we
have treated CHF as being of one of two etiologies, ischemic versus non-ischemic,

denoted by $\theta = 1$ or 0, respectively. However, that may be a simplification. Patients may have simultaneously both ischemic and non-ischemic CHF; one need not occur to the exclusion of the other. Thus we may consider θ not just as a single value, but a continuum of values between 0 and 1. Small values of θ indicate a primarily non-ischemic etiology, large values of θ indicate almost exclusively ischemic CHF, and intermediate values indicate a substantial presence of both etiologies in the same heart (Figure 12.5).

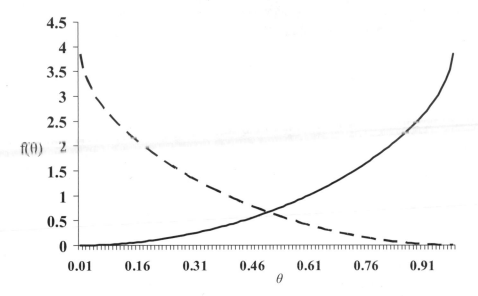

Figure 12.5. Hypothetical distribution of nonischemic and ischemic causes of CHF in the same heart. This indicates the presence of intermediate values signifying a mixture of ischemic and nonischemic etiology of CHF in the population.

This development permits the investigator to focus on regions of the value of θ. Small values of θ, (i.e., $\theta \leq 0.30$) indicate that the cause of the patient's CHF is primarily non-ischemic, perhaps suggesting one therapeutic approach. Intermediate values of θ indicate a mixed etiology, suggesting another therapeutic modality, and large values of θ (i.e., $\theta \geq 0.70$) point to a primary ischemic etiology for the patients heart failure, suggesting yet another therapeutic option.

In this case, θ has a continuous range of values, and the distribution of θ has a particular new meaning. From this point of view, any value of θ between 0 and 1 is possible. This distribution is termed the prior distribution as is denoted by $\pi(\theta)$. From the above example, the distribution of $\pi(\theta)$ is readily obtainable (Figure 12.6). The investigator is no longer interested in whether the value of θ is merely 0 or 1, but, instead focuses on the range of values in which θ falls.

In this circumstance, the probability of ischemic CHF based on a positive test result can be written as

$$P[\theta \geq 0.70 \,|\, x \geq 0.85] = \frac{P[x \geq 0.85]\,P[\theta \geq 0.70]}{P[x \geq 0.85]\,P[\theta \geq 0.70] \;+\; P[x \geq 0.85]\,P[\theta < 0.70]}.$$

Now, the investigators update the prior distribution $\pi(\theta)$ with the conditional distribution (i.e., the sensitivity and specificity of the test) to compute the posterior distribution of θ given the test result $\pi(\theta \,|\, x)$.

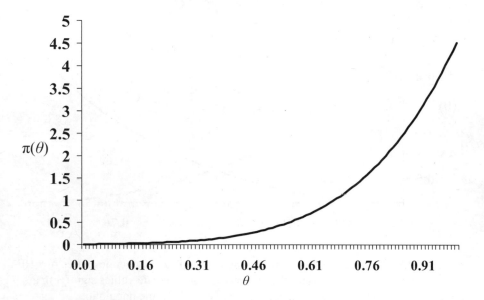

Fig. 12.6. Distribution of the probability of ischemic CHF in the population. The larger the value of θ, the greater the likelihood of an ischemic cause. The area under the curve indicates the probability of θ falling within a range of values.

The evolution of the problem from variables x and θ that could only have values zero or one to continuous variables requires us to modify the mathematics. The formal statement of this is written as

$$\pi(\theta \,|\, x) = \frac{f(x \,|\, \theta)\,\pi(\theta)}{f(x)}. \tag{12.6}$$

This is just a generalization of the formula that we have utilized thus far in this chapter. In realistic problems e.g., the last scenario of the previous example, the posterior distribution commonly requires calculus to identify.

To the Bayesian, information concerning the parameter of interest θ goes through a series of stages. With no observation from which to work, our best information for θ is expressed as $\pi(\theta)$, the prior distribution of θ. After x is observed, we combine the information learned about θ from the research with the information known about θ obtained from $\pi(\theta)$ and assemble the posterior distribution of θ, denoted by $\pi(\theta \,|\, x)$. In this way, the posterior distribution contains information from prior knowledge of θ and information gathered from observing the data (Figure 12.7).

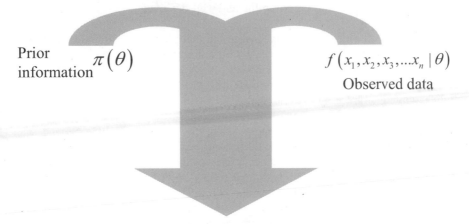

Prior information $\pi(\theta)$

$f(x_1, x_2, x_3, \ldots x_n \,|\, \theta)$
Observed data

Posterior Information
$\pi(\theta \,|\, x_1, x_2, x_3, \ldots x_n)$

Fig. 12.7. In Bayes procedures, the prior information about the unknown parameter θ and the observed data combine to produce the posterior distribution θ.

12.4 Feasibility of Prior Distributions

The incorporation of a prior distribution is one of the hallmarks of a Bayesian analysis. The concept that the population parameter has its own variability stands in stark contrast to the perspective of the classical (frequentist) approach, in which no consideration is given and no allowance made for variability in the population parameters. The only source of variability the frequentists consider is sampling variability (the variability that comes from the sample).

However, the flexibility of prior distribution interpretation is quite useful to the Bayesian. For example, consider blood glucose measurements. If we apply comments about sampling schemes from Chapter One, we would say that if the investigator could measure everybody's blood glucose everywhere, he would have determined the blood glucose measurement exactly. However, this admittedly impossible task may itself be something of a simplification. The blood glucose measurement for an individual is not a constant but a quantity that varies. It changes with time of day, activity level digestive state, hormonal status, etc. This intrinsic, biologic variability is better approximated by applying a probability distribution to it, and not assuming it is a fixed, unmovable target.

The use of prior distributions can have important implications in clinical research. Healthcare consumers are not seen as contributors to, but as consumers of, large clinical research programs. Earlier we pointed out that the nature of the practitioner's focus on individual patients limits that practitioner's ability objectively to discern the benefits and hazards of a particular intervention.[*] Practitioners must embrace the tools of population sampling and well-designed experiments in order to gain this objectivity.

However, although we have suggested that physicians embrace the results of well-designed experiments, we have said nothing about the possible contributions they could make. Of course, clinical researchers do use these practitioners' patients, working hard to randomize those who meet the trial entry criteria to their studies, while guaranteeing that the clinical trial will not completely take the patient away from the practitioner. This patient contribution must not be minimized, because if the trial results are to be generalizable, the trial must include patients who are representative of the population. This contribution by practicing physicians is invaluable. Also, the clinician provides strategies on how to help patients stay on the study medication and comply with their follow-up visits.

However, we also know that the concepts of community protection, the tools used by physician-scientists in designing trials, are different from the tools used by practitioners in their day-to-day treatment of individual patients. Is this difference so great that it precludes any intellectual contribution by practitioners to a well-designed clinical trial? Is there no room for the possibility that these practitioners may be able to contribute at a more central level, providing insight into event rates of disease and the degree to which the intervention may be effective? Does their experience count for nothing in the research process, beyond ignition of the initial idea and the valuable contribution of their patients?

One way to incorporate the experience of physicians into the design of a clinical trial is through the Bayesian approach. Such a procedure would permit physicians to contribute their own prior information concerning the underlying treatment rate, as well as their expectation of the efficacy of the intervention being evaluated. The mathematics of this process is not complicated. It is fairer to say that the organization of the process (i.e., collecting the individuals' assessments of prior information and efficacy from community physicians who are not themselves researchers) would be more daunting then the calculations. However, this process would allow the inclusion of the vital insight of practitioners. Designing a clinical study without due consideration of the experience of the practitioners who have been seeing patients for years before the trial's inception is at best squandering a useful resource, and perhaps is also somewhat unrepresentative. The notion of translational research, i.e., having clinical research results be presented in a format that the community can easily identify and assimilate, begins with the practitioner

---

[*] See Chapter One.

community's involvement in the research construction, thereby adding to the clinical trial cognitive repository

12.5 The Loss Function

We have seen that in the Bayes paradigm, prior information about a quantity is combined with new information from a research effort to construct the posterior distribution of the parameter. However, the end of the Bayesian computation is not the determination of the posterior distribution; once one has it, one must decide what to do with it. How Bayesians manipulate the posterior distribution depends on the loss function they use.

The Bayesian constructs the loss function to reflect the true consequences of correct and incorrect decisions. Once the loss function is defined, it tells the investigator how to use the posterior distribution to take an action. The loss function is denoted as $L(\theta, \delta)$, where θ is the parameter to be estimated and δ is the estimator to be used. The loss function determines what loss the user sustains when she attempt to take an action. That action may be to identify an estimator for the parameter θ, or it may be to make a decision about the location of θ (i.e., decide that $\theta = 0$).

For example, if the purpose of the analysis is to estimate a continuous parameter, a commonly used loss function is squared error loss. In this case, we write $L(\theta, \delta) = (\theta - \delta)^2$. This loss function is smallest when $\delta = \theta$, i.e., when the estimate is equal to the parameter. However, it also says that the further the estimator is from the parameter θ (i.e., the worse our estimate is), the loss we incur increases, and increases quadratically. A second implication of this loss function is that the penalty is the same for underestimating θ as for overestimating θ.

The Bayesian estimator is the quantity that minimizes the average loss. This averaging is taken over the updated information for θ i.e., from the posterior distribution. Thus, the loss function is used in combination with the posterior density to identify the estimator that reduces the expected values of the loss function or the risk. If the loss function is squared error loss, the Bayes estimator θ is the mean of the posterior distribution. Alternatively, if the loss function is absolute error loss i.e., $L(\theta, \delta) = |\theta - \delta|$, then the Bayes estimator is the median of the posterior distribution. Thus, it is the loss function that determines how the posterior distribution is to be used to find θ.

12.6 Example of Bayesian Estimation

For example, let's assume that the prior probability distribution of total cholesterol follows a normal distribution with mean μ and variance τ^2. The investigator wishes to update this information for the mean cholesterol value, collecting a random sample of individuals from the population, measuring their cholesterol values. He assumes that the cholesterol values obtained from his sample follow a normal distribution as well, but with mean θ and variance σ^2. If the investigator were to use the frequentist approach, he would simply estimate θ, the mean cholesterol value by the sample mean of his data. Although there is variability associated with this estimate (σ^2/n), it is important to note that this variability is associated with only the sampling scheme, i.e., variability associated with the sample mean, not the population mean. The population mean is fixed. The sample mean, because of sampling error contains all of the variability.

However, the Bayesian doesn't just take the mean cholesterol level of his sample, he combines his data with the prior distribution to construct the posterior distribution. In this case when the prior distribution is normal with mean μ and variance τ^2 and the conditional distribution is normal with mean θ and variance σ^2, the posterior distribution of θ given x is also normal. The mean of this posterior distribution, μ_p is

$$\mu_p = \frac{\tau^2}{\tau^2 + \sigma_{\bar{x}}^2} \bar{x} + \frac{\sigma_{\bar{x}}^2}{\tau^2 + \sigma_{\bar{x}}^2} \mu \qquad (12.7)$$

and variance v_p

$$v_p = \frac{1}{\dfrac{1}{\tau^2} + \dfrac{1}{\sigma_{\bar{x}}^2}}. \qquad (12.8)$$

Using squared error loss the Bayes estimator δ_B is the posterior mean. The posterior mean μ_p depends not just on the distribution of x, but also depends on the parameters μ and τ^2 from the prior distribution as well. The posterior mean is a weighted average of the mean of the prior distribution and the sample mean obtained from the data. The prior mean μ has been updated to the posterior mean μ_p by the sample data. Similarly, the prior variance τ^2 has been updated to the posterior variance v_p^2 by the incorporation of $\sigma_{\bar{x}}^2$.

As an example, suppose an investigator is interested in a Bayesian assessment of total cholesterol values in her clinic. She believes that the total cholesterol level will be normally distributed. Her prior assessment is that the mean is 175 mg/dl and the standard deviation is 10. However, she collects the data and observes that the mean of her sample is 200 and the standard deviation of 15. Application of equations (12.7) and (12.8) reveals that the posterior mean is 180 mg/dl and the standard deviation is 7. Comparison of the three distributions is revealing (Figure 12.8).

The posterior distribution of total cholesterol is located between the positions of the prior distribution and the conditional distribution, representing the updated understanding of the total cholesterol levels. The position is not the midpoint between the prior and posterior distribution. Its actual location depends on the standard deviations from the prior and posterior distribution. The posterior distribution will be closest to the distribution with the greatest precision (i.e., smallest standard deviation.)

12.7 Bayesians and *P*-values

Significance testing is easily within the Bayesians' reach. In earlier chapters we have argued for the arbitrary choice of type I and type II errors. We have argued that they should be chosen prospectively, we have argued that they should be chosen thoughtfully, but we have always argued that they should be chosen. The Bayesian approach is not so preoccupied with the arbitrary choice of alpha levels.

Classical statisticians talk about significance testing. Bayesians talk about taking *action*. In hypothesis testing, the Bayesian acts, taking an action to either accept or reject a hypothesis.

In the classical approach, we are concerned with making a decision about an unknown parameter θ (e.g. the mean of a distribution, or a cumulative incidence rate). We obtain a collection of observations from the population. This collection of observations has a probability distribution that depends on θ. Since the probability distribution of the data depends on θ, this can be viewed as each observation in the data containing some information about θ. Thus, in estimation, we find a function of the x's that allows us to estimate θ. In significance testing, we identify a function of the x's that allow us to make a decision about the location of θ (e.g. $\theta = 0.25$ versus. $\theta \neq 0.25$).

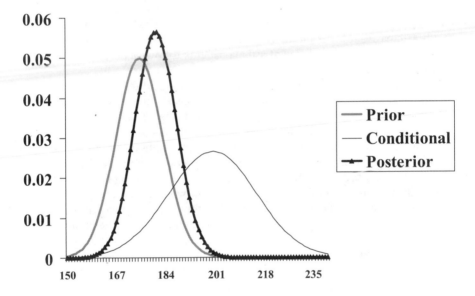

Fig. 12.8. Comparison of prior, conditional, and posterior distribution of total cholesterol values.

The Bayesian approach uses the posterior distribution of θ to generate its *p*-values. These quantities are termed posterior probabilities

12.8 Bayes Testing: Asthma Prevalence

Consider the example of a clinic whose administrator needs to decide whether the proportion of patients it sees with asthma is greater than 5% during the summer months. If the proportion is larger, the clinic administrator will need to invest resources in the clinic so that it may better serve its community. This will involve both an education program for the clinic staff as well as the provision of ample medical supplies to treat asthma. In his quest to determine the proportion of asthma patients seen in the summer months, the administrator approaches the clinic doctors, learning that they are not at all sure of the prevalence of this problem in their patients. They do agree that its prevalence is greater than 1% and less than 20%, but can reach no consensus on a more refined estimate.

The administrator wishes to take a Bayesian action. Let θ be the prevalence of asthma. In order to take a Bayesian action in this problem of testing for the location of θ, the administrator must be armed with the following three items:

1. the prior distribution of θ,
2. the distribution of the data obtained in his sample, and
3. the loss function.

He uses the information provided by the physicians to estimate the prior distribution of θ. If no one value in this range of 0.01 to 0.20 is more likely than any other, he can spread the prior probability uniformly over this region.*

He also identifies the distribution of the estimated proportion of patients with asthma from a sample of clinic data. If the number of patients who visit the clinic is n, then the prevalence of asthma patients follows a normal distribution with mean θ and variance $\theta(1 - \theta)/n^\dagger$.

Having identified the prior distribution of θ and the distribution of the data from the sample, the administrator now must consider the loss function. He begins by considering the possible actions he can take (Table 12.1).

The administrator can make one and only one decision about the location of θ and recognizes that this decision will be either right or wrong. Let the first action (a_1) be the decision that $\theta < 0.05$, and the second action (a_2) the decision that θ is ≥ 0.05. Let's say the administrator takes action a_1, deciding that $\theta < 0.05$. If he is right, then he incurs no loss. However, if he is wrong, then the clinic will incur a cost. That cost is not being prepared for the asthma patients that will visit the clinic. This means patients lost to the clinic and some diminution of the clinic's reputation in the community. The administrator denotes this cost by k_1, setting $k_1 = \$10,000$.

Alternatively, the administrator could take action a_2, deciding that θ is greater than 0.05. Again, he could be right or wrong. If he is correct, the cost is zero. If he is wrong, then he has invested more money into the clinic staff training and supplies than was necessary. Call that cost k_2, and set $k_2 = \$1,500$.

---

* Some critics would argue that assuming probability is equally distributed across this region is assuming knowledge about the location of θ. Here we use it to provide an example, not to justify the approach.

† If θ is the prevalence of asthma, then the number of cases X follows a binomial distribution, $P[X = k] = \binom{n}{k} \theta^k (1 - \theta)^{n-k}$. The variance of the estimate of θ is $\theta(1 - \theta)/n$. This is used as the variance of the distribution of the sample estimate in this example.

Table 12.1. Loss function for asthma prevalence decision rule

	Possible Actions	
	a_1 decide $\theta < 0.05$	a_2 decide $\theta \geq 0.05$
$\theta < 0.05$	0	$k_2 = \$1,500$
$\theta \geq 0.05$	$k_1 = \$10,000$	0

The Bayesian action is the action that produces the smallest expected loss. Thus, the administrator begins by computing his expected loss for each of his actions. If he takes action a_1 his expected loss is

$$E_P\left[L(\theta, a_1)\right] = L(\theta < 0.05, a_1)P[\theta < 0.05] + L(\theta \geq 0.05, a_1)P[\theta \geq 0.05].$$

From Table 12.1, the administrator sees that $L(\theta < 0.05, a_1)$ is zero, since concluding that $\theta < 0.05$ when that is the case is a correct decision. However, taking action a_1, i.e., concluding that $\theta < 0.05$ when it is greater than or equal to 0.05 is an incorrect decision and incurs a cost of $L(\theta \geq 0.05, a_1) = \$10,000$. Thus, we may simplify the expression for the expected loss to

$$E_P\left[L(\theta, a_1)\right] = 10,000P[\theta \geq 0.05].$$

Analogously, the expected posterior loss for action a_2 is

$$E_P\left[L(\theta, a_2)\right] = L(\theta < 0.05, a_2)P[\theta < 0.05] + L(\theta \geq 0.05, a_2)P[\theta \geq 0.05]$$
$$= 1500P[\theta < 0.05].$$

The administrator assessed these losses using the posterior probability distribution for θ and chooses action a_2 when its expected or average loss is less than that for action a_1 or $1,500P[\theta < 0.05] \leq 10,000P[\theta \geq 0.05]$.

Now if we let $p = P[\theta \geq 0.05]$, and the application of some algebra reveals that the administrator should take action a_2 if $p > 1,500/11,500 = 0.1304$.

The administrator needs to identify the distribution of θ in order to choose the Bayes action. He already has the distribution of θ based on the prior distribution; the beliefs of the clinic physicians suggested that the proportion of asthma cases was between 1% and 20%. However, he cannot base his judgment solely on their beliefs, since these beliefs are based on their own experiences and are subject to bias and distortion. He assesses the proportion of patients identified in the clinic during the past summer and finds that this proportion is 0.065. The administrator can now compute (or have computed for him) p using the posterior probability distribution. For our problem, the mathematics lead to

$$= \frac{\int_{0.05}^{0.20} \sqrt{\frac{n}{2\pi\theta(1-\theta)}} e^{-\frac{n}{2\theta(1-\theta)}(\theta-x)^2} d\theta}{\int_{0.01}^{0.20} \sqrt{\frac{n}{2\pi\theta(1-\theta)}} e^{-\frac{n}{2\theta(1-\theta)}(\theta-x)^2} d\theta}, \qquad (12.9)$$

which is the ratio of two normal probabilities. Using the value $x = 0.065$ in equation (12.9), he computes that $p = 0.929$. Since this quantity is greater than 0.1304, he concludes that θ is greater than 0.05, and proceeds with the additional training and supply procurement

It is useful to consider the implications of this rule for different values of x. If x were 0.050, then $p = 0.541$ and the decision would have been to expand the asthma service. If $x = 0.040$, then $p = 0.541$, and the decision would have again been to expand the asthma service. Only when $x < 0.036$ would the decision have been to keep the asthma service unchanged, begging the question, "If $x < 0.05$, why is p still greater than 0.05?"

The answer resides in the loss function. This function is built on the premise that the worst error would be not to expand the services when they should be expanded. This is transmitted directly to the decision rule, that advocates for expansion even with asthma prevalence values of 0.04.

Note that this exercise in stating a problem, drawing a sample, and making a decision based on that sample was carried out without a single statement about significance testing or type I or type II error. The administrator computed a single posterior probability. However, this probability has the look and feel of a p value even it is not derived from a classical hypothesis test. Admittedly, it is based on a loss function, which is new to frequentists. The paradigm was different. In this case, the administrator's reliance on experience was tempered by the conditional probability distribution. He simply estimated the costs of the possible mistakes he could make, then followed a procedure to minimize these costs.

Also note that administrator could have taken the approach of going only by the physician beliefs i.e., the prior distribution. While this is useful, it is commonly mistaken since, as pointed out in Chapter One, the focus of practicing physician's on the patient distorts their perception of the true proportion of events. It is easy and correct to justify the need for a more objective measurement of the proportion of patients with asthma by taking a sample of data from the clinic.

However, we must examine the other side of this coin. Once the administrator has collected his sample of data and obtained a sample estimate of 0.065 for the proportion of patients with asthma, why not just discard the physician opinions? In fact, if the administrator had consulted a frequentist statistician, this is precisely what would have happened. The frequentist would have constructed a binomial test of proportions covered in an elementary statistics course and carry out a straight-forward hypothesis test, using only the data and discarding the physician beliefs.

By sticking with the Bayesian approach, the administrator wisely allowed the opinions of the physicians who see the patients into the decision process. We have seen the havoc sampling error has raised with estimates.[*] It is possible that the sample estimate obtained from the clinic would be very different from the true proportion of asthma patients. The opinions of the physicians have provided some anchor for the estimate of the proportion of asthma patients to be seen at the clinic. By including the physician estimates, the administrator reaps the benefit of clinic physician experience and the sample estimate.

This does not yet commonly occur in large clinical trials. Because such a trial is designed using the frequentist approach, there is no way formally to incorporate the opinions of the many physicians who contribute their patients into its intellectual repository. These physician opinions we acknowledge as being by necessity biased. However, they provide useful information about the clinical event rate of interest and the efficacy of the intervention. Bayesian procedures admit the experiences of these physicians into the estimates of the vital parameters of the trial.

It is important to emphasize this point. A physician's biased opinion should not be rejected out of hand. Biased estimates can be good estimates, just as unbiased estimates can be bad estimates. As a simple example of this principle, consider the problem of computing the average cholesterol level of subjects in a cholesterol screening program for one day. Observer 1 decides to take the cholesterol level of each individual, and before taking the average, adds five mg/dl to each patient measurement. This is clearly a biased estimate. Observer 2 chooses to compute the usual average cholesterol, and then flip a coin. If its heads, he adds 50 mg/dl to the result. If it is tails, he subtracts 50 mg/dl. Observers 2's estimate of the average cholesterol is unbiased, while that of observer 1 is biased, but on any given day, we would be more comfortable with the biased estimate. In this example, the long-term behavior of the estimate is unhelpful.

12.9 Conclusions

The Bayesian approach to statistical analysis makes unique contributions. It explicitly considers prior distribution information. It allows construction of a loss function that directly and clearly states the loss (or gain) for each decision. It has admirable flexibility where traditional p–values are murky, e.g., on the level of loss and community protection to be provided by the test.

However, Bayesian p–values are not manna from heaven. The requirement of a specification of the prior distribution can be a burden if there is not much good information about the parameter to be estimated. What should that prior distribution be. What shape should it have? Should it be normally distributed, or follow some other distribution like a χ^2 distribution? What are the parameters of this distribution? This should be determined before any conclusions are drawn. Since the results will be based on this assumption, it is often useful to consider how the results change if the underlying prior distribution changes. Also, as we have seen, with very simple prior distribu-

---

[*] See Chapter Two.

tions and familiar conditional distributions, computations for the posterior distribution can be problematic. Computing tools have eased this pain, but to the non-statistician, the underlying mathematics can be intimidating. Similarly, a detailed loss function is required before the Bayesian action can be computed. Bayesian statisticians fret over this specification, while frequentists ignore it. Of course, retrospective Bayesian prior distributions and retrospective loss functions, chosen when the research program is over, are just as corruptive and just as worthless as retrospective alpha level thresholds.

Perhaps both the Bayes approach and the frequentist approach to statistical inference each should be viewed as mere tools in a toolkit. One should use the approach that fits the problem. If there is good prior information, and high hopes of constructing a defensible loss function, it is difficult to argue against the Bayesian approach to statistical inference. However, if there is little or no prior information and no hope for consensus on a loss function, the worker might be best served by staying with the classical perspective. In any event, the worker must decide, and decide prospectively.

References

1.   Berger James O (1980) *Statistical Decision Theory. Foundations, Concepts, and Methods*. New York: Springer-Verlag.
2.   Lindley DV (1976) Inference for a Bernoulli process (a Bayesian view) *The American Statistician* **30**:112–118.
3.   Pratt JW (1962) Discussion of A. Birnbaum's "On the foundations of statistical inference" *Journal of the American Statistical Association* **57**:269–326.

Conclusions:
Good Servants but Bad Masters

Drawing conclusions based on a sample of data is a thinking person's business. Yet I am often asked for simple rules or guidelines for interpreting medical research. The best rule I can give is this: Use your head! While this deliberative thought process will produce its own share of mistakes, it is my thesis that we are worse off if we let p-values do our thinking for us.

Correct interpretation of a research effort is not as simple as reading from a rulebook. Every effort is unique, requiring us carefully to sift and weigh information about the prospective nature of the research design, its concordant execution, the state of healthcare in the community, and the appropriateness of the analysis plan before we can make decisions. Nevertheless, the principles of research design, execution, and analysis are simple.

This doctrine begins with the acknowledgment that, for ethical, fiscal, logistical and administrative reasons, researchers can only study a tiny fraction of the targeted population of subjects in which they are interested. However, they are extremely interested in extending their sample results from the relatively small collection of patients they have observed to thousands or millions that they have not. This extension is both necessary and hazardous. It is made more dangerous by the recognition that several competent researchers can each independently evaluate different samples from the same population, generating different "generalizable" results. The sample-to-sample variability weakens the claim that any particular sample is the one whose results are generalizable. Researchers who ignore the effect of sampling error while drawing conclusions from sample-based research are like pilots who ignore the effect of gravity while flying aircraft. The impact of these predictable but unaccounted for forces can be grievous.

The ability to extend a research effort's results from a sample to a population depends on whether the research was designed to answer the question. P-values jointly interpreted with effect size are most helpful in determining the influence of sampling error on the confirmatory analyses drawn from research programs.

As important as p-values are for measuring sampling error, we are reminded that that is all that they do. P-values are not the sole arbiter for the study. They do not measure effect size, nor do they convey the extent of study discordance. A small p-value does not in and of itself mean that the sample size was adequate, that the effect size is clinically meaningful, or that there is clear attribution of effect to the exposure or intervention of interest.

Many research findings in healthcare are not generalizable. They occur simply by the random aggregation of subjects in small samples, commonly refereed to as the freak of chance. Commonly these "findings" are unanticipated. It is inappropriate for the researcher to elevate these unanticipated exploratory findings, replacing the prospectively declared evaluations with these "surprise results." The fisherman is suspect when he returns from a fishing trip not with fish but with boots and claims that he was "fishing for boots all along." So too is the researcher who claims that he has identified an important answer from his sample when in fact he never intended to ask that research question of his sample. The sample supplied an answer that he never thought to ask.

The tendency among many researchers and their advocates to "analyze everything, and report what is favorable to our belief" is a process that mixes the relatively unstructured "search and exploration" aspect of science with the tight discipline required of research and confirmation. Combining the two confuses the view of the population landscape because it mixes in with the small number of good, prospectively planned evaluations many more false findings commonly generated by a small sample full of sampling error.

The medical community is commonly flummoxed by these reports. Some findings are reliable, most are not, and the investigator provides no methodologically sound discriminator, relying instead only on the *p*-value. The readership, confronted with this confusing situation, must work its way through this mixture of reliable an unreliable evaluations like soldiers traversing a mine field with a false map based on misleading *p*-values; they learn the hard way (as in ELITE I/II, and PRAISE I/ II) which results are trustworthy and which are not.

This problem is avoided by reporting research results at two levels. The highest level is occupied by those questions asked by the investigator before any data were obtained. These questions are often small in number, well considered, and, more specifically, are the inquiries around which the research was designed. The maxim "first say what you plan to do, then do what you say" leads to the clearest extension of the research's results from the small sample to the large population. It is in this well-defined circumstance that *p*-values are most useful, and their joint consideration with effect size, effect size variability and confidence intervals provide the clearest reflection of the population effects in the sample.

The second-tier questions are exploratory or hypothesis-generating questions. The definitive answers provided to this second group of questions must wait until the next research effort, because the research that spawned them was not designed to answer them. *P*-values are rarely helpful in these circumstances.

There are other destructive influences that distort research results as well. The wrong exposure duration, inferior inclusion/exclusion criteria, or poor selection of the endpoints can produce non-responsive research programs that shed no useful life on the scientific question at hand. Statistical hypothesis tests are of limited use in this setting; small *p*-values cannot save poorly designed studies.

In addition, *p*-values cannot rescue a research effort from its own poor execution. Concordantly executed research (i.e., a research effort that is executed according to the prospectively specified protocol) allows the cleanest and clearest interpretation of *p*-values, while discordant research (i.e., research efforts that undergo a midcourse change in analysis plan or endpoint) can be impossible to interpret. Because the findings are so difficult for us to integrate into our fund of knowledge, these discordant programs accomplish little more than squandering precious resources. Attempting to view a population effect through a discordant research effort is like trying to learn about your appearance by studying your reflection in muddy water. It is an effort bound to mislead and must ultimately be set aside.

These factors of research design and execution must be considered separately from the statistical analysis of the data. P-values do not cover a host of methodologic sins. Bradford Hill (speaking of the chi-square test) described them as good servants, but bad masters. Reflexively responding to p-values to the exclusion of these other issues is shortsighted thought evasion.

The appropriate role of p-values is to measure the effect of sampling error on the research results. They are most useful when 1) they are the product of a well-designed, well executed research program and 2) are interpreted jointly with effect size, the variability of the effect size, and confidence intervals. In these circumstances, type I and type II error control are an important part of the research design process. Fortunately, their calibration is under the complete control of the investigators, and the acceptable levels of these errors must be chosen with care. I have provided several strategies that produce conservative, tightly controlled type I error levels and lead to clear interpretation of a concordantly executed research program with multiple endpoints. These strategies allow the investigator to choose a level of type I error symmetrically or asymmetrically. They are not the only available strategies, and of course no investigator should be compelled to use them. However, investigators should choose something. They should be plain about their choice, stick with their choice, and report the results of their choice. Readers of clinical research should continue to insist on this standard.

Physician investigators cannot understand alpha error concepts unless they understand the sampling error principles. Statisticians cannot provide the best advice on experimental design unless they understand the medical framework and underlying theory of the intervention or exposure. Statisticians and physician investigators must understand each other, investing the time and effort to communicate effectively, learning to appreciate the nuances of each other's language. Liking each other is preferable – understanding each other is essential.

In addition, we physicians must control our inclination to explain any research result simply because we read it in a manuscript or heard it in a lecture. We must instead first ask if these results are due to sampling error. If they are, we need not go forward with interesting theories about the research findings; our time could be better spent elsewhere. Just as we would not squander our time on trying to explain why a 7 appeared as the result of throwing a pair of dice, so we should not exert great effort in attempting to explain results that are likely to be due to chance.

Since the written and visual media quickly convey new research findings for consumption to an increasingly health-conscious community, there is even less time and room for error. We should uphold community health by ensuring that we do not expose it to the corrosive influences of misleading results. Even with adequate precautions, sampling error still produces misleading conclusions from well-designed research efforts. By standing now for community protection through tight type I error control, we can help to shape the future rather than be stampeded in the wrong direction by results that are themselves driven by sampling error.

Finally, I believe there are three important principles of research. They are simple, and, by and large, nonmathematical.

1. Provide for the general welfare of your patients.

This should not be reduced to a truism. Patients volunteer their time, their energy, and quite frankly, their health by taking part in the studies that we researchers design and execute. Researchers are honor bound and obligated to ensure that the participants in their studies receive the best available treatment. These research subjects are a precious resource that must never be taken for granted or squandered.

I have pointed out several areas where the ethics and the mathematics of clinical experiments collide, but this is not one of them. Consider, a 4,000 patient clinical trial, designed to test the effect of therapy to reduce total mortality. If we assume the cumulative event rate for the placebo group is 20%, then we expect $(2,000)(0.20) = 400$ deaths in the placebo group. If we anticipate that the cumulative mortality rate in the treatment group is 0.16, we would expect $(2,000)(0.16) = 320$ patients to die during the course of the trial in the treatment group. Out of the four thousand patient trial, the entire measure of therapy effectiveness is reduced to the experiences of $400 - 320 = 80$ patients. The results on this large, multimillion dollar clinical trial hinge on the findings in only 80 participants (Figure 13.1).

4,000 patient, multi-million dollar study

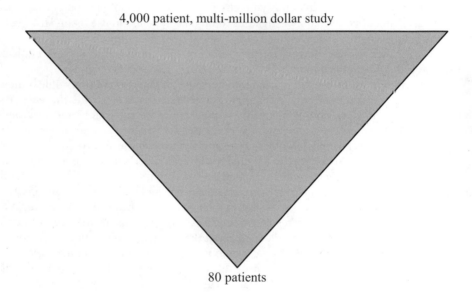

80 patients

Fig. 13.1. The results of a multimillion dollar study teter precariously on the findings in 80 patients.

Clearly, if the investigators knew who these 80 patients were at the trial's inception, these patients would be singled out for very special care. For example, they would ensure that these participants understood the importance of the protocol. The investigators would see to it that these patients attended each follow-up visit. Any complaints these patients had would be addressed at once. Of course the investigators do not know the identities of these 80 patients. Therefore the investigator must treat *each* patient in the study as if *that* patient is *the* patient that will make the difference in the trial.

2. Promote collegial relationships with co-investigators

Issues of publication policy, doses of medication, and the characteristics of the patients to be included in the study are critical, and strong-willed scientists can vehemently disagree on these fundamental trial characteristics. Investigators should expect this. However, they must actively work to ensure that the communication between investigators does not become choked with anger, resentment, or hostility. If these are permitted to occur, the research effort is weakened and its survival threatened.

Each investigator makes a unique contribution of personality, intellect and perspective and deserves full expression and consideration. Investigators must remember that their quiet answers to wrathful questions from their strongly opinionated colleagues can blunt this anger, turning it aside.

Research efforts experience external, centrifugal forces (e.g., opposing points of few in the medical community, politically charged scientific issues, contrary findings in other research programs) that threaten to tear the research effort apart. These destructive forces are counterbalanced by the centripetal force of investigators who are able to put their differences of opinion aside and hold their common effort together.

3. Preserve, protect, and defend the protocol

Prospective statements of the questions to be answered by the research effort and rejection of tempting data-based changes to the protocol preserve the best estimates of effect size, standard errors, and measures of sampling error. In a clinical trial, carrying out a well-designed protocol as it was initially and carefully planned is one of the best ways to protect vulnerable patient communities from exposure to harmful placebos. By following the enunciated principles of this book, investigators will be able to recognize the menace of type I error to both the patient and scientific communities, while simultaneously controlling and accurately reporting it. Adjustments to type I error are unavoidable. However, we must be ever vigilant, avoiding the corrupting influences of having the data determine the analysis plan.

Following these principles promotes the prosecution of a successful research program, i.e., the construction and protection of a research environment that permits an objective assessment of the therapy or exposure being studied. If there is any fixed star in the research constellation, it is that sample-based research must be hypothesis-driven and concordantly executed to have real meaning for both the scientific community and the patient populations that we serve.

Appendix A
Standard Normal Probabilities

The standard normal distribution is perhaps the most commonly used distribution in probability and statistics. Its ubiquity is due to its wide spread applicability and its ease of use, despite the fact that one must have access to a table in order to compute the probabilities associated with it.

Assume that an observation follows a normal distribution. We must specify its mean μ and its standard deviation σ in order to identify its location and variability. In this case, we say that x follows a $N(\mu, \sigma^2)$. This is enough for us to know that, for example, $P[\mu - 1.96\sigma \le x \le \mu + 1.96\sigma] = 0.95$. The value of this probability is the same regardless of what μ and σ happen to be.

However, other probabilities will depend on the values of these parameters. For example, if x is blood glucose level, and we wish to compute the probability that x is less than 60 mg/dl, then the solution will depend on whether we think the blood sugar level follows a normal distribution with $\mu = 70$ and $\sigma = 20$ or if its parameters are $\mu = 220$ and $\sigma = 30$.

The implication of this observation is that we would need to have a normal distribution for each combination of μ and σ. Fortunately this is not the case. As pointed out in Chapter Three, each normally distributed random variable can be converted to a standard normal distribution. This standard normal distribution has $\mu = 0$ and $\sigma = 1$. This permits one table to be used to compute the values of events whose probabilities are governed by this distribution.

For example, in order to compute the probability that $x < 60$, we write $P[x < 60] = P\left[(x-70)\big/20 < (60-70)\big/20 \right] = P[z < -0.5]$. We write the last probability in terms of z, where $z = (x-70)\big/20$ follows a standard normal distribution. Using the table we find that $P[z < -0.5] = 0.480$.

In a similar computation of this probability, if $\mu = 220$ and $\sigma = 30$, then $P[x < 60] = P\left[(x-220)\big/30 < (60-220)\big/30 \right] = P[z < -5.33]$. Using the same table from this appendix we see that the probability of this value is quite small (<0.001).

Using the symmetry of the normal distribution, we can compute $P[z > a] = P[z < -a]$ when a is a positive number. Additionally we can also write $P[a < z < b] = P[z < b] - P[z < a]$. These relationships increase the utility of the following table.

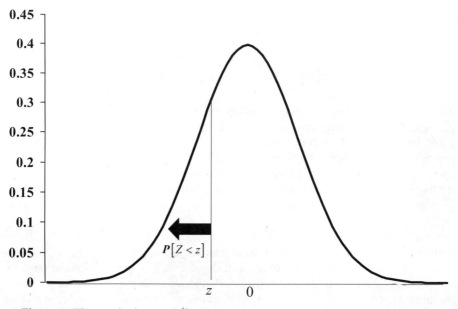

Figure A. The standard normal distribution.

z	P(Z < z)	z	P(Z < z)	z	P(Z < z)	z	P(Z < z)
-3.90	0.0000	-1.95	0.0256	0.00	0.5000	1.95	0.9744
-3.85	0.0001	-1.90	0.0287	0.05	0.5199	2.00	0.9772
-3.80	0.0001	-1.85	0.0322	0.10	0.5398	2.05	0.9798
-3.75	0.0001	-1.80	0.0359	0.15	0.5596	2.10	0.9821
-3.70	0.0001	-1.75	0.0401	0.20	0.5793	2.15	0.9842
-3.65	0.0001	-1.70	0.0446	0.25	0.5987	2.20	0.9861
-3.60	0.0002	-1.65	0.0495	0.30	0.6179	2.25	0.9878
-3.55	0.0002	-1.60	0.0548	0.35	0.6368	2.30	0.9893
-3.50	0.0002	-1.55	0.0606	0.40	0.6554	2.35	0.9906
-3.45	0.0003	-1.50	0.0668	0.45	0.6736	2.40	0.9918
-3.40	0.0003	-1.45	0.0735	0.50	0.6915	2.45	0.9929
-3.35	0.0004	-1.40	0.0808	0.55	0.7088	2.50	0.9938
-3.30	0.0005	-1.35	0.0885	0.60	0.7257	2.55	0.9946
-3.25	0.0006	-1.30	0.0968	0.65	0.7422	2.60	0.9953
-3.20	0.0007	-1.25	0.1056	0.70	0.7580	2.65	0.9960
-3.15	0.0008	-1.20	0.1151	0.75	0.7734	2.70	0.9965
-3.10	0.0010	-1.15	0.1251	0.80	0.7881	2.75	0.9970
-3.05	0.0011	-1.10	0.1357	0.85	0.8023	2.80	0.9974
-3.00	0.0013	-1.05	0.1469	0.90	0.8159	2.85	0.9978
-2.95	0.0016	-1.00	0.1587	0.95	0.8289	2.90	0.9981
-2.90	0.0019	-0.95	0.1711	1.00	0.8413	2.95	0.9984
-2.85	0.0022	-0.90	0.1841	1.05	0.8531	3.00	0.9987
-2.80	0.0026	-0.85	0.1977	1.10	0.8643	3.05	0.9989
-2.75	0.0030	-0.80	0.2119	1.15	0.8749	3.10	0.9990
-2.70	0.0035	-0.75	0.2266	1.20	0.8849	3.15	0.9992
-2.65	0.0040	-0.70	0.2420	1.25	0.8944	3.20	0.9993
-2.60	0.0047	-0.65	0.2578	1.30	0.9032	3.25	0.9994
-2.55	0.0054	-0.60	0.2743	1.35	0.9115	3.30	0.9995
-2.50	0.0062	-0.55	0.2912	1.40	0.9192	3.35	0.9996
-2.45	0.0071	-0.50	0.3085	1.45	0.9265	3.40	0.9997
-2.40	0.0082	-0.45	0.3264	1.50	0.9332	3.45	0.9997
-2.35	0.0094	-0.40	0.3446	1.55	0.9394	3.50	0.9998
-2.30	0.0107	-0.35	0.3632	1.60	0.9452	3.55	0.9998
-2.25	0.0122	-0.30	0.3821	1.65	0.9505	3.60	0.9998
-2.20	0.0139	-0.25	0.4013	1.70	0.9554	3.65	0.9999
-2.15	0.0158	-0.20	0.4207	1.75	0.9599	3.70	0.9999
-2.10	0.0179	-0.15	0.4404	1.80	0.9641	3.75	0.9999
-2.05	0.0202	-0.10	0.4602	1.85	0.9678	3.80	0.9999
-2.00	0.0228	-0.05	0.4801	1.90	0.9713	3.85	0.9999

Appendix B
Sample Size Primer

The purpose of this appendix is to provide a brief discussion of the underlying principles in sample size computations for a clinical trial. In the process, one of the simplest and most useful formulas for the sample size formulations will be reproduced. These basic formulas are the source of several of the calculations in Chapters Four through Eleven. First we will provide the solution and proceed to a discussion that both motivates and derives the sample size and power formulas.

B.1 General Discussion of Sample Size

Assume that a clinical trial has been designed to measure the effect of a randomly allocated intervention on a prospectively defined primary endpoint. Let θ_c be the cumulative incidence rate of the primary endpoint in the control group and let θ_t be the cumulative incidence rate of the primary endpoint in the treatment group. Then the statistical hypothesis for the primary endpoint in this clinical trial is

$$H_0 : \theta_c = \theta_t \quad \text{versus} \quad H_a : \theta_c \neq \theta_t. \tag{B.1}$$

Let Z_a be the ath percentile from the standard normal distribution. The investigators have chosen an a priori test-specific type I error level α, and the power of the statistical hypothesis test is $1 - \beta$. The hypothesis test will be two-sided. Let p_c be the cumulative incidence rate of the primary endpoint in the control group of the research sample, and let p_t be the cumulative incidence rate of the active group in the research sample. Then the trial size, or the sample size of the clinical trial,[*] N may be written as

$$N = \frac{2\left[p_c\left(1-p_c\right)+p_t\left(1-p_t\right)\right]\left[Z_{1-\alpha/2}-Z_\beta\right]^2}{\left(p_c-p_t\right)^2}. \tag{B.2}$$

Analogously, the power of the study may be calculated as a function of N,

$$1-\beta = P\left[N(0,1) > Z_{1-\alpha/2} - \frac{p_c - p_t}{\sqrt{\dfrac{p_c\left(1-p_c\right)}{N/2}+\dfrac{p_t\left(1-p_t\right)}{N/2}}}\right]. \tag{B.3}$$

---

[*] This is the total number of patients in the study (number of patients in the placebo group plus the number of patients in the control group).

There are many different treatises on sample size calculations in clinical trials. A representative group is [1– 5]. Several of these sources discuss important and useful nuances of the sample size computation that are useful in complex clinical trial design. The focus of the discussion here, however, will be on the most basic sample size computation, since that formula demonstrates most clearly the influence of the design parameters of the study (cumulative primary endpoint event rate in the control group, the anticipated effect of the intervention, the magnitude of the statistical errors, and test sidedness) on the resulting sample size.

For these discussions, assume that patients are randomized to receive either a new intervention or to receive control group therapy. In this example, there is one primary endpoint that occurs with a cumulative event rate θ_c. In the intervention group the cumulative event rate for the primary endpoint is θ_t. The investigator does not know the value of θ_c, since he does not study every patient in the population. He therefore selects a sample from the population and uses that sample to compute p_c, which will serve as his estimate of θ_c. If the clinical trial has been executed concordantly, then p_c is a good estimator of θ_c; this means that the investigator can expect that p_c will be close to the value of θ_c. Analogously p_t is the estimate from the investigator's sample of the cumulative incidence of the endpoint in the population θ_t.

Thus, if the trial was executed according to its protocol (and not subject to the destabilizing influences of random research), then $p_c - p_t$ can be expected to be an accurate estimate of $\theta_c - \theta_t$. If the null hypothesis is true, then $\theta_c - \theta_t$ will be zero and we would expect $p_c - p_t$ to be small. If the alternative hypothesis is correct, and the investigator's intuition that the therapy being tested in the clinical trial will reduce the cumulative event rate of the primary endpoint is right, then θ_c is much greater than θ_t, and $p_c - p_t$, the best estimate of $\theta_c - \theta_t$ will be large as well.

A key point in understanding the sample size formulation is the critical role played by the number of endpoint events produced by the sample. The research sample produces primary endpoints—the rate at which these endpoints are accumulated is directly linked to the cumulative event rate in the control group. This cumulative event rate therefore plays a central role in the sample size calculations. If the primary endpoint of a clinical trial is total mortality, then recruiting 1,000 patients into the study provides no useful information for the evaluation of the effect of therapy on total mortality if at the end of the study none of the 1,000 recruited patients die.

Therefore, the more primary endpoint events that occur during the course of the trial, the greater the volume of germane data available to answer the scientific question of whether the occurrence of those endpoint events are influenced by the intervention being studied. It follows that the larger the cumulative control group event rate is, the greater the number of primary endpoint event rates that will be generated. The greater the rate at which primary endpoints are produced, the smaller the required sample size for the clinical trial will be, assuming that everything else (effect of therapy, test sidedness, magnitude of the statistical errors) is equal, (or *ceteris paribus*).

A second measure that is critical in sample size considerations is the effectiveness of the therapy. This is often measured by the difference between the cumulative incidence rate of the primary endpoint in the population θ_c and the cumulative incidence of the primary event rate in the population if everyone in the population were to receive the treatment being studied in the clinical trial, θ_t. This difference is commonly referred to as "delta" or $\Delta = \theta_c - \theta_t$.[*] The greater the difference between θ_c and θ_t, then the fewer the number of patients required to obtain a reliable estimate of that difference.

To understand this principle, it may be helpful to think of the two primary sources of variability involved in the estimation of the treatment effect in a clinical trial. The test statistic used to test the statistical hypothesis that $\theta_c = \theta_t$ versus the alternative hypothesis that these events are not equal is

$$\frac{p_c - p_t}{\sqrt{Var[p_c - p_t]}}. \tag{B.4}$$

The first source of this variability is systematic; it is induced by the intervention being studied by the clinical trial and is an estimate of Δ, the difference between the treatment and control group event rates that are seen in the sample. This variability is estimated by $p_c - p_t$ and resides in the numerator of (B.4). This is the "signal."

The denominator of (B.4) is the second source of variability or the "noise"; it is an expression of the fact that, since the research is sample-based, estimates of $p_c - p_t$ will vary from sample to sample. Since this sampling variability "noise" should not be confused with the systematic, intervention-induced "signal" measured by $p_c - p_t$, this noise must be removed from the estimate of the therapy's effect. Therefore using these characterizations, the greater the signal–to–noise ratio, the larger the expression in (B.4) will be.

The greater the signal–to–noise ratio as represented by (B.4), the easier it is to detect a genuine population effect of the intervention. If the magnitude of the difference $\theta_c - \theta_t$ is small in the population, then $p_c - p_t$ is also likely to be small. In this circumstance where the magnitude of the signal is small, the noise must be co-incidently reduced to detect the weak signal with precision. One useful tool the investigator has to reduce the background noise is to increase N, the sample size of the clinical trial. Part of the genius of choosing the reliable estimate $p_c - p_t$ of $\theta_c - \theta_t$ is that this estimate's sampling variability decreases as the sample size increases.[†]

B.2 Derivation of Sample Size

It if useful to consider the sample size computation as a three phased calculation. For each demonstration, there will be three phases of the computation.

Phase I – under the null
Phase II – under the alternative

---

[*] Sometimes it is useful to refer to the percent reduction in events attributable to the therapy, otherwise known as the therapy's efficacy.
[†] This indispensable property of the estimates of effect size can be lost if the experiment is not executed concordantly (see Chapter Two).

Phase III – consolidation

We will step through each of these phase as we compute the sample size for the clinical trial as outlined earlier in this appendix.

B.2.1 Phase 1: Under the Null Hypothesis
Note that the test statistic

$$\frac{p_c - p_t - (\theta_c - \theta_t)}{\sqrt{Var[p_c - p_t]}} \tag{B.5}$$

follows a normal distribution. Under the null hypothesis that $\theta_c - \theta_t = 0$ reduces to

$$\frac{p_c - p_t}{\sqrt{Var[p_c - p_t]}}. \tag{B.6}$$

One useful way to think of this test statistic is as a normed effect size. Under the null hypothesis, we expect this normed effect size to have a mean of zero and a variance of one. It will follow the normal or bell shaped distribution. Then, the null hypothesis will be rejected when[*]

$$\frac{p_c - p_t}{\sqrt{Var[p_c - p_t]}} > Z_{1-\alpha/2} \tag{B.7}$$

or,

$$p_c - p_t > Z_{1-\alpha/2}\sqrt{Var[p_c - p_t]}. \tag{B.8}$$

B.2.2 Phase 2: Under the Alternative Hypothesis
We now consider what should have if the alternative hypothesis was true. In this case, we start with the definition of statistical power.

Power = Probability [the null hypothesis is rejected | alternative hypothesis is true]

---

[*] This is not the only circumstance under which the null hypothesis will be rejected. It will also be rejected when harm is caused by the intervention or when $p_t - p_c$ is very much less than zero. However, in the sample size computation, attention is focused on the tail of the distribution in which the investigators are most interested.

The null hypothesis is rejected when the test statistic falls in the critical region or when $p_c - p_t > Z_{1-\alpha/2}\sqrt{Var[p_c - p_t]}$. The alternative hypothesis is true if $\theta_c - \theta_t = \Delta \geq 0$. This allows us to write

$$Power = 1-\beta = P\left[p_c - p_t > Z_{1-\alpha/2}\sqrt{Var[p_c - p_t]} \mid \theta_c - \theta_t = \Delta\right]. \qquad (B.9)$$

We now standardize the argument in the probability statement of (B.9) so that the quantity on the left follows a standard normal distribution. This requires subtracting the population mean effect under the alternative hypothesis (i.e., Δ) and dividing by the square root of the variance of $p_c - p_t$. These operations must be carried out on both sides of the inequality in the probability expression in (B.9) as follows.

$$1-\beta = P\left[\frac{p_c - p_t - \Delta}{\sqrt{Var[p_c - p_t]}} > \frac{Z_{1-\alpha/2}\sqrt{Var[p_c - p_t]} - \Delta}{\sqrt{Var[p_c - p_t]}}\right]$$

$$= P\left[\frac{p_c - p_t - \Delta}{\sqrt{Var[p_c - p_t]}} > Z_{1-\alpha/2} - \frac{\Delta}{\sqrt{Var[p_c - p_t]}}\right] \qquad (B.10)$$

$$= P\left[N(0,1) > Z_{1-\alpha/2} - \frac{\Delta}{\sqrt{Var[p_c - p_t]}}\right].$$

By the definition of a percentile value from a probability distribution, we can now write

$$Z_\beta = Z_{1-\alpha/2} - \frac{\Delta}{\sqrt{Var[p_c - p_t]}}. \qquad (B.11)$$

B.2.3 Phase 3: Consolidation

We are now ready to conclude this computation, by solving for N, the size of the trial. The sample size is embedded in the variance term in the denominator of expression (B.11).

$$Var[p_c - p_t] = \frac{p_c(1-p_c)}{n_c} + \frac{p_t(1-p_t)}{n_t}. \qquad (B.12)$$

where n_c is the number of patients to be recruited to the control group in the clinical trial and n_t is the number of patients to be recruited to the active group. The sample size or trial size is the total number of patients required for the experiment $= N = n_c + n_t$. If we assume that the number of patients in the control group will equal the number of patients in the treatment group, then $n_c = n_t = n$ and $N = 2n$. Then (B.11) can be rewritten as

$$Z_\beta = Z_{1-\alpha/2} - \frac{\Delta}{\sqrt{\dfrac{p_c(1-p_c)}{n} + \dfrac{p_t(1-p_t)}{n}}}. \qquad (B.13)$$

We only need solve this equation for n

$$n = \frac{\left[p_c(1-p_c) + p_t(1-p_t)\right]\left[Z_{1-\alpha/2} - Z_\beta\right]^2}{\Delta^2}. \qquad (B.14)$$

The trial size $N = 2n$ may be written as

$$N = \frac{2\left[p_c(1-p_c) + p_t(1-p_t)\right]\left[Z_{1-\alpha/2} - Z_\beta\right]^2}{\Delta^2}. \qquad (B.15)$$

To compute the power we only need to adapt the following equation from the last line of expression (B.10),

$$1-\beta = P\left[N(0,1) > Z_{1-\alpha/2} - \frac{\Delta}{\sqrt{Var[p_c - p_t]}}\right] \qquad (B.16)$$

and rewrite the Var $[p_c$ - $p_t]$ to find

$$1-\beta = P\left[N(0,1) > Z_{1-\alpha/2} - \frac{\Delta}{\sqrt{\dfrac{p_c(1-p_c)}{N/2} + \dfrac{p_t(1-p_t)}{N/2}}}\right]. \qquad (B.17)$$

B.3 Example

If the experiment is designed for a two–sided α of 0.05, 90 % power ($\beta = 0.10$), $p_c = 0.20$, and $\Delta = 0.03$, then $p_t = 0.17$ (corresponding to a $(0.20 - 0.17)/0.20 = 0.15$, or a 15% reduction in events attributable to the intervention. The trial size can be computed from

$$N = \frac{2\left[p_c(1-p_c) + p_t(1-p_t)\right]\left[Z_{1-\alpha/2} - Z_\beta\right]^2}{\left[p_c - p_t\right]^2}. \qquad (B.18)$$

Inserting the data from this example reveals

$$N = \frac{2\ [(0.20)(0.80)+(0.17)(0.83)]\ [1.96-(-1.28)]^2}{[0.20-0.17]^2} = 7024 \quad (B.19)$$

or 3,512 subjects per group. If only 2,000 subjects per group can be identified, the power can be formulated from

$$Power = P\left[N(0,1) > Z_{1-\alpha/2} - \frac{\Delta}{\sqrt{\dfrac{p_c(1-p_c)}{N/2} + \dfrac{p_t(1-p_t)}{N/2}}} \right] \quad (B.20)$$

and including the data from this example

$$Power = P\left[N(0,1) > 1.96 - \frac{0.03}{\sqrt{\dfrac{(0.20)(0.80)}{2000} + \dfrac{(0.17)(0.83)}{2000}}} \right] = 0.69. \quad (B.21)$$

B.4 Continuous Outcomes

Many clinicial trials have outcome measures that are continuous. Consider a clinical experiment that is designed to test the effect of an intervention on the change in left ventricular end diastolic volume (EDV). Patients are recruited using a random-sampling plan and have their baseline EDV measured. They are then randomized to receive placebo care or the intervention, and followed for three months, at the end of which they have their EDV measured again. The investigator assumes that the EDVs will be normally distributed, and wishes to analyze the change in EDV over time across the two groups. He believes that there will be a large increase in EDV in the placebo group, reflecting the natural progression of the disease. It is his hope that the EDV change will be smaller in the treatment arm of the experiment.

Let $\mu_d(c)$ be the population mean change in the end diastolic volumes for the placebo group and $\mu_d(t)$ be the population mean change in the end diastolic volume in the active group. Let's begin with the null hypothesis,

$$H_0 : \mu_d(c) = \mu_d(t) \text{ versus } H_a : \mu_d(c) \neq \mu_d(t).$$

Clearly, the investigator does not believe the alternative hypothesis as stated, he believes that $\mu_d(c)$ the population mean change in EDV in the placebo group, will be greater than $\mu_d(t)$, the population mean change in EDV in the active group. However, since he recognizes that he does not know the effect of therapy, he states the alternative hypothesis as two–sided.[*] However, his true belief in the ability of the treatment to affect the change in EDV will be reflected in phase II.

B.4.1 Phase I : The Null Hypothesis

The purpose of phase I is simply to construct the test statistic and identify its critical region. The distribution of the test statistic is the distribution under the null hypothesis, i.e., under the assumption that there is no treatment effect on the mean change in EDV. As was stated before, the investigator believes the difference in EDVs will follow a normal distribution. Let d_c be the sample mean change in the placebo group, and d_t is the sample mean change in the active group, and $Var[d_c - d_t]$ be the variance of the difference in chance of the EDVs We note that under the null hypothesis the quantity

$$\frac{d_c - d_t}{\sqrt{Var[d_c - d_t]}} \qquad\qquad (B.22)$$

follows a normal distribution. Then the null hypothesis will be rejected when

$$\frac{d_c - d_t}{\sqrt{Var[d_c - d_t]}} > Z_{1-\alpha/2}, \qquad\qquad (B.23)$$

where $Z_{1-\alpha/2}$ is the $1 - \alpha/2$ percentile value from the standard normal distribution with mean zero and variance one. We may rewrite equation (B.23) to see that we will reject the null hypothesis in favor of the alternative if

$$d_c - d_t > Z_{1-\alpha/2}\sqrt{Var[d_c - d_t]}. \qquad\qquad (B.24)$$

This ends phase I.

B.4.2 Phase II: The Alternative Hypothesis

This next phase incorporates the result of phase I with the notion of power. Begin with the definition of power:

Power = Prob[The null hypothesis is rejected | the alternative hypothesis is true]

---

[*] This notion of test oidedness is discussed in Chapter Five.

The null hypothesis is rejected when the test statistic falls in the critical region. The alternative hypothesis is true if $d_c - d_t = \Delta \geq 0$. This quantity Δ is the difference that the investigator hopes to see between the changes in the two groups. This consideration is not two-sided at this point, and is the opportunity for the investigator to state precisely state the magnitude of efficacy he believes this treatment will produce.

Using the result of Phase I we can write the power equation as

$$Power = P\left[d_c - d_t > Z_{1-\alpha/2}\sqrt{Var[d_c - d_t]} \mid \Delta\right]. \tag{B.25}$$

We now standardize this so that the quantity on the left follows a standard normal distribution. Under phase II, the alternative hypothesis the mean of the treatment difference $d_c - d_t = \Delta \geq 0$. This leads to

$$Power = P\left[\frac{d_c - d_t - \Delta}{\sqrt{Var[d_c - d_t]}} > \frac{Z_{1-\alpha/2}\sqrt{Var[d_c - d_t]} - \Delta}{\sqrt{Var[d_c - d_t]}}\right], \tag{B.26}$$

which can be simplified to

$$= P\left[\frac{d_c - d_t - \Delta}{\sqrt{Var[d_c - d_t]}} > Z_{1-\alpha/2} - \frac{\Delta}{\sqrt{Var[d_c - d_t]}}\right] \tag{B.27}$$

$$= P\left[N(0,1) > Z_{1-\alpha/2} - \frac{\Delta}{\sqrt{Var[d_c - d_t]}}\right].$$

These steps are simply algebra. At this point, we can use the fact that $P\left[N(0,1) \geq Z_\beta\right] = 1 - \beta$ to write

$$Z_\beta = Z_{1-\alpha/2} - \frac{\Delta}{\sqrt{Var[d_c - d_t]}}. \tag{B.28}$$

This concludes Phase II

B.4.3 Phase III: Consolidation

Phase II concluded with an equation, that we must now solve for n. We assume that there were be an equal numnber of subjects in the treatment group and the intervention group. The sample size n is embedded in the variance term in the denominator of equation (B.28).

$$Var[d_c - d_t] = \frac{\sigma_D^2}{n} + \frac{\sigma_D^2}{n} = \frac{2\sigma_D^2}{n}, \tag{B.29}$$

where σ_D^2 is the variance of an intrasubject difference. The trial size (i.e. the total number of subjects needed for the experiment) $= N = 2n$. Replacing the denominator of the expression on the right–hand side of equation (B.28) with the right hand size of (B.29), we have

$$Z_\beta = Z_{1-\alpha/2} - \frac{\Delta}{\sqrt{Var[d_c - d_t]}}. \tag{B.30}$$

We need only solve this equation for n

$$n = \frac{2\sigma_D^2 \left[Z_{1-\alpha/2} - Z_\beta \right]^2}{\Delta^2}, \tag{B.31}$$

and the trial size[*] N, is

$$N = \frac{4\sigma_D^2 \left[Z_{1-\alpha/2} - Z_\beta \right]^2}{\Delta^2}. \tag{B.32}$$

To compute the power one need only adapt the following equation from Phase II,

$$1 - \beta = P \left[N(0,1) > Z_{1-\alpha/2} - \frac{\Delta}{\sqrt{Var[d_x - d_y]}} \right], \tag{B.33}$$

and rewrite the variance to find

$$1 - \beta = P \left[N(0,1) > Z_{1-\alpha/2} - \frac{\Delta}{\sqrt{\dfrac{2\sigma_D^2}{n}}} \right] \tag{B.34}$$

B.4.4 Example

If, for this experiment, the investigator chooses a two-sided alpha of 0.05, 90% power (beta = 0.10), delta = 10 and $\sigma_D = 18$, the trial size is

---

[*] The trial size is the total number of patients required for the experiment; here it is the number of patients randomized to the placebo group plus the number of patients randomized to the intervention group.

$$N = \frac{4\sigma_D^2 \left[Z_{1-\alpha/2} - Z_\beta \right]^2}{\left[\Delta \right]^2} = \frac{4(18)^2 \left[1.96 - (-1.28) \right]^2}{\left[10 \right]^2} = 136. \qquad \text{(B.35)}$$

Or 68 subjects per group. If the delta of interest is 5 rather than 10, the power is

$$1 - \beta = \boldsymbol{P} \left[N(0,1) > Z_{1-\alpha/2} - \frac{\Delta}{\sqrt{\dfrac{2\sigma^2}{n}}} \right]$$

$$= \boldsymbol{P} \left[N(0,1) > 1.96 - \frac{5}{\sqrt{\dfrac{2(18)^2}{68}}} \right] \qquad \text{(B.36)}$$

$$= \boldsymbol{P}[N(0,1) > 0.34] = 0.37.$$

References

1. Lachim, J.M (1981) Introduction to sample size determinations and power analyses for clinical trials. *Controlled Clinical Trial* **2**:93–114.
2. Sahai, H., Khurshid, A (1996) Formulae and tables for determination of sample size and power in clinical trials for testing differences in proportions for the two sample design. *Statistics in Medicine* **15**:1–21.
3. Davy, S.J., Graham, O.T.(1991) Sample size estimation for comparing two or more treatment groups in clinical trials. *Statistics in Medicine* **10**:3–43.
4. Donner, A (1984) Approach to sample size estimation in the design of clinical trials – a review.*Statistics in Medicine* **3**:199–214.
5. George, S.L., Desue M.M (1974) Planning the size and duration of a clinical trial studying the time to some critical event. *Journal of Chronic Disease* **27**:15–24.

Daubert and Rule 702 Factors

Daubert hearings are discussions that place before the court in cases involving the determination of causation between an exposure and a disease. To assist the court, the federal court system provided the following gudiance.

C.1 The *Daubert* Factors

The expert's general and specific causation methods should be scrutinized pursuant to amended FRE Rule 702 and the *Daubert* factors. Amended Rule 702 provides additional areas of inquiry and each factor applicable to the testimony should be included in the motion. The *Daubert* factors are —

Testing: Has the theory or methodology been tested or can it be?

Rate of Error: What is the known or potential rate of error in an expert's methodology? High rates of error detract from the reliability of the methodology and conclusions. See *United States v. Dorsey*, 45 F.3d 809, 815 (4th Cir.), *cert. denied*, 515 US 1168 (1995).

Peer Review: Has the theory or technique been published in a peer reviewed journal? Such publication is a relevant consideration in accessing the scientific validity of a particular technique or methodology on which an opinion in premised

General Acceptance: Has the theory or methodology gained "general acceptance" in the relevant scientific community?

C.2 The 702 Factors

1. Are the experts proposing to testify about matters growing naturally and directly out of research they have conducted?
2. Has the expert unjustifiably extrapolated from an accepted premise to an unfounded conclusion?
3. Has the expert adequately accounted for obvious alternative explanations (other causes)?
4. Is the expert being as careful as he/she would be in his regular professional work outside of his paid litigation consulting?

Federal Rule of Evidence 702 provides some general standards the trial court must use to access the reliability and helpfulness of proffered expert testimony:

If scientific, technical, or other specialized knowledge will assist
the trier of fact to understand the evidence or to determine a fact

in issue, a witness qualified as an expert by knowledge, skill, experience, training, or education, may testify thereto in the form of an opinion or otherwise, if (1) the testimony is based upon sufficient facts or data, (2) the testimony is the product of reliable principles and methods, and (3) the witness has applied the principles and methods reliably to the facts of the case.

Failure of plaintiff's expert to meet any one of the above factors is fatal to the plaintiff's expert, and hence the case. Plaintiffs often argue that the amendments to Rule 702 mean that the courts should be more flexible and not rely on *Daubert* exclusively. See Michael H. Graham, *The Expert Witness Predicament: Determining "Reliable" Under the Gatekeeping Test of Daubert, Kumho and Proposed Amended Rule 702 of the Federal Rules of Evidence*, 54 U. Miami L. Rev. 317 (2002).

Index

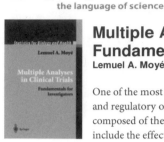

Multiple Analyses in Clinical Trials:
Fundamentals for Investigators

Lemuel A. Moyé

One of the most challenging issues for clinical trial investigators, sponsors, and regulatory officials is the interpretation of experimental results that are composed of the results of multiple statistical analyses. These analyses may include the effect of therapy on multiple endpoints, the assessment of a subgroup analysis, and the evaluation of a dose-response relationship in complex mixtures. *Multiple Analyses in Clinical Trials: Fundamentals for Clinical Investigators* is an essentially nonmathematical discussion of the problems posed by the execution of multiple analyses in clinical trials. It concentrates on the rationale for the analyses, the difficulties posed by their interpretation, easily understood solutions, and useful problem sets.

2003. 436 p. (Statistics for Biology and Health Hardcover ISBN 0-387-00727-X

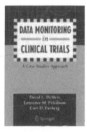

Data Monitoring in Clinical Trials:
A Case Study Approach

David DeMets, Curt Furberg, and Lawrence Friedman (Editors)

Randomized clinical trials are the gold standard for establishing many clinical practice guidelines and are central to evidence based medicine. Obtaining the best evidence through clinical trials must be done within the boundaries of rigorous science and ethical principles. This book, through a series of case studies presented by many distinguished clinical trial experts, illustrates the complexity of this monitoring process. The editors provide an overview of the process and a summary of a multitude of the lessons learned from the cases presented.

2005. 288 p. Softcover ISBN 0-387-20330-3

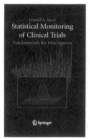

Statistical Monitoring of Clinical Trials

Lemuel A. Moyé

Statistical Monitoring of Clinical Trials: Fundamentals for Investigators introduces the investigator and statistician to monitoring procedures in clinical research. Clearly presenting the necessary background with limited use of mathematics, this book increases the knowledge, experience, and intuition of investigations in the use of these important procedures now required by the many clinical research efforts.

2005. 280 p. Softcover ISBN 0-387-27781-1